Fourth Edition

THE
CERVICAL SYNDROME

By

RUTH JACKSON, B.A., M.D., F.A.C.S.

Assistant Clinical Professor
of Orthopaedic Surgery
Southwestern Medical School of
The University of Texas, Dallas
Consulting Orthopaedic Surgeon
Baylor Medical Center
Consultant, Parkland Memorial Hospital
Formerly, Chief of Orthopaedic Surgery
Parkland Hospital and
Instructor in Orthopaedic Surgery
Baylor University College of Medicine
Dallas, Texas

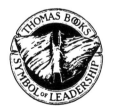

CHARLES C THOMAS · PUBLISHER
Springfield · Illinois · U.S.A.

Published and Distributed Throughout the World by
CHARLES C THOMAS • PUBLISHER
Bannerstone House
301-327 East Lawrence Avenue, Springfield, Illinois, U.S.A.

© *1956, 1958, 1966, 1971, and 1978 by* CHARLES C THOMAS • PUBLISHER
ISBN 0-398-03696-9 (cloth) ISBN 0-398-06178-5 (paper)
Library of Congress Catalog Card Number: 77-22261

First Edition, 1956
Second Edition, First Printing, 1958
Second Edition, Second Printing, 1963
Second Edition, Third Printing, 1965
Third Edition, First Printing, 1966
Third Edition, Revised Second Printing, 1971
Third Edition, Third Printing, 1976
Fourth Edition, 1977

*With THOMAS BOOKS careful attention is given to all details of
manufacturing and design. It is the Publisher's desire to present books that
are satisfactory as to their physical qualities and artistic possibilities and
appropriate for their particular use. THOMAS BOOKS will be true to those
laws of quality that assure a good name and good will.*

Library of Congress Cataloging in Publication Data

Jackson, Ruth.
    The cervical syndrome.

    (American lecture series)
    Bibliography: p.
    Includes index.
    1. Cervical syndrome. I. Title. [DNLM:
1. Cervical vertebrae—Injuries. 2. Cervico-
brachial neuralgia. 3. Whiplash injuries. WE708 J13c]
RC422.C4J33   616.7'3   77-22261
ISBN 0-398-03696-9. — ISBN 0-398-06178-5 (pbk.)

Printed in the United States of America
C-1

THE CERVICAL SYNDROME

Publication Number 1014
AMERICAN LECTURE SERIES®

A Monograph in
The BANNERSTONE DIVISION *of*
AMERICAN LECTURES IN ORTHOPAEDIC SURGERY

FOREWORD

THERE ARE FEW PROBLEMS of greater complexity than what the author calls the cervical syndrome. It is truly kaleidoscopic in its ramified clinical manifestations. Many men might have yielded to the temptation of a purely descriptive approach and to handcuff the subject by extensive subdivisions on purely observational grounds. It is in this particular aspect that Dr. Jackson's monograph is notably different. In her quest to give the mass of symptoms which meet the eye interpretative meaning, she not only draws heavily upon information furnished by the basic sciences, but the whole structure of the work is built upon basic and recognized factors in the field of anatomy and kinetics. In her attempt to establish the causal connections between basic facts and clinical manifestations, she succeeds uncommonly well.

One of these facts is the relation of the much-ignored uncovertebral articulation to foraminal compression. Another is the anatomical relations which the sympathetic nervous system of the cervical spine bears to certain projected localizations of pain.

In perusing the book carefully as the writer has done, one cannot help but credit Dr. Jackson with having developed on the foundation of basic facts a clear cut pattern of logical coherence between the manifestation and background which should do much for the understanding of a most difficult clinical entity.

This present monograph is preceded by a number of publications and instructional courses pertaining to this subject which Dr. Jackson has given for a number of years. Her very large clinical experience, well-documented in this book, enjoins the reader to give serious consideration to her statements.

It has been my privilege to know Dr. Jackson for many years and to follow the keen interest she has taken in this subject and the earnest and intensive studies she has devoted to it. They have made her one of the foremost authorities in this specific field.

Iowa City, Iowa   A. STEINDLER, M.D.

PREFACE

I BECAME INTERESTED in disorders of the cervical spine in 1936. This interest grew as the number of patients with neck problems increased. The first neck injury which was the result of a sudden acceleration in a rear-end collision was seen in 1937. It has been my privilege to follow this patient through subsequent neck injuries and to observe the progressive changes which have occurred in her cervical spine. Numerous other patients have been followed for many years, and they have contributed greatly toward making the studies of the cervical spine of significant importance.

There was a dearth of medical information concerning the cervical spine in 1936. This in itself was a stimulating factor in the attempt to understand the symptoms and clinical findings which the neck patients presented. The answers were not immediately available. Many unnecessary radiographs of the thoracic spine were made in an effort to find some pathology which might explain the cause of interscapular pain and muscle spasm. Psychiatric consultations were requested when the origin of the pain could not be established, only to find that the symptoms were not of psychoneurotic origin. However, with continued research and study of the anatomy of the very complex cervical spine, progress was made toward the clarification of some of the diagnostic problems. Many of the answers were found in what might be called antiquated writings.

The original monograph on *The Cervical Syndrome* emanated from Instructional Course Lectures I gave at the annual meetings of the American Academy of Orthopaedic Surgeons in 1953, 1954 and 1955. An expression of gratitude is due Dr. Charles N. Pease, Dr. Thomas Beath, Dr. Robert Joplin, Dr. Charles W. Goff, the late Dr. Arthur Steindler and many other good friends for their encouragement and inspiration to continue the work in this field.

During the past twenty-five years, the medical literature has been flooded with writings concerning the cervical spine. Many of these are repetitious, as so frequently happens when a sudden interest develops in a specific medical problem, whereas some have presented fresh concepts in diagnostic and treatment technics.

As the fourth edition of *The Cervical Syndrome* is in preparation, I have been surrounded completely by books, journals and reprints relating to this subject. Reviewing these writings has been a monumental task and it is impossible in this small volume to make reference to each and every author. The third edition will become the fourth edition with few changes in the basic concepts, but additions must be made as experience and knowledge increase.

My many patients have contributed much to this fourth edition. One patient suggested the illustration for the book jacket and I would like to acknowledge her at this point: Miss Cathy E. Newman, Editor of "Lifestyle" of the *Miami News,* now a member of the Editorial Staff, National Geographic.

R.J.

CONTENTS

THE CERVICAL SYNDROME

Chapter 1

INTRODUCTION

C URRENT MEDICAL LEXICOGRAPHERS define the *Cervical Syn-drome* as a condition caused by irritation or compression of cervical nerve roots marked by pain in the neck radiating into the shoulder, arm and forearm, depending upon which nerve roots are affected. This is an inadequate definition which gives no indication of the many ramifications of this most complex syndrome. It is true the cervical nerve roots are irritated or compressed within or near their intervertebral foramina through which they pass as they leave the spinal canal and before they divide into their anterior and posterior primary rami; however, the other structures within the foramina may be involved. These include the recurrent spinal meningeal nerves, the spinal branches of the vertebral arteries and their accompanying veins, the sympathetic fibers contained within the anterior roots of the fifth, sixth, seventh and eighth nerve roots and perhaps the other nerve roots, although it has not been definitely established that those above the fifth nerve roots do contain sympathetic fibers.

The first two nerve roots do not pass through intervertebral canals but they, too, are vulnerable to injuries and disorders involving the upper portion of the cervical spine, as are their accompanying vascular and sympathetic structures.

The term *syndrome* has been used frequently with other descriptive words to indicate special conditions at specific locations, when in reality the true pathology involves the nerve roots and their adjacent structures. *The scalenus anticus syndrome* is a typical example of this, and it is used today to describe a separate entity, although Nachlas, in 1942, refuted its possibility and showed conclusively that the true causative factor was involvement of the cervical nerve roots. *The thoracic outlet syndrome,* a frequently heard term, has been used to designate a conglomerate of clinical manifestations. As a diagnostic term, it is uninformative and leaves unsolved the identification of the true causative factor.

3

The scapulocostal syndrome and the costoclavicular syndrome are examples of other phrases used to designate symptoms rather than clinical entities.

An understanding of the anatomy of the cervical spine and of the mechanism involved in cervical nerve root irritation will clarify some of the confusion and will assure treatment directed toward the true causative factors and, hopefully, will prevent precipitous operations.

It is important to know the embryonic and fetal development of the cervical spine for a clear understanding of the many anomalies which are found in the cervical region of the spine. This problem is well documented by Hadley in his book *The Spine* and in his article *Development and Congenital Anomalies of the Cervical Spine; The Upper Cervical Spine* by V. Torklus and Gehle and *Functional Pathology of the Cervical Spine* by L. Penning are other books of value concerning anomalies.

The *Interpretation of Pain in Orthopedic Practice* by Steindler should be studied by all who are interested in disorders of the cervical spine, inasmuch as pain is the symptom which most frequently brings the patient to the doctor and an analysis and interpretation of pain is often neglected or ignored completely, or many unnecessary tests are done.

Head Injuries by Gurdjian and Webster, *The Intervertebral Disc* by Rabinovitch, *The Human Spine in Health and Disease* by Schmorl and Junghaus, *Luschka's Joint* by Hall, *Injuries of the Cervical Spine* by Braakman and Penning, as well as many other books, should be of value in the study of cervical spine disorders.

Chapter 2

ANATOMY

THE CERVICAL SPINE has certain definite characteristics which make it more subject to injury than any other portion of the vertebral column. It is vulnerably placed between the dorsal spine, which is relatively immobile, and the skull, which is a weight that must be balanced on the cervical spine and is held in place by the supporting capsular, ligamentous, cartilaginous and muscular structures. It is necessary because of the special sense organs of sight and hearing that the neck have a great range of motion in all directions. The position and the mobility of the neck are, therefore, two important factors in its vulnerability to injury.

MOBILITY

The mobility of the cervical spine is dependent upon the composite motion between all the vertebrae and not upon the small amount of motion which occurs between any two of them. The slight flexibility of the intervertebral discs, the shape and inclination of the primary articular processes and their incomplete apposition, as well as the slight laxity of the ligamentous and capsular structures, determine the range of normal motion.

The special architectural design of the atlas and axis, or the first two cervical vertebrae, permits nodding, rotation and lateral bending movements of the head. The head and atlas move primarily as one unit on the axis in rotation and lateral bending movements. Due to the shape of the atlanto-occipital articulations and the laxness of their joint capsules, nodding movements are fairly free. The range of backward movement is greater than the range of forward movement.

The motion between the atlantoaxial joints takes place around transverse, anteroposterior and vertical axes. Nodding, or bending the head forward and backward, occurs about the transverse axis. Bending the head sideways occurs about an anteroposterior axis which is inclined upwards and forwards so that when the head is

5

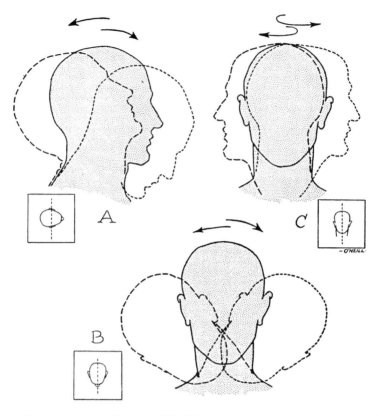

Figure 1. Axes of motion. A: Nodding occurs about a transverse axis. B: Lateral bending occurs about an anteroposterior axis. C: Rotation occurs about a vertical axis.

bent to one side the face is slightly turned toward the opposite side. Rotation of the head occurs around a vertical axis (Fig. 1).

As rotation of the head and atlas takes place upon the axis, the inferior facets of the atlas slip forward and backward over the superior facets of the axis. As one watches this rotatory movement, it can be seen that the lateral masses of the atlas change their relationship to the odontoid process. Turning the head to the left, let us say, causes the anteromedial surface of the right lateral mass, or articular process of the atlas, to approach the odontoid process, while on the left side the posteromedial surface of the

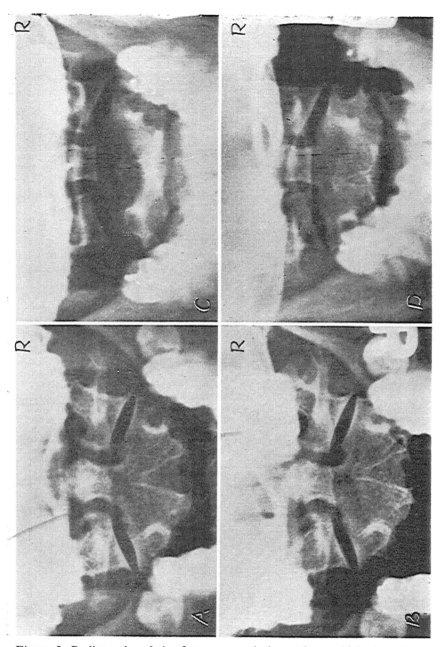

Figure 2. Radiographs of the first two cervical vertebrae which show the relationship of the lateral masses of the atlas to the odontoid process of the axis. The heads are straight in A and C. The head is rotated to the left in B, and in D the head is rotated to the right. There is no change in the relationship of the atlantoaxial joints, and the lateral masses maintain a constant relationship with the odontoid process in radiographs. The axis appears to rotate to the side opposite the rotation of the head because the atlantoaxial ligaments are intact.

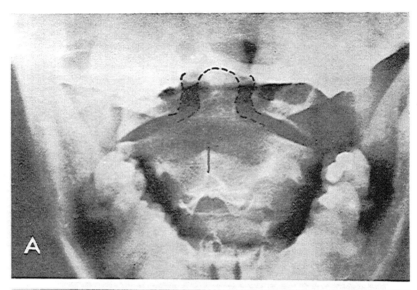

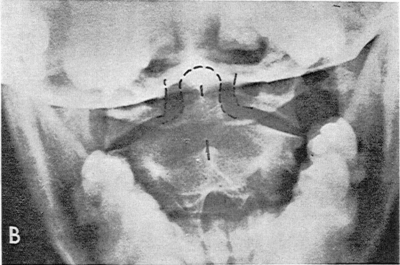

Figure 3. Lateral tilting of the head does not change the atlantoaxial relationship. In A the head is straight. In B the head is tilted to the right, showing a constant relationship between the lateral masses of the atlas and the odontoid and rotation of the axis to the side opposite the tilt, indicating that the alar and atlantoaxial ligaments are intact.

left lateral mass approaches the odontoid process. In radiographic films, the relationship of the lateral masses of the atlas to the odontoid process appears the same as if the head and atlas had not been rotated (Fig. 2). When the head is flexed forward, the

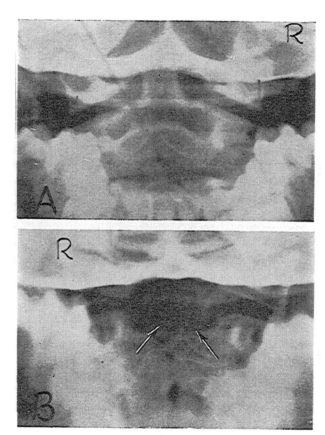

Figure 4. Fracture of the base of the odontoid process with lateral tilting toward the left lateral mass of the atlas is shown in radiograph A. This patient, age nine, was hit in the back of the neck with a stick when he was in a stooped position. It was necessary eventually to fuse the first and second vertebrae. A rudimentary disc between the odontoid process and the body of the axis is shown in B. This patient, age eight, and a brother of patient shown in A, fell out of bed. He had symptoms of cord injury. Note the line of decreased density at the base of the odontoid, the shape of the odontoid and the relationship of the lateral masses to the odontoid and to each other.

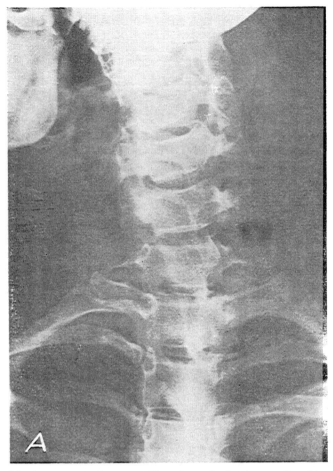

Figure 5A. Anteroposterior x-ray film of cervical spine made with the neck in rotation. Rotation is accompanied by lateral bending.

odontoid process maintains its constant relationship to the anterior arch of the atlas unless there is relaxation of the transverse ligament of the atlas. Lateral tilting of the head does not alter the atlanto-odontoid relationship unless there is undue relaxation of the alar ligaments (Fig. 3). Any appreciable disproportion between the lateral masses of the atlas and the odontoid process of the axis as seen in radiographs is due to a lateral subluxation of the atlas on the axis because of ligamentous instability (Fig. 83),

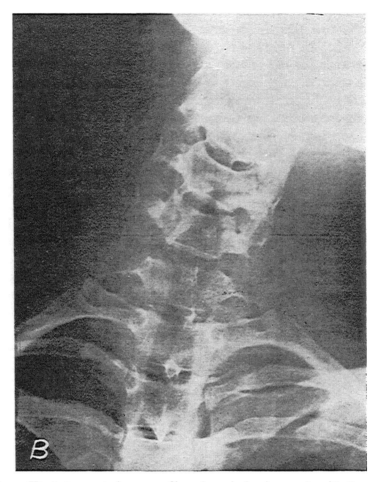

Figure 5B. Anteroposterior x-ray film of cervical spine made with the neck in lateral bending. Lateral bending is accompanied by rotation.

to a fracture-displacement of the odontoid process or to a congenital anomaly (Fig. 4).

The articular surface of the lateral masses of the atlas and the superior articular processes of the axis are not at full apposition when the head is facing straight forward, so that slight tilting of the head to one side is the position of greatest ease and stability.

Motion in the other cervical joints consists of forward flexion, hyperextension, lateral bending and rotation. Here, also, the primary or posterior articulations are not in true apposition when the head faces straight ahead, so that the position of ease and stability occurs when the head and neck are tilted slightly to one side.

Movement in the cervical area is very free when that portion of the spine is considered as a whole. The plane of the articular surfaces facilitates flexion and hyperextension but prevents lateral bending from occurring without some degree of rotation, or prevents rotation from occurring without some degree of lateral bending (Fig. 5). Forward bending of the neck causes each of the spinous processes to separate from each other, whereas hyperextension causes them to approximate each other, giving rise to smooth uninterrupted backward and forward curves, in the absence of any abnormality (Fig. 6). Fielding has shown by cinéradiography that there appears to be a gliding movement between the vertebral bodies, which is due, of course, to the elasticity of the nucleus pulposus of the intervertebral discs, which tends to equalize the pressure in each disc as the bending movements take

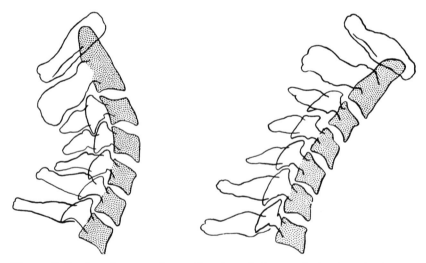

Figure 6. In the absence of any disorder of the cervical spine, backward bending produces a smooth forward curve and flexion produces a smooth backward curve. In extension the spinous processes approach each other and in flexion they separate; although in some instances C6 and C7 show less approximation than do the other spinous processes, as shown here in the hyperextension view.

place. The annulus fibrosus does, because of its elasticity, contribute to these movements. The arrangement of the fibers within the discs and their attachments to the adjacent bony and ligamentous structures definitely restrict movement between adjacent vertebral bodies, but a minimum amount of motion does occur in all directions.

The ligamentous and capsular structures are somewhat lax to permit a normal range of motion. Undue laxness gives rise to subluxations of the articulations, or allows an abnormal range of motion or slipping between the articular surfaces.

THE VERTEBRAE

Descriptions of the cervical vertebrae can be found in all text books of anatomy but certain characteristics of them should be considered here.

The Atlas and the Axis

The first two vertebrae are of special architectural design. The atlas, upon which the skull sits, has no body and only a rudimentary spinous process. The body became detached during its embryological development and fused with the body of the axis to form the odontoid process. The fusion is usually complete by the sixth year, although a rudimentary fibrocartilage disc may, in some instances, persist between the body of the axis and the odontoid process. The atlas is a solid ring of bone consisting of two lateral masses, on the upper and lower surfaces of which are the articular facets; a short anterior arch which articulates with the odontoid process of the axis; and a somewhat longer posterior arch which forms the posterior wall of the vertebral foramen. The superior facets are ellipsoidal in shape and they are cupped for receiving the occipital condyles. The inferior facets are somewhat round in shape; they are concave and face laterally and downward to fit the superior facets of the axis. Extending laterally from the lateral masses are the transverse processes, which are longer and stronger than those of the other vertebrae because they give attachment and leverage for the muscles which rotate the head. Each process encloses a foramen for the vertebral artery, a network of veins and sympathetic fibers. Immediately posterior to the superior facets are grooves for the vertebral arteries and the first cervical nerves, as shown in Figure 7.

The axis is characterized by the odontoid process, which rises perpendicularly from the midportion of its upper surface as a pivot. The odontoid process has an articular facet on its anterior surface for articulating with the anterior arch of the atlas, and one on its posterior surface for articulating with the transverse ligament of the atlas. On each side of the body of the axis is a superior and an inferior facet for articulating with the atlas above and with the third vertebra below. There are no pedicles, therefore. The superior facet faces upward and outward and its surface is convex, whereas the inferior facet faces downward and for-

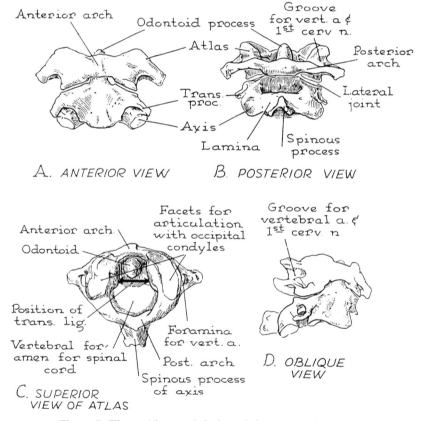

Figure 7. The architectural design of the atlas and the axis.

ward with varying degrees of inclination. The axis has very thick laminae or posterior arch, with a large bifid spinous process. The transverse processes are small and have single rounded tubercles at their ends, as well as foramina for passage of the vertebral arteries with their accompanying postganglionic sympathetic nerve fibers and veins.

The inferior surface of the body of the axis is beveled on its posterolateral margins for articulating with the upward lips on the adjacent surfaces of the third vertebra. The anterior and inferior margin is somewhat rounded and juts downward and slightly forward.

These special characteristics of the upper two vertebrae leave them without intervertebral foramina for the first and second nerve roots, as shown in Figure 17. The nerve roots lie upon the posterior surfaces of the lateral masses.

The blood supply of the odontoid process has been studied by Schiff and Parke in an attempt to clarify the pathological processes involving the odontoid process which may be related to its arterial supply. They showed that the odontoid is supplied on each side by ascending anterior and posterior arteries which arise from the vertebral arteries at or near the lower portion of the axis. The right and left posterior ascending arteries meet in the midline to form an apical arcade at the apex of the odontoid to supply it, the apical and alar ligaments and the periarticular structures. At the base of the odontoid, perforating arteries from the internal carotid arteries afford anastomosing branches with the anterior and posterior ascending branches of the vertebral arteries.

Injuries or some involvement of the upper portion of the cervical spine can be anticipated to cause sclerotic or necrotic changes in the odontoid process as well as changes in the immediate ligamentous structures.

The Lower Five Vertebrae

These vertebrae have characteristics in common. They possess bodies, vertebral arches, pedicles, superior and inferior facets, laminae and spinous processes.

The vertebral bodies are distinctive. Their transverse diameters are nearly twice the anteroposterior diameters. Their posterior surfaces are flattened, whereas their anterior surfaces are rounded, and the vertical diameters are greater posteriorly than anteriorly, which contributes to the difference between the vertical diameters of the anterior and posterior portions of the intervertebral discs.

The upper surfaces of the bodies are somewhat concave and at the margins are the "vertebral rims" which give attachments for Sharpey's fibers of the intervertebral discs. At the posterolateral margins there are upward curved lips or projections, often called uncinate processes, for articulating with the corresponding beveled areas on the inferior surfaces of the vertebrae above them. These upward projections are clearly visible at the age of nine or ten as shown in radiographs. The lower surfaces are somewhat concave from the front to the back but slightly convex from side to side (Fig. 8).

The vertebral arches arise from the cartilaginous plates, as do the pedicles with their superior and inferior articulating facets,

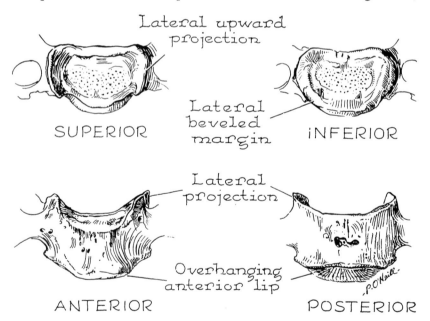

Figure 8. The anatomic characteristics of the bodies of the lower five cervical vertebrae, except the inferior surface of the body of the seventh which simulates a thoracic vertebra.

which face at a forty-five degree angle to the bodies. The laminae arise from their own centers of ossification and arch backward to meet in the midline where the spinous processes are formed and which jut downward and become bifid at their ends, except the seventh which is longer than the others and is not bifid.

The articular masses are called pillars, and the portion of bone between the facets is called the interarticular isthmus. The articular masses are placed posterior to the transverse processes. The transverse processes project laterally, slightly anteriorly and downward. Their upper surfaces are grooved or troughlike and the cervical nerves with their accompanying structures lie in these grooves.

Each of these vertebrae has three primary centers of ossification —one for the body or the centrum and one for each neural or vertebral arch. At birth each vertebra is in three pieces—the centrum of the body and one neural arch on either side. The centrum is joined to each posterolateral part (or neural arch) by a plate of cartilage which has been called the *neurocentral joint*. The neurocentral joints disappear in the cervical spine in the third year. Each upward lateral projection on the sides of the vertebral bodies, or the uncus if you prefer, is derived from the center of ossification of the neural arch and is fused with the center of ossification of the vertebral body at the age of three.

The transverse processes arise from the cartilaginous plates beween the vertebral bodies and the neural arches. Each transverse process has two distinct parts or roots—an anterior and a posterior. The posterior root is the true transverse process and it arises from the anterior portion of the articular pillar and ends laterally as the posterior tubercle. The anterior root corresponds to a rib and is called the costal process. It arises at the side of the vertebral body and ends laterally as the anterior tubercle.

The posterior tubercles provide attachments of origin for the middle and posterior scalene muscles: the middle, two through six; posterior, four through six. The anterior tubercles from the third to the sixth provide attachments of origin for the anterior scalene and longus capitis muscles, and the superior oblique portion of the longus cervicis muscles arise from the third, fourth and fifth. The inferior oblique portions of the longus cervicis muscles are inserted into the fifth and sixth anterior tubercles.

The anterior and posterior roots are united near their free ends by a curved bar of bone called the costotransverse lamella. The plane of the two roots and of the transverse lamella varies from the third to the sixth vertebra. The two roots of each transverse process, the transverse lamella, and the pedicle at the side of the vertebral body form the boundaries of a somewhat oval-shaped foramen which is called the *foramen transversarium.* In some instances a spicule of bone divides the foramen, thus producing two foramina. Through each transverse foramen, except the seventh, passes the vertebral artery and its plexus of veins, a tangled web of sympathetic fibers and on the posterior aspect of the vertebral artery, at least as high as the fourth vertebra, a plexus of sympathetic ganglia. Each transverse foramen of the seventh cervical vertebra is an empty hole through which, for some unknown reason, nothing passes.

The cervical nerves, three through eight, as they leave the intervertebral foramina, lie between the middle and anterior scalene muscles, as does the subclavian artery as it passes over the first rib between the insertion of these muscles.

The vertebral arches, which are joined to the posterolateral aspects of the vertebral bodies midway between the upper and lower margins, consist of pedicles with inferior and superior facets for articulation with the proximate vertebrae. The superior articulating processes do face upward at a near forty-five degree angle to the bodies. The portion of the bone between the facets is called the interarticular isthmus. These articulating masses when in a column form rounded pillars behind the transverse processes.

The posterior portion of the vertebral bodies, the pedicles and the neural arches, or laminae, form the spinal canal, or vertebral foramen, which is somewhat triangular in shape and is larger in comparison to the foramen in the thoracic and lumbar areas to accommodate the largest portion of the spinal cord and to protect the spinal cord from compression by the normal movements of the neck.

Each lamina fuses with its partner posteriorly to form the spinous process at the early part of the second year of life. Each spinous process, except the seventh, is bifid for the attachment of the deep posterior neck muscles; even the sixth, as well as the seventh, spinous process may not be bifid. The spinous processes slope downward and may overlap the adjacent distal spinous process. Certainly they vary in size and strength and in their downward inclination in each individual.

THE JOINTS AND THEIR LIGAMENTS

The Atlantoaxial Joints

There are four synovial joints between the atlas and the axis— two lateral and two median. The lateral joints are formed by the opposing articular surfaces on the lateral masses. The median joints are formed by the articulation of the odontoid process with the anterior arch of the atlas and by the articulation of the odontoid process with the transverse ligament of the atlas, which is called a bursa rather than a joint by some authors.

The plane of the lateral joints is inclined laterally and downward. The inferior articular surface of each lateral mass of the atlas is somewhat concave to conform with the superior articular surface of the axis which is convex. This design permits a great amount of rotation between these two vertebrae, in fact the greatest amount which can occur between any two vertebrae (Fig. 7).

The capsules of these lateral joints and their ligamentous structures have sufficient laxness to permit the great range of motion found here. However, the special arrangement of the ligaments and their unusual design prevent movement beyond a specific range and assure the maintenance of a constant relationship of the axis and the atlas so that the head and the atlas do not fall off the neck, aided, of course, by the capital muscles.

These ligaments deserve special attention (Fig. 9A, B, C, D). The internal or deep ligaments are important checking structures in the prevention of trauma to the upper portion of the cervical spinal cord. The transverse ligament of the atlas, which arises from small tubercles on either side of the anterior arch of the atlas on its posterior surface and from the lateral masses of the atlas, forms a sling behind the odontoid process to hold it firmly against

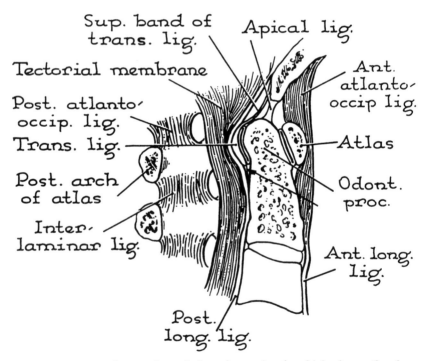

POSTERIOR VIEW WITH POSTERIOR ARCHES REMOVED

Foramen magnum

Alar lig.

Apical lig.

Occipital condyle

Atlas

Trans. lig.

Accessory atlanto-axial ligs.

Axis

Post. long. lig.

Figure 9A. The deep posterior ligamentous structures of the atlas and the axis. The small arrow points to the sectioned superior band of the transverse ligament and the large arrow points to the inferior band of the transverse ligament.

MEDIAN SECTION

Sup. band of trans. lig.

Apical lig.

Tectorial membrane

Ant. atlanto-occip lig.

Post. atlanto-occip. lig.

Trans. lig.

Atlas

Post. arch of atlas

Odont. proc.

Inter-laminar lig.

Ant. long. lig.

Post. long. lig.

Figure 9B. A median section of the atlas and axis which shows the deep ligaments and the superficial ligaments of this very complex portion of the cervical spine. Arrow points to the inferior band of the transverse ligament.

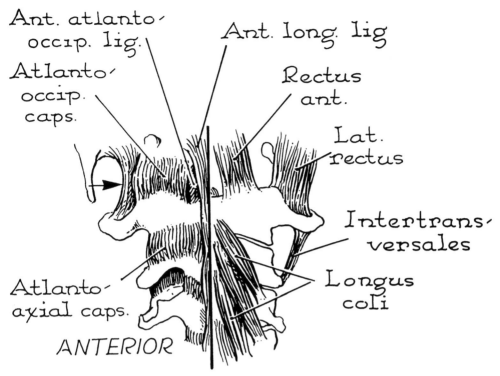

Figure 9C. The ligaments, capsules and suboccipital muscles as seen from the front of the upper portion of the cervical spine. The arrow points to the lateral atlantoaxial ligament.

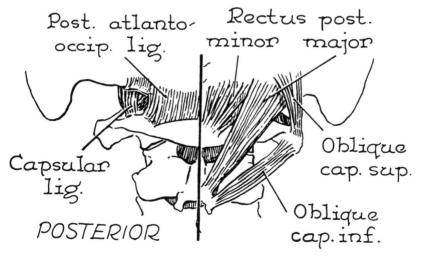

Figure 9D. The suboccipital capsules, superficial ligaments and muscles, as seen from behind.

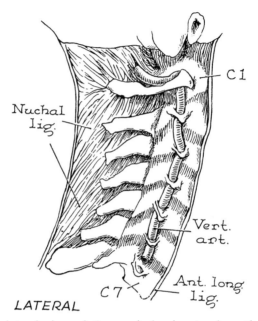

Figure 9E. A lateral view of the cervical spine to show the interspinous ligament, or the nuchal ligament, which forms an intermuscular septum in the posterior midline of the cervical spine.

the midportion of the anterior arch. If the odontoid is fractured, the transverse ligament will prevent posterior dislocation of the odontoid, but it does not prevent forward dislocation without the aid of other intact ligaments.

Extending upward from the midportion of the transverse ligament, there is a band which is attached to the margin of the foramen magnum, and extending downward there is another band which is attached to the midportion of the body of the axis. This gives the transverse ligament the appearance of a cross. These vertical extensions of the transverse ligament add to its strength and are of definite assistance in preventing luxation forward.

Beneath the transverse ligament, and arising from the tip of the odontoid, there is another small ligament which extends vertically beneath the superior band to attach to the midanterior surface of the foramen magnum. It is called the apical or suspensory ligament of the odontoid (Fig. 9B).

Extending from the medial aspect of the condyles of the occipital bone downward and medially, are two very strong ligamentous bands which have their medial attachments to the upper lateral portions of the odontoid (alar ligaments) as shown in Figure 9A. These are very important check ligaments which limit rotation of the skull and the atlas on the axis and prevent lateral subluxation of the skull and the atlas on the axis. In this connection, it must be kept in mind that the skull and atlas move very much as one unit and that there is only a little side to side gliding movement between them because the condyles of the skull fit snugly into the elliptical cuplike superior facets of the lateral masses of the atlas, forward and backward movements are free, backward more than forward.

Two other important check ligaments extend from the inner aspect of the lateral masses of the atlas obliquely downward and slightly inward to become attached to the lateral aspects of the posterior surface of the body of the axis (the accessory atlanto-axial ligaments). These two ligaments check excessive rotation of the atlas and the head on the axis (Fig. 9A).

The tectorial ligament, which is the upper portion of the posterior longitudinal ligament, is somewhat fan-shaped at its attachment to the basilar groove of the occipital bone. It extends downward over the posterior surface of the vertebral bodies and covers the other ligaments described above giving them additional strength and reinforcement (Fig. 9B).

The other ligamentous structures can be considered as superficial or external ligaments. Anteriorly there is a broad dense band of ligament which extends from the anterior margin of the foramen magnum to the upper border of the anterior arch of the atlas and it is continuous laterally with the capsules of the atlanto-occipital joints (the anterior atlanto-occipital ligament–Fig. 9C). It is reinforced in its midportion by a round ligament which extends from the basilar portion of the occipital bone to a tubercle on the anterior surface of the anterior arch of the atlas. The articular capsules are reinforced by the lateral atlanto-occipital ligaments which extend from the jugular process of the occipital bone to the transverse process of the atlas on each side.

Another strong ligamentous band extends from the anterior

arch of the atlas to the anterior surface of the body of the axis. Overlying this and the anterior atlanto-occipital ligament is the narrow anterior longitudinal ligament, which reinforces actually only the midportion of these two structures.

The posterior atlanto-occipital ligament connects the margins of the foramen magnum with the upper margin of the posterior arch of the atlas (Fig. 9D). The vertebral arteries pierce this ligament to enter the cranium. The first cervical nerve pierces it also. In some instances the posterior portion of the ligament becomes ossified and forms a bony arch behind the artery on one or both sides, as seen in Figure 69.

The ligamentum flavum extends from the inner surface of the posterior arch of the atlas to the margin of the superior surface of the lamina of the axis, and it aids in preventing the head and atlas from forward displacement on the axis, as well as giving protection to the spinal cord.

The interspinous ligament in the cervical area is of special design to lend further support to the other ligaments. It is a somewhat fan-shaped structure which extends from the external occipital protuberance and median nuchal line downward and between the spinous processes of all the cervical vertebrae and forms a septum in the midline between the muscles on the posterior aspect of the neck (Fig. 9E). It is much stronger in quadripeds than in bipeds because it must help hold the head forward and upward against the force of gravity.

From the foregoing discussion of the joints and the ligamentous structures of the upper portion of the cervical spine, one wonders why we were endowed with so much movement at this area and were deprived of sufficient structural stability to protect adequately the so vital structures which connect the brain with the body. It is true that few people lose their heads, and hence their lives, as compared to other causes of death. However, in this era of increased traumatic experiences, one should keep in mind that even unstable joints and ligamentous structures which are secondary to trauma or disease can result in a variety of disabilities. Therefore, let us tear away some of these stabilizing structures to see what happens.

If the transverse ligament of the atlas is cut, torn or stretched, or in any way weakened, the head and atlas luxate forward on the axis to narrow the vertebral foramen and thus cause compression of the spinal cord. The amount of cord damage will depend upon the amount of luxation and upon how well the other supporting ligaments are functioning. Even a small amount of luxation can be detected in lateral, forward-bending radiographs. If the superior band is severed, the head may have a tendency to slip forward; if the inferior band is weakened, the head and the atlas will slip forward on the axis (Fig. 10).

Cutting or stretching the alar ligaments will permit luxation of the head and atlas to the side. If the left alar ligament is not functioning, the slipping will be to the right side, as seen in Figure 11.

If one of the accessory atlantoaxial ligaments is stretched or severed, rotation of the axis occurs because these ligaments check rotation when intact. If, at the same time, the alar ligament and

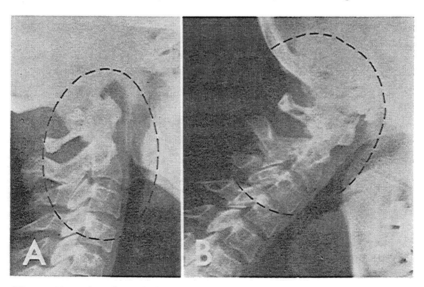

Figure 10. Relaxation of the transverse ligament of the atlas permits forward slipping of the atlas on the axis when the head is placed forward as shown in B. In the straight position, the anterior arch of the atlas is not separated from the odontoid process as seen in A. This relationship does not change when the head is placed forward unless the transverse ligament is stretched or relaxed.

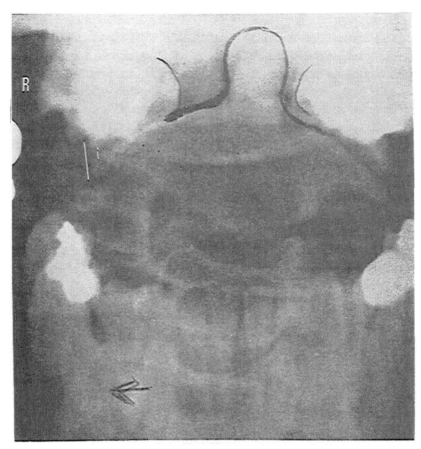

Figure 11. Note the marked disproportion between the lateral masses of the atlas and the odontoid process. The atlas is subluxated to the right because the alar ligament on the left side is torn or stretched.

the accessory atlantoaxial ligament are cut on the same side, subluxation of the head and the atlas on the axis and rotation of the axis occur because both guy wires are broken on the same side, as illustrated in Figure 12. Under normal conditions, when the head and first cervical vertebra are rotated to one side the second vertebra rotates to the opposite side, as shown in Figure 2, or so it appears in the radiograph. Stretching or tearing of these ligaments can occur when the neck is forcefully flexed. If the head is

rotated and tilted to one side, stretching or tearing of the ligaments on the opposite side may occur. The short ligaments which
bridge two bony parts are most susceptible to stretching or tearing.

If one places the atlas upon the axis and then rotates the atlas
on the axis, the posterior arch of the atlas slips over the posterior
arch or lamina of the axis and thus encroaches on the vertebral
foramen. If the spinal cord were within the foramen, it would be
compressed by the posterior arch of the atlas. However, when the

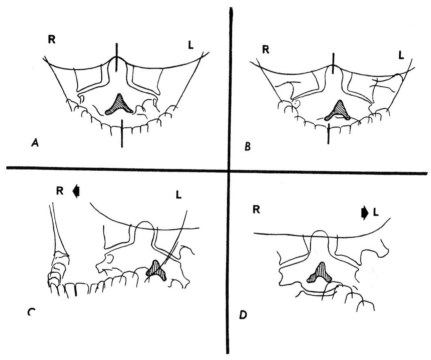

Figure 12. Tracings of radiographs. In A there is a normal relationship between the axis and the atlas. In B the axis is rotated to the left side because
the right accessory atlantoaxial ligament is torn or stretched. In the latter
instance, when the head is rotated to the right, the axis rotates to the left
because the left accessory atlantoaxial ligament is intact as shown in C.
However, when this neck and head are rotated to the left side, the axis does
not rotate to the right because the right accessory ligament is torn and the
right alar ligament is torn or stretched which allows subluxation of the
atlas on the axis to the left side.

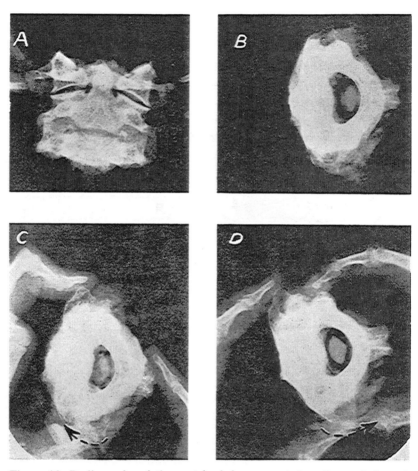

Figure 13. Radiographs of the vertebral foramen at the atlas and the axis with the ligaments and capsules intact. With rotation of the atlas on the axis there is very little, if any, encroachment on the canal by the posterior arch of the atlas.

ligamentous and capsular structures are intact there is little if any encroachment of the vertebral foramen by the posterior arch of the atlas, as demonstrated in Figure 13. It is true that the vertebral foramen is larger in the cervical area than in the other areas of the spine which is for accommodation of the largest part of the spinal cord, but it is not large enough to permit the marked encroachment of the posterior arch of the atlas, as demonstrated by Fielding, without compression of the spinal cord.

The Other Joints

The joints below the atlantoaxial articulations are of special design, also, as compared with the joints of the thoracic and lumbar areas. There are three joints between each two adjacent vertebrae in the latter areas: the posterior, or apophyseal joints, the secondary fibrocartilaginous joint (or the joint which is made by the fibrocartilaginous disc) and the adjacent surfaces of the vertebral bodies. In the cervical area between the second and third and each subsequent vertebrae, there are in addition two small lateral joints between the vertebral bodies, as shown in Figure 14.

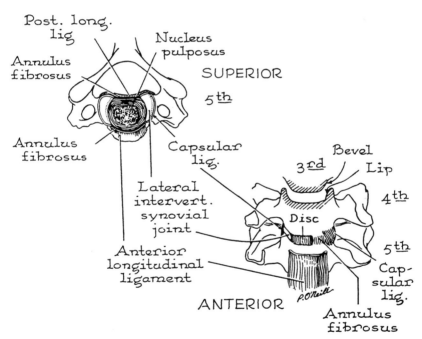

Figure 14. Intervertebral disc and lateral interbody joints. Disc does not extend to the lateral side of the vertebral bodies because of the lateral intervertebral joints. The annulus is thicker posteriorly than anteriorly, and it has a very narrow exposure posteriorly as compared to its anterior exposure.

Angle of Inclination (Apophyseal Joints)

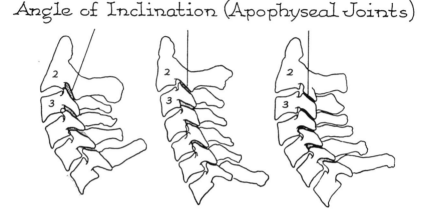

Figure 15. The angle of inclination of the posterior joints varies.

The Posterior Joints

The posterior joints, as elsewhere in the movable portion of the spine, are formed by the articular processes of the vertebral arches. The articulating surfaces are flat and the plane of the joints faces upward at a near forty-five degree angle, although the angle of inclination varies between the second and third vertebrae (Fig. 15).

The Lateral Interbody Joints

The lateral interbody joints are formed by the upward lateral projections, or lips, on the postero-superior surfaces of the vertebral bodies and the corresponding beveled areas on the infero-lateral surfaces of the bodies. The upper lip and the corresponding beveled area are covered with articular hyaline cartilage, as are all other articulating surfaces.

According to medical literature, these articulating surfaces were described as true joints with capsules and synovial linings by von Luschka in 1858. He called them "hemiarthroses interverte-brales laterales." This is an excellent descriptive term but, as so frequently happens when something new or different is described, they now bear his name–the joints of "Luschka." Trolard, in 1892, called them "articulations uncovertebrales." It has been pointed out in *Cunningham's Text Book of Anatomy* that these small joints are analogous to the joints between the lateral masses of the atlas and axis which are placed on the body and pedicles rather than at the junction of the pedicles with the laminae as they are in the other vertebrae. I have preferred to call these small articulations *the lateral interbody joints,* which leaves no doubt concerning their anatomical position and gives them a more definite identity.

In recent years, there has been much controversy over these particular articulations. In 1950, Bovill attempted to show that they are not true synovial joints but only brusae. Compere, in 1959, demonstrated all of the elements of a true joint in microscopic sections of these lateral interbody articulations. However, one year later Sherman and her coworkers attempted to show that these are not true synovial joints but are the result of degenerative processes occurring within the disc joints resulting in osteophytic growth at the margins of the adjacent vertebral bodies.

Other authors, including Cunningham, Brain, Bull and Cave, have referred to these joints as "Neurocentral Joints," which, as Hall has stated, is unfortunate and confusing inasmuch as this term has been used to indicate the cartilaginous plate which joins the ossification centers of the vertebral body to the vertebral arches in infants and which disappears at the age of three years. The upward lateral projection (or uncus if you prefer to think of it as a hook) is, as previously stated, derived from the center of ossification of the vertebral arch and fuses with the ossification center of the vertebral body; as Hall has stated, this refutes the suggestion that the upward lateral projections occur only as a postnatal development or that they are the result of degenerative processes occurring within the disc joints and represent osteophytic formations at the margins of the vertebral bodies, or that they are simply adaptive processes.

Despite the controversies which have arisen, certain facts are evident: (1) The adjacent surfaces at the sides of the bodies of the vertebrae are plated with articular cartilage. (2) Capsular ligaments are present. (3) There is a definite space between the adjacent articular surfaces (Fig. 16). (4) These articulations do

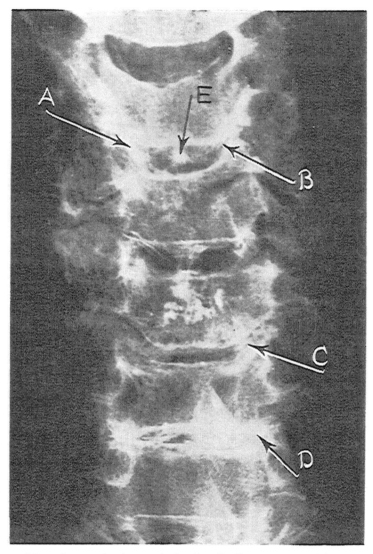

Figure 16. Arthrograph of a cervical spine. Radiopaque material was injected into the lateral interbody joints at A, B, C and D. The material has remained within the joints at A, B and C. At D the material has spread into
the crevices of the degenerated disc. The material was injected into the disc
at E.

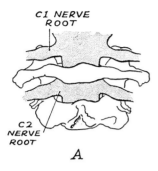

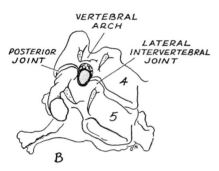

Figure 17. Intervertebral foramina. A: First and second nerve roots have no foramina. B: Typical foramen showing the boundaries of the other nerve roots.

satisfy the standard definition of synovial joints. (5) Osteophytic formations do occur at the margins of the articulations which is characteristic of synovial joints. (6) They are of great significance in the cervical spine because of the proximity of the cervical nerve roots as they lie within their intervertebral canals, as shown in Figure 17B. (7) They act as barriers to the extrusion of cervical disc material because they are placed posterolaterally between the vertebral bodies, as shown in Plate 3-1, hence preventing pressure upon the cervical nerve roots from extruded disc material, which occurs in the lumbar area especially and to a lesser extent in the thoracic area (Fig. 18). (8) Grossly and microscopically, chondromalacic changes are found in the articular cartilages of these joints such as occur in other synovial joints. (9) They do, as suggested by Luschka, account for the greater mobility of the cervical spine as compared to other areas of the spine. (10) The annulus fibrosus of the cervical discs does not extend to the lateral margins of the vertebral bodies but ends at the medial boundaries of the lateral interbody joints.

The presence of a space between the articular surfaces of the posterolateral areas of the vertebral bodies is shown in Figure 16. A radiopaque material was injected into some of the interbody articulations of a specimen and then radiographs were made of the specimen. Marked degenerative changes of the disc between the sixth and seventh vertebrae can be seen. Here the radiopaque material has spread through the crevices of the disc, indicating that marked degenerative changes in a disc disrupt the medial boundaries of the corresponding interbody joints. Later dissection of this area revealed the marked degeneration of the disc and of the interbody joints. The articular surfaces of the joints presented a typical gross picture of chondromalacia, and there were spur formations at the margins of the joints.

It is possible that these lateral interbody joints are remnants of the synovial joints which are found between the cervical vertebrae of some of the lower vertebrates such as birds. They do not occur

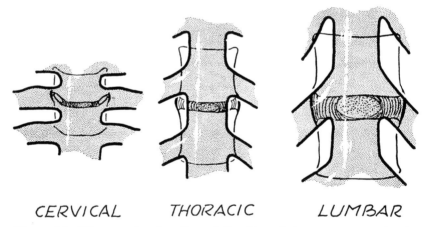

CERVICAL   THORACIC   LUMBAR

Figure 18. Diagram showing the relationship of the nerve roots in the cervical, thoracic and lumbar areas of the spine. In the cervical area, the nerve roots do not pass over the intervertebral discs and are protected from the discs, which in most instances extrude posteriorly. In the thoracic area, the nerve roots lie above the intervertebral discs, whereas in the lumbar area the nerve roots lie directly over the posterolateral portions of the discs and are, therefore, extremely vulnerable to disc extrusion.

in the canidae, but they are present in primates, marsupials and rodents, as shown by Hall.

The Secondary Fibrocartilaginous Joints

The secondary fibrocartilaginous joints in the cervical spine are distinctive. The vertical diameter, or the height, of the anterior portion of the disc is approximately two to three times greater than the posterior diameter. This design normally assures a forward curve in the cervical area and permits the discs to conform to the contour of the superior and inferior surfaces of the adjacent vertebral bodies, as illustrated in Figure 19. In most instances, the nucleus pulposus of the disc is slightly anterior to the midportion of the disc, and the annulus fibrosus is thicker posteriorly in its anteroposterior diameter than it is anteriorly, as seen in Figure 19. There is some controversy concerning this, but in my dissections this has been found to be true.

The discs do not extend to the posterolateral margins of the

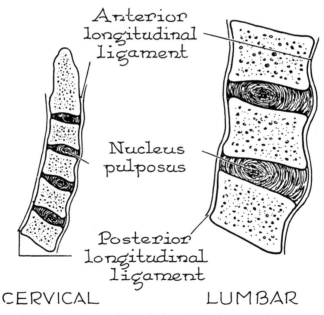

Figure 19. Median section of cervical and lumbar vertebrae to show the position of the nucleus pulposus and the vertical diameter of the discs which is greater anteriorly than posteriorly.

adjacent vertebral bodies because it is at this location that the lateral interbody joints are found, so that the discs form the medial boundaries of these joints.

Clefts or fissures may appear in the disc and extend laterally through the annulus fibrosus to connect the disc with the lateral interbody joint or joints, as shown in Figure 16 at D. The cause of such fissuring is somewhat controversial. My dissections of cervical spines have shown that these clefts appear only when there is evidence of disc prolapse, disc narrowing or loss of nuclear substance. Chronic stress and strain, acute trauma of a disc or of the lateral interbody joints may cause a breakthrough between these structures. Tondry has demonstrated fissuring or clefts in the middle portion of the intervertebral discs and states that they always originate first in the upper discs and that they form in the lower more movable part of the cervical spine later or are missing entirely. He believes that the lateral interbody joints are only clefts and not true joints. He believes that the clefts in the lateral interbody joints have a tendency to break through the discs transversely, dividing the discs into two parts, and that because these clefts are connected with the nucleus pulposus of each disc the nuclear material is able to escape laterally. As a result of the loss of the insufficient intervertebral disc, the so-called uncinate processes act as load carriers and become thickened and are transformed into clublike swollen appendages of the vertebral bodies. He contends that the fibrous cartilaginous coating of the uncinate processes disappears little by little, inasmuch as they cannot for long serve a supporting function.

My dissections and the injection of radiopaque material into the discs of cervical spines have not revealed such findings. Plates 1-1 and 1-2 show fissuring extending laterally through the interbody joints only where there is evidence of osteophytic changes about the lateral interbody joints and narrowing or degeneration of the proximate discs. One wonders, therefore, if perhaps the clefts or fissures as shown by Tondry are the result of sectioning the cervical spine.

Each disc with its adjacent vertebral bodies and their processes should be considered as a single motor unit; under normal conditions, each unit possesses definite dynamic and mechanical functions. Any disturbance in any one motor unit has an effect upon the adjacent motor units, which is true in all areas of the spine and is due to the interrelationship of all the individual components of the motor segments.

The lower five cervical vertebrae are held apart and at the same time are held together by the fibrocartilaginous discs. However, the ligamentous structures are of significant importance in the maintenance of the proper relationship between the vertebrae. The anterior longitudinal ligament is a fibrous band which extends from the base of the skull over the anterior arch of the atlas to which it is attached and proceeds downward over the anterior surfaces of the vertebral bodies. It is firmly attached to the bodies and loosely attached to the intervening discs. It is a single layered structure and is fairly weak as compared to the posterior longitudinal ligament.

The posterior longitudinal ligament is a strong, two-layered ligament, although most anatomists do not recognize this as being true; however, the cervical portion of this ligament does present two very distinct layers. The superficial layer is the continuation of the tectorial membrane or ligament and it is a dense broad structure which is attached to the vertebral bodies and to the deep layer of the ligament which it overlies. The deep layer is denticulated in appearance as seen in the thoracic and lumbar areas. It is narrow over the vertebral bodies and fans outward as it passes over the intervertebral discs. It is firmly attached to the bones and to the discs, which in all probability prevents posterior extrusion of disc material and accounts for the low incidence of such occurrence in the cervical area. The capsular ligaments of the lateral interbody joints take origin from the deep layer, as well as the vertebral body, as they pass obliquely downward and laterally to gain attachment to the margins of the upward projections on the posterolateral aspects of the superior surfaces of the vertebral bodies, as illustrated in Figure 20.

The interlaminar ligaments, or the ligamenta flava, bridge the intervals between the laminae. Each one is attached above to the front of the lower border of the lamina and below to the back of

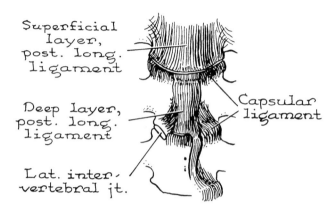

Figure 20. The two-layered posterior longitudinal ligament and the capsular ligaments of the lateral intervertebral joints.

the upper border of the adjacent lamina. The ligament is actually divided in the midline by a cleft through which pass veins that connect the venous plexus within the vertebral canal to the posterior venous plexus.

Each ligament extends laterally to the capsules of the apophyseal joints but does not blend with the capsules. These ligaments are the most elastic ligaments in the body and they permit separation of the laminae in flexion of the cervical spine. On hyperextension of the cervical spine, because of their elasticity they shorten, which prevents their folding into the vertebral canal or to be caught between the laminae they connect. Their elastic tension aids the posterior neck muscles in holding the head and neck erect.

In the neck, the supraspinous ligament which connects the tips of the spinous processes merges with the interspinous ligaments to form the *nuchal ligament,* which is a fibrous partition between the posterior muscles at each side of the neck. In man, the nuchal ligament is much less elastic than in quadrupeds and lends very little support to the posterior muscles.

The nerve supply to the capsular and ligamentous structures of the cervical spine is of great significance in the interpretation of painful conditions. The capsules of the atlantoaxial joints and of the posterior or apophyseal joints are supplied by the capsular branches of the medial divisions of the posterior primary rami of the cervical spinal nerves. The posterior longitudinal ligament and the capsular structures of the lateral interbody joints receive their nerve supply from the recurrent spinal meningeal nerves (the sinuvertebral nerves) which contain afferent somatic sensory and efferent sympathetic fibers. The nerve supply to the anterior longitudinal ligament has never been adequately defined.

Jung and Brunschwig, in 1932, were able to demonstrate the presence of nerve endings in the ligament and they found that these endings were much more numerous in the central portion of the ligament than at the lateral margins. They were unable to demonstrate nerve endings in the annulus fibrosus, nor did they determine the origin of the nerve supply to the ligament.

Roofe, in 1940, described nerve endings in the posterior portion of the annulus which emanate from the nerve supply to the posterior longitudinal ligament—the recurrent spinal meningeal nerves. Cloward believes that branches of the spinal meningeal nerve from each side pass around the disc, that the terminal fibers extend a short distance across the midline and decussate with those from the opposite side, and that the terminal fibers probably enter the anterior longitudinal ligament where it crosses the disc. He postulates that the ligament as a whole has a very insignificant nerve supply.

Inasmuch as the actual origin of the nerve supply to this ligament is not known, one can postulate further that the ligament is supplied by the nerves of the adjacent muscles, which is true of other joints. In this event, the nerve supply would derive from the anterior primary rami of the cervical nerves. The muscular branches carry both somatic efferent fibers and somatic afferent proprioceptive fibers, or sensory endings. The former are motor fibers and the latter serve sensations of pain, a common accompaniment of injury or disorder of the structures supplied.

The nerve supply to the other ligamentous structures, although not specifically defined in the anatomic literature, must be pre-

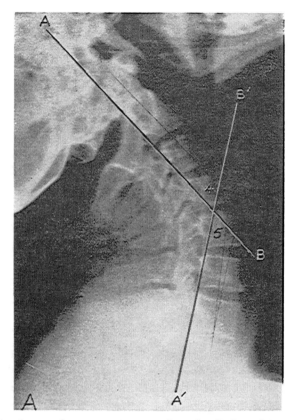

Figure 21A. Areas of greatest stress and strain. Point of intersection of lines AB and A'B' indicates level of greatest stress and strain in hyperextension.

sumed to derive from the muscular branches supplying the overlying or adjacent muscles.

THE AREAS OF GREATEST STRESS AND STRAIN

The joints between the sixth and seventh cervical vertebrae are the first freely movable joints above the dorsal area, but the joints between the sixth and fifth and between the fifth and fourth vertebrae are more vulnerable to stress and strain and to injury than are any of the other joints. This can be illustrated on lateral x-ray films made with the neck in hyperextension and in flexion (Fig. 21). In the position of hyperextension, the joints between

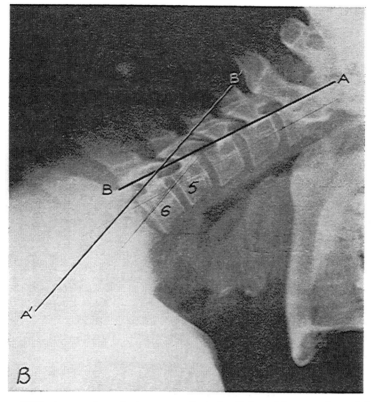

Figure 21B. Areas of greatest stress and strain. Point of intersection of lines AB and A'B' indicates level of greatest stress and strain in flexion.

the fourth and fifth vertebrae are at the apex of the forward curve of the cervical spine, whereas the joints between the fifth and sixth vertebrae are at the apex of the backward curve of the cervical spine when the neck is in flexion. In the hyperextended position, a line AB drawn parallel to the posterior surface of the body of the second cervical vertebra and a line A'B' drawn parallel to the posterior surface of the body of the seventh cervical vertebra intersect each other at the level of the interspace between the fourth and fifth vertebrae. This indicates that the point of greatest stress and strain occurs at the level of the fourth and fifth articulations in hyperextension. In the flexed position, the line AB and the line A'B' intersect each other at the level of the interspace between the

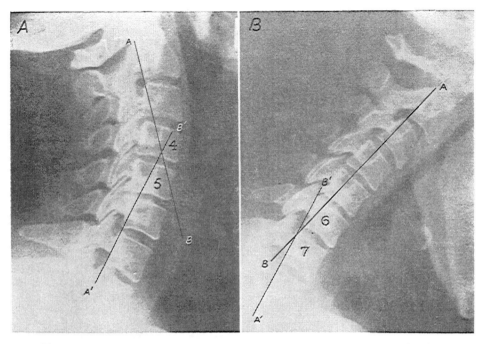

Figure 22A and B. Areas of maximum stress and strain altered by fixation of vertebrae. Films A and B were made in 1946. Note progressive hypertrophic and degenerative changes and alteration in the points of maximum stress and strain as further fixation has occurred.

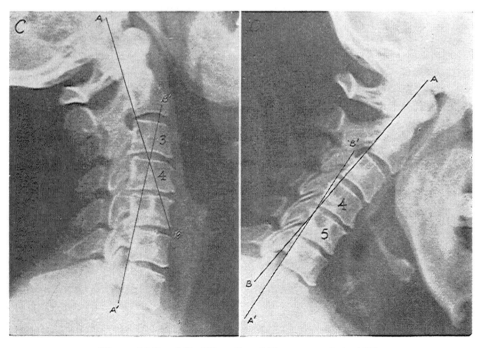

Figure 22C and D. Films C and D were made in 1953.

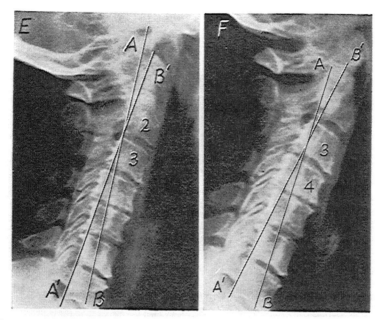

Figure 22E and F. Radiographs E and F, made in 1957, demonstrate that points of maximum stress have shifted upward in hyperextension (E) and in flexion (F) with the increased fixation or altered motion. Note the increased osteophytic changes which have occurred in spite of the minimal amount of motion which occurs below the second and third vertebrae.

fifth and sixth cervical vertebrae, which indicates that the greatest amount of stress and strain occurs at this level when the neck is in flexion.

Limitation of motion of the cervical spine from muscle spasm or fixation, however, will alter the point of greatest stress and strain depending on the degree and level of motion and the area of fixation. In Figure 22A and B it can be seen that there is degeneration of the intervertebral discs between C4 and C5, and C5 and C6, with narrowing of the discs and hypertrophic changes. In hyperextension, the apex of the forward curve is at the body of C4. There is fixation of C4, 5 and 6 which decreases the backward curve when the neck is in flexion so that the point of greatest stress and strain falls at the level of C6 and 7. However, as the degenerative processes progress, one can see that the points of

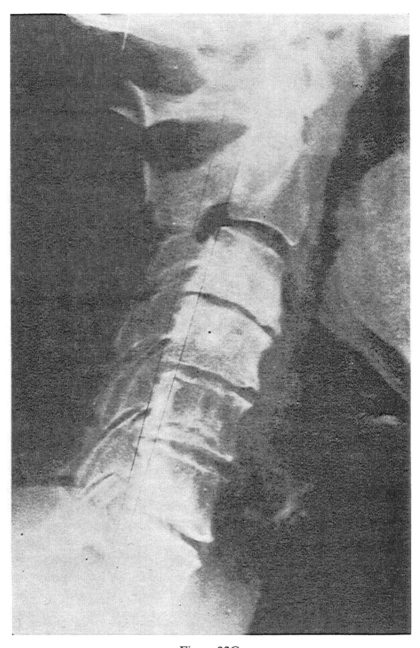

Figure 22G

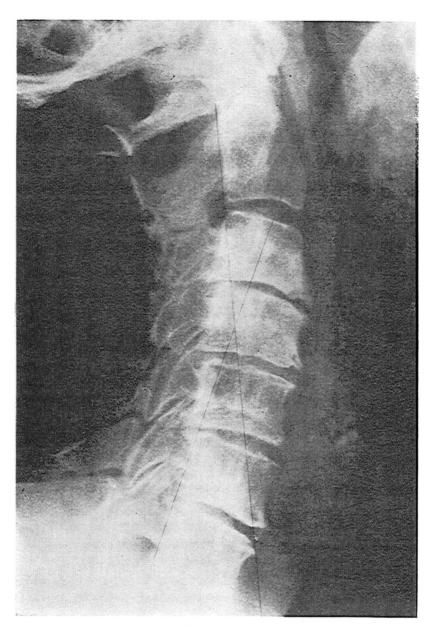

Figure 22H

Figure 22G and H. The radiographs in G and H are of the same cervical spine made in 1965 following a severe rear-end collision which caused a fracture of the upper portion of the odontoid process. The points of maximum stress have shifted downward in hyperextension (H) and downward to the upper thoracic area in flexion (G). There now appears to be some motion between the other vertebrae indicating spraining of the ligamentous and capsular structures and the severity of the injury.

greatest stress and strain are altered again, and ligamentous instability is demonstrable above the area of fixation (Fig. 22C and D). This may be due to sprain of the ligamentous and capsular structures at this area, as was true in this case, or it may be due to a compensatory mechanism resulting from an attempt by these joints to take over the function of the fixed areas of the neck.

Radiographs of this cervical spine made in 1957 illustrate further degenerative changes and fixation. The only demonstrable motion present occurs between the atlanto-occipital joints and perhaps a very minimal amount between the atlantoaxial joints. The points of maximum stress and strain with further fixation have shifted upward (Fig. 22E and F). Radiographic studies made in 1965 demonstrate other changes in the points of maximum stress, as shown in Figure 22G and H.

THE VERTEBRAL CANAL AND THE SPINAL CORD

The vertebral canal, which is formed by the vertebral foramina in series, is triangular in shape; the base of the triangle is its anterior boundary, which is formed by the posterior longitudinal ligament overlying the posterior portion of the vertebral bodies and the intervertebral discs. The sides of the triangle are formed by the pedicles and the laminae with their interlaminar ligaments, or the ligamenta flava.

The vertebral foramen of the atlas is more rounded than the foramina of the other cervical vertebrae and it is slightly larger to accommodate the origin of the spinal cord. Its anterior boundary is the posterior longitudinal ligament overlying the special ligaments at this level posterior to the odontoid process of the axis.

The spinal cord is a continuation of the medulla oblongata into the vertebral canal. It is slightly flattened anteriorly and posteriorly. The diameter of the cord is much less than that of the vertebral canal which provides for free movements of the vertebral joints with little chance, normally, of any contact between the spinal cord and the surrounding ligamentous and bony structures.

The spinal cord is invested with three membranes–the pia mater, the arachnoid mater and the dura mater. The pia mater forms the immediate covering of the spinal cord and is a vascular membrane of trabecular tissue; from its inner surface fine septa penetrate the substance of the cord. The arachnoid, the next layer, is a very thin transparent membrane surrounding the cord loosely, which leaves an appreciable interval between it and the pia mater. This is called the subarachnoid space, which contains a certain amount of cerebrospinal fluid. The third membrane, the dura mater, is a dense fibrous sheath, and the cord is suspended within this sheath by the denticulate ligaments, which extend from the sides of the spinal cord to the inner surface of the dura mater (Fig. 24).

Between the vertebral canal and the dura mater there is a narrow interval called the extradural space, which is filled with areolofatty tissue and many thin-walled veins.

The spinal dura, which is a continuation of the dura mater of the brain, is attached to the margins of the foramen magnum and to the second and third vertebrae. It has no other attachment to the vertebral column until it reaches the back of the coccyx, where it blends with the periosteum. These attachments do not interfere with the free movement of the vertebral column. On either side of the spinal cord the spinal nerve roots pierce the dura separately and carry with them tubular coverings of the dura mater spinalis, which are called the dural sleeves of the nerve roots.

Injuries or inflammatory reactions within the dural sleeves of the nerve roots, or within the nerve roots themselves, and in their adjacent structures may result in the formation of adhesions between the dural sleeves and the proximate structures, which is an important factor in the consideration of the mechanism of cervical nerve root irritation.

The blood supply of the spinal cord is derived from the vertebral arteries or their branches, as explained in the description of the vertebral arteries.

THE INTERVERTEBRAL FORAMINA

The absence of posterior articulations between the head and atlas and between the atlas and axis leaves the first two nerves without actual intervertebral foramina, as stated above. However, their relationship to adjacent bony structures is important.

The first nerve root leaves the dura at right angles and the nerve passes immediately over the lateral portion of the posterior arch of the atlas. It lies directly beneath the vertebral artery for a short distance, as the artery courses around the base of the lateral mass of the atlas to enter the dura. It then lies behind the artery before it turns backward to supply the suboccipital muscles (Fig. 23). The superior articulation of the atlas overhangs the artery and nerve root posteriorly–an important anatomical fact to be considered under the mechanism of cervical nerve root irritation.

The second cervical nerve, as it leaves the dura, passes laterally for a short distance of approximately one quarter of an inch. Here it rests on the midportion of the medial margin of the atlantoaxial articulation. It then follows the margin of this joint laterally and slightly downward. It lies beneath the posterior arch of the atlas until it turns posteriorly within the upper neck muscles. Its close proximity to the lateral joint and the posterior arch make it potentially vulnerable to irritation or compression, as can be seen in Figures 23 and 17A.

The intervertebral foramina formed by the other cervical verte-

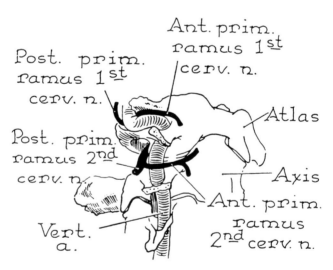

Figure 23. Relationships of first and second nerve roots which have no intervertebral canals.

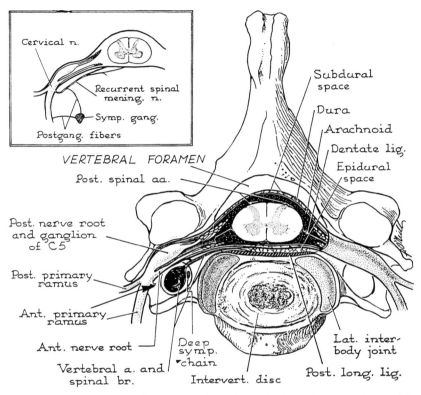

Figure 24. A diagrammatic cross section of a typical cervical vertebra which shows the contents of an intervertebral canal. The arrow points to the origin of the recurrent spinal meningeal nerve and the insert at the upper left shows this nerve in detail.

brae are bony canals which are somewhat ovoid in shape and which have greater vertical diameters than anteroposterior diameters. The roofs and floors of the foramina are formed by the grooves in the roots of the adjacent vertebral arches. The inferior groove of the proximal root is wider than the superior groove of the inferior root so that the roofs are definitely wider than the floors (Fig. 17B). The posterior walls of the canals are formed by the adjacent posterior articular processes, but primarily by the superior articular processes of the distal vertebrae. The anterior walls are formed by the lateral portion of the bodies of the adjacent vertebrae and the margins of the intervening interbody articulations. The anterior walls are of great significance from a mechanical standpoint, inasmuch as the nerve roots pass directly over and are in intimate contact with the margins of the lateral interbody joints. The gliding motion which occurs between these joints whenever the head and neck are turned or moved in any direction subjects the nerve roots to irritation if there is any mechanical derangement present.

The nerve roots and their accompanying structures lie on the floor of the canals and fill their anteroposterior diameter completely. The upper one-eighth to one-fourth of the foramina, or the canals, is filled with areolar and fatty tissues and small veins. Small spinal arteries, branches of the vertebral artery, pass back through the intervertebral foramina to enter the vertebral canal. Minute branches from the nerve trunks, the recurrent meningeal nerves, pass back through the intervertebral foramina anterior to the nerve roots (Fig. 24).

THE CERVICAL NERVES

The cervical nerves are formed by the union of dorsal and ventral fibers, or roots, which arise on the corresponding surfaces of the spinal cord. These fibers, for the most part, leave the cord within the spinal canal on a level with the body of the corresponding vertebra. This means that there is not usually a continuous flow of nerve fibers from the cord but a short interval between each group of fibers. These short intervals, or spaces, are on a level with the intervertebral discs.

Figure 25 is a sketch of the ventral and dorsal surfaces of the cervical spinal cord and the corresponding nerve roots. It can be seen that the upper fibers of each nerve root pass obliquely downward with decreasing degrees of obliquity to join the lower fibers at the lateral portion of the spinal canal where the ventral and dorsal fibers pierce the dura mater separately. Both sets of fibers are invested with a common dural sheath as they leave the spinal canal. The third to eighth, inclusive, enter the intervertebral foramina immediately. As they enter the openings of the intervertebral canals they are at right angles to the cord. The ventral

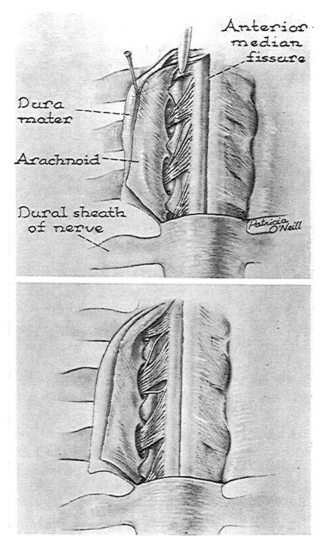

Figure 25. Ventral (upper sketch) and dorsal (lower sketch) nerve roots. Note intercommunication of nerve root fibers. Note exit of nerve roots from spinal canal.

fibers, or the ventral nerve roots, are in intimate contact with the margins of the lateral interbody joints. The posterior fibers, or the posterior nerve roots, are in intimate contact with the posterior superior articular processes of the adjacent distal vertebrae.

Often there are intercommunicating fibers between two and three nerve roots, as seen in Figure 25. This makes the actual localization of nerve root irritation difficult.

Because of their close proximity to the anterior and posterior walls of the intervertebral foramina, the cervical nerve roots are extremely vulnerable to compression or to irritation from any mechanical derangement or inflammatory condition in or about the foramina. Such irritation or compression may cause pain and/or sensory and motor disturbances anywhere along the segmental distribution of the nerves.

The Anterior Cervical Plexus

The anterior primary rami of the upper four cervical nerves are concerned in the formation of the anterior cervical plexus. Each nerve is joined by one or more gray rami communicantes from the superior cervical sympathetic ganglion on each side of the vertebrae. The plexus is formed by a series of irregular loops from each of the nerves, and loops from the fourth nerve root to the fifth nerve root connect the cervical plexus with the brachial plexus.

From the loops of the plexus, ascending and descending cutaneous branches are formed. The ascending branches are derived from the second and third nerves. The *lesser occipital* communicates with the greater auricular, greater occipital and facial nerves. The *greater auricular* communicates with the greater occipital, posterior auricular and facial nerves. *The anterior cutaneous nerve of the neck* communicates with branches of the facial nerves (Fig. 26).

The descending branches are derived from the third and fourth nerves as the *medial, intermediate* and *lateral supraclavicular nerves.* The medial branches give branches to the sternoclavicular joints and the lateral branches supply the acromioclavicular joints.

The other branches from the cervical plexus are muscular and

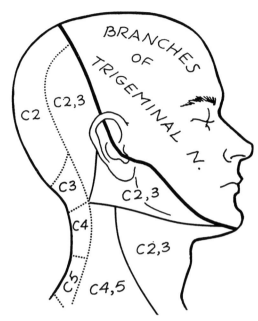

Figure 26. Diagram to show the areas supplied by the ascending and descending cutaneous branches of the cervical plexus. The area posterior to the dotted line is supplied by the medial branches of the posterior rami of the cervical nerves. C2 is the greater occipital nerve which communicates with the ophthalmic division of the trigeminal nerve. C3 is the third occipital nerve.

are divided into medial and lateral branches. The medial branches from the first through the fourth supply the prevertebral muscles and the branches from the first and second nerves supply the rectus capitis anterior, the rectus capitis lateralis and the longus capitis muscles. The intertransverse, longus cervicis and longus capitis muscles are supplied by the second, third and fourth nerves. The third and fourth nerves supply the posterior and middle scalene muscles. The descending cervical nerve is formed by two slender trunks from the second and third nerves, and it forms a communication with the descending branch of the hypoglossal nerve. This loop of communication is called the *ansa hypoglossi* and from it branches are given to the sternohyoid and sternothyroid muscles and to both bellies of the omohyoid muscle. The hypoglossal nerve which derives fibers from the first two cervical nerves supplies the thyrohyoid and geniohyoid muscles.

Branches of the fourth nerve, reinforced by fibers from the third and fifth nerves, form the *phrenic nerve* which gives muscular branches to the diaphragm, pleural branches to the mediastinal and diaphragmatic pleura, pericardial branches to the pericardium, abdominal branches to the diaphragmatic peritoneum, inferior vena cava and liver via the phrenic and hepatic plexuses, as well as communications to the subclavius muscle, the fifth and sixth cervical nerves, the cervical sympathetics, the coeliac plexus and the suprarenal gland.

The medial branches from the first to the third cervical nerves give communicating branches to the vagus nerves.

The *lateral branches* of distribution consist of muscular and communicating nerves located primarily in the posterior triangle. From the second nerve, a branch is given to the sternomastoid muscle where it communicates with the accessory nerve. From the third and fourth nerves, branches supply the trapezius, the levator scapulae and the middle and posterior scalene muscles (anterior scalene muscles are supplied by the anterior rami of C_2 to C_8). The second, third and fourth nerves communicate with the accessory nerve and give some nerve supply to the sternomastoid and trapezius muscles.

The Posterior Cervical Plexus

The posterior primary rami of the cervical nerves form a very simple plexus. With the exception of the first, each ramus divides into medial and lateral branches. The medial branches are sensory or cutaneous and the lateral branches supply muscles and the adjacent joint structures.

The posterior rami of the first cervical nerves are very small or they may be absent. They have no cutaneous branches, but they give lateral or muscular branches to the semispinalis capitis, rectus capitis posterior major, the rectus capitis minor and the superior and inferior oblique capital muscles. Branches supply the adjacent capsular structures, and communicating branches descend to the second cervical nerve.

The posterior rami of the second nerves are larger than the anterior branches. The medial cutaneous branches accompany the occipital arteries as the greater occipital nerves which provide the chief sensory supply for the posterior part of the scalp. They communicate with the great auricular and the third cervical nerves, as well as the lesser occipital and the posterior auricular nerves. The medial or muscular branches supply the semispinalis capitis, inferior oblique, semispinalis cervicis and multifidus muscles, and branches supply the adjacent joint structures.

The third nerves have smaller posterior rami which communicate with the second and fourth nerves. The medial branches become cutaneous as the third occipital nerves. The lateral branches supply the deep intervertebral contiguous muscles and the joints.

The posterior primary rami of the fourth, fifth and sixth nerves are very small and the medial branches supply the skin at the back of the neck near the midline. The lateral branches supply the neighboring muscles and joints. In some instances the fourth and third nerves form a communication from which adjacent muscles are supplied.

The seventh and eighth posterior rami have no cutaneous branches. They end in the deep muscles of the upper back.

The brief description of the cervical plexus and its many communications with the cranial nerves and with the sympathetic nerves should aid in the clarification of symptoms resulting from injuries or disorders of the upper portion of the cervical spine.

THE AUTONOMIC NERVOUS SYSTEM

The autonomic nervous system is a dependent of the central nervous system and linked to it by afferent and efferent fiber systems. It has been described as that part of the nervous system concerned with regulation of the internal environment of the body and the maintenance of its stability; it is divided topographically into the sympathetic and parasympathetic systems.

The parasympathetic system is connected with the central nervous system in the cervical area through the oculomotor, facial, glossopharyngeal and vagus cranial nerves.

The sympathetic system originates in the mediolateral gray matter of the base of the anterior horns of the spinal cord from C4 through C8 in the cervical area.

The fibers of both systems run side by side to the same structures where there is normally a harmonious interaction between them which maintains a balance, but they are capable of producing antagonistic effects.

Their reactions are dependent on chemical substances liberated at their ganglia or at their endings. The sympathetic fibers, with few exceptions, release an adrenalinelike substance and are known as adrenergic fibers, whereas the parasympathetic fibers release acetylcholine and are called cholinergic fibers. These two systems respond differently to certain drugs.

We must remember, however, that the autonomic system is not a separate system but is an integral part of the somatic and visceral peripheral nervous systems and of the central nervous system.

The Sympathetic Nervous System

The sympathetic nervous system plays a definite role in the picture of cervical nerve root irritation. It has been held by most anatomists that the cervical nerve roots are composed of motor and sensory fibers only, whereas the dorsal and upper two lumbar nerve roots contain white rami communicantes of the sympathetic nervous system as well. The cervical nerves have their connection with the sympathetic nervous system through the white rami communicantes of the upper two dorsal nerves which join the sympathetic trunk by way of their anterior primary rami and proceed upward to the cervical ganglia. Gray rami communicantes or postganglionic fibers pass from the cervical ganglia to the anterior primary rami of the cervical nerves and are distributed with the divisions of the nerves. Other gray rami communicantes pass directly or indirectly to most of the cranial nerves and peripheral branches pass to the pharynx, to the heart as cardiomotor nerves, and to the arteries of the head, neck and arms (Plate 2).

Laruelle, however, has demonstrated the presence of sympathetic cell bodies in the cervical portion of the spinal cord where they are located in the mediolateral gray matter of the base of the anterior horns from C4 through C8 levels as shown in Plate 2. The preganglionic sympathetic fibers leave the spinal cord with the somatic motor nerve fibers in the ventral roots of C5 through T1. One part of the preganglionic neurons forms a synaptic connection with postganglionic neurons in the small ganglia of a deep sympathetic chain, which has been described by Delmas and his associates. The other preganglionic neurons traverse the deep chain of small sympathetic ganglia situated in the transverse canals and join the vertebral nerve, with which they reach the cervicothoracic group. The deep chain consists of a tangled web of sympathetic fibers and of macroscopically visible ganglia. It ascends along the posterior aspect of the vertebral artery from C7 to C4. It is the continuation in the neck of the thoracolumbar ganglionated trunk.

The classic sympathetic trunk in the cervical area is composed of the superior, middle and inferior ganglia which are connected by intervening cords. The efferent branches proceed to the viscera of the neck and chest and the afferent branches form the vertebral nerve. Communicating rami connect the superior cervical ganglion with the ninth and twelfth cranial nerves. Gray rami communicantes join the anterior rami of the upper four cervical nerves. The internal carotid nerve passes upwards with the artery to form the internal carotid plexus. Pharyngeal branches pass to the side of the pharynx, communicate with the superior laryngeal nerve and join the pharyngeal plexus. The external carotid nerve forms a plexus around the external carotid artery. Cardiac branches follow the carotid artery into the thorax on the left side and on the right side they follow the trachea to end in the deep cardiac plexus.

From the middle ganglion, branches are given to the inferior thyroid artery and to the thyroid gland. A cardiac branch ends in the cardiac plexus. Another branch, the ansa subclavius, descends to the subclavian artery and then ascends to join the inferior ganglion.

The inferior ganglion sends fine filaments to the subclavian plexus and larger filaments form the vertebral plexus around the vertebral artery. A cardiac branch reaches the deep cardiac plexus.

According to Tinel, the fifth cervical spinal nerve root carries sympathetic fibers which join the carotid plexus giving sympathetic innervation to the arteries of the head and neck, the sixth root carries sympathetic fibers which go to the subclavian artery and the brachial plexus and from the seventh root, fibers reach the cardioaortic plexus and the subclavian and axillary arteries as well as the phrenic nerves.

The sympathetic fibers which surround the internal carotid arteries give branches to the back of the orbit, the orbital muscles, the dilator muscles of the pupils and the smooth muscle of the upper eyelids. Those which surround the vertebral arteries and the basilar artery within the cranium reach the vestibular portion of the ears.

Stimulation of the cervical portion of the sympathetic nervous system gives rise to the clinical manifestations, as described by Barré in 1926 and later by one of his pupils, Lieou. Symptoms of such irritation include vertigo, blurring of vision, tinnitus and transitory deafness, pharyngeal and laryngeal paresthesias as well as many other symptoms involving the shoulder, arm and hand.

Other postganglionic fibers make communications with the recurrent spinal meningeal nerves before these nerves pass back through the intervertebral foramina to supply the dura and ligamentous structures (Fig. 27).

It must be remembered that pain-conducting afferent spinal nerve fibers from the blood vessels of the head, neck and upper

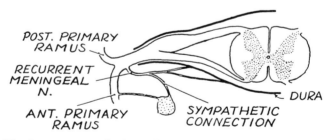

Figure 27. A recurrent spinal meningeal nerve and its sympathetic communication.

extremities traverse the sympathetic trunk and communicating rami, also. The close association of the parasympathetics to the sympathetic system makes it imperative that one understands the functions of both systems in the production of pain and the changes which occur as the result of irritative factors.

In view of these newer anatomic concepts, one can more readily interpret the symptoms and clinical findings of cervical nerve root irritation, which have been difficult to explain.

THE VERTEBRAL ARTERY

The anatomy of the vertebral artery should be considered in this study because of its close relationship to the cervical nerves and to the cervical vertebrae. It is the first branch from the subclavian trunk. It reaches the transverse foramen of the sixth cervical vertebra by passing upwards and backwards between the scalenus muscle and the lateral border of the longus anterior cervicis muscle. As it passes through the transverse foramina of the sixth to the second cervical vertebrae, it lies directly anterior to the trunks of the cervical nerves and medial to the intertransverse muscles. As soon as the artery has passed through the transverse foramen of the atlas, it turns sharply backwards and runs medially around the posterolateral aspect of the superior articular process of the atlas which overhangs it. It then lies in the groove on the upper surface of the posterior arch of the atlas, enters the vertebral canal, and runs upward through the foramen magnum into the cranial cavity where it pierces the arachnoid and passes to the lower border of the pons to unite with its mate from the opposite side to form the basilar artery.

Opposite each intervertebral canal each artery gives off spinal branches to supply the ligaments, the dura, the nerve roots and the bones and to communicate with the posterior spinal arteries which are branches of the vertebral arteries that are given off near the lateral margins of the medulla oblongata and which descent on the dorsolateral surfaces of the spinal cord. At the level of the foramen magnum a branch is given off each vertebral artery to form the anterior spinal arteries which descend on the anterior surface of the spinal cord.

The vertebral arteries supply the posterior half of the brain and the cervical spinal cord. They are vulnerable to injury throughout their course in the cervical area when any trauma to the cervical spine occurs. Inasmuch as they are surrounded by plexuses of postgangliotic sympathetic nerve fibers and on their back surfaces, at least from C4 to C8, are small ganglia which derive their pre-ganglionic fibers from sympathetic cell bodies in the cervical spinal cord, injury to them may give rise to what might seem confusing symptoms.

Chapter 3

THE MECHANISM OF CERVICAL
NERVE ROOT IRRITATION

THE FOREGOING BRIEF but pertinent anatomical review of the cervical portion of the spine provides a background of knowledge for interpretation of the mechanisms involved in irritation of the cervical nerve roots.

Irritation of the cervical nerve roots may give rise to pain, sensory changes, muscle atrophy, muscle spasm and to alteration of the tendon reflexes anywhere along their segmental distribution.

Any condition causing narrowing of the intervertebral canals may cause compression of the nerve roots, the spinal branches of the vertebral arteries, venous congestion and irritation or compression of the recurrent spinal meningeal nerves and of the sympathetic fibers within the anterior portion of the nerve roots, C5 through C8.

ENCROACHMENT OF THE INTERVERTEBRAL CANALS

Encroachment or narrowing of the intervertebral canals may be the result of some involvement of the proximate soft tissue structures and/or the bony structures. Any condition which causes inflammation or swelling of the dural sleeves of the nerve roots may cause neural compression, also.

Inflammation

Acute inflammatory reactions within the capsules of the apophyseal and interbody joints and of the superficial layer of the posterior longitudinal ligament overlying the lateral interbody joints give rise to swelling of these structures and, therefore, foraminal encroachment. If the inflammation persists and becomes a chronic condition, hyperplasia of the capsular and ligamentous structures occurs to cause continued narrowing of the intervertebral canals.

Hemorrhage

Following an acute traumatic incident, bleeding from torn structures may occur to cause spacial narrowing and pressure upon the nerve roots. If the hemorrhagic products are not mobilized by cellular activity, adhesions may form between the dural sleeves of the nerve roots and the adjacent capsular structures. In this event, extremes of neck motion produce a tug upon the adherent dural sleeves, which have an excursion of approximately one-quarter to one-half an inch within their canals normally, to give rise to added irritation of the nerve roots.

Ligamentous and Capsular Instability

The capsular and ligamentous structures, as described in the previous chapter, have sufficient laxity, elasticity and tensile strength to permit a normal range of motion. Any unusual laxness of these important structures allows subluxations of the joints, especially with extremes of motion, which alter the size and shape of the intervertebral canals. The cervical nerve roots and their accompanying structures are subjected to irritation or compression within their canals which may be manifested by radicular symptoms and findings.

Backward slipping of one vertebra in its relationship to the adjacent distal vertebra occurs when the neck is hyperextended, if there is instability of the binding structures of the joints. Such backward slipping or subluxation causes narrowing of the anteroposterior and vertical diameters of the intervertebral foramina in the following manner: The posteroinferior margins of the beveled posterolateral portions of the body of the upper vertebra approach the anteromedial portions of the superior facets of the adjacent lower vertebra to produce anteroposterior narrowing of the intervertebral canals near their midportions. The nerve roots within the canals are compressed anteriorly and posteriorly as if they were being squeezed by a pincher. The posterior facets subluxate or override to produce a decrease in the vertical and anteroposterior diameters of the intervertebral canals, as shown in Figure 28.

If two adjacent spinous processes override or are kissing, hyperextension of the neck may cause posterior subluxation because of the leverlike action which is produced.

Forward slipping of one vertebra on the adjacent distal vertebra when the neck is flexed may occur if the posterior ligamentous structures are stretched or torn. This results in anteroposterior narrowing of the intervertebral foramina as the anteromedial margins of the inferior facets of the upper vertebra approach the posterolateral margins of the upward lips on the superior surface of the posterolateral portions of the adjacent lower vertebra. However, there is not the same pincherlike effect on the proximate nerve roots inasmuch as the compression forces do not approximate each other in the same plane. The vertical diameter of the intervertebral canals is increased as the inferior facets of the upper vertebra are elevated on the superior facets of the adjacent lower vertebra (Fig. 28).

Lateral bending and rotation in the cervical joints, which occur simultaneously, cause some alteration of the anteroposterior and

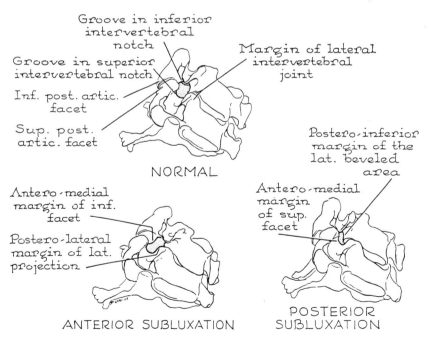

Figure 28. The effect of subluxations on the intervertebral foramina.

vertical diameters of the intervertebral canals and may give rise to irritation of the proximate nerve roots, if ligamentous instability is present.

The vertebral arteries within the transverse foramina anterior to the cervical spinal nerves may be subjected to traumatic insults as subluxations occur. Vascular trauma may result in marked vasoconstriction to give rise to symptoms of vertebral artery insufficiency which may extend far beyond the point of insult.

Ligamentous instability between the atlas and axis is often overlooked or not recognized, but such instability is of great importance. Tearing or relaxation of the transverse ligament of the atlas permits forward subluxation of the head and atlas on the axis when the head is placed forward in flexion of the neck. This causes narrowing of the vertebral foramen and may result in pressure upon the spinal cord itself to give rise to symptoms and findings of cord compression. Relaxation or stretching of the guy ligaments may allow lateral subluxation of the head and atlas on the axis and excessive rotation of the axis in its relationship to the head and atlas, and may be responsible for irritation of the second nerve roots and for actual constriction of the vertebral arteries as they wind around the atlantoaxial joints and the superior facets of the atlas (Fig. 23).

Osteophytic Formations

Following traumatic inflammatory reactions imposed upon the joints of the cervical spine, cartilage cells may appear at the margins of the joints which become ossified to form spurs or osteophytes. (Perhaps certain other inflammatory reactions may be responsible for osteophytic formations.) Osteophytic formations at the margins of the lateral interbody joints and at the margins of the posterior joints project into the intervertebral canals to cause spacial narrowing and pressure upon the nerve roots. Inasmuch as these changes occur slowly over a varying period of time, the nerve roots may have an opportunity to adjust somewhat to their narrowed canals and they may be able to tolerate such encroachment forces until some other insult is imposed upon them by an apparently trivial traumatic incident.

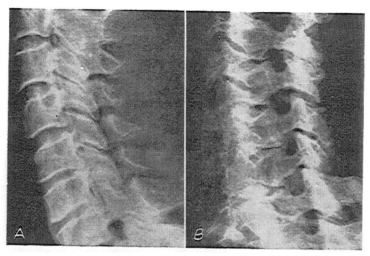

Figure 29. Lateral x-ray view (A) of a specimen which appears to have spur formations on the posterior margins of the vertebral bodies of C5 and 6. Oblique view (B) shows narrowing of the intervertebral foramen by the formation of spurs at the margins of the lateral interbody joint. Dissection of this specimen revealed no spur formations on the posterior margins of the vertebral bodies.

These osteophytic changes are found most frequently at the margins of the lateral interbody joints, especially between the fifth and sixth and between the fourth and fifth vertebrae (Fig. 29). However, they may be found at any level as demonstrated in Figures 30 and 31. Lateral radiographic views may give the impression that these changes occur at the adjacent posterior margins of the vertebral bodies when in reality they are at the margins of the posterolateral interbody joints (Fig. 31). Of course, they do occur at the posterior vertebral margins, but less frequently than they form at the anterior margins and at the anterolateral margins of the vertebral bodies.

Radiographs may not reveal the true condition nor the extent of the osteophytic changes. The radiographs may appear to be normal when there is definite pathology present which cannot be demonstrated in the radiographs. Figure 32A represents a lateral view of an anatomic specimen. A pin was placed posteriorly into

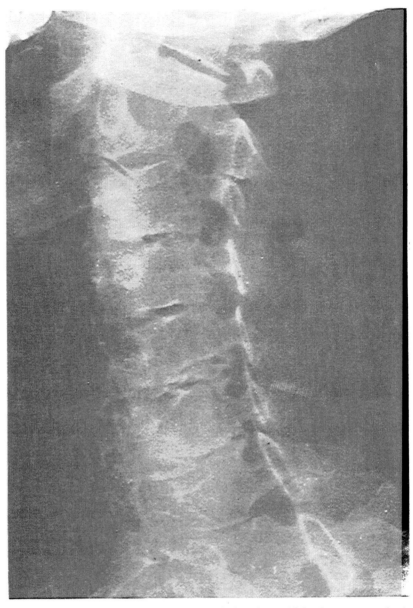

Figure 30. An oblique view of a cervical spine which shows osteophytic formations at the margins of the lateral interbody joints causing narrowing of the third, fourth, fifth and sixth canals.

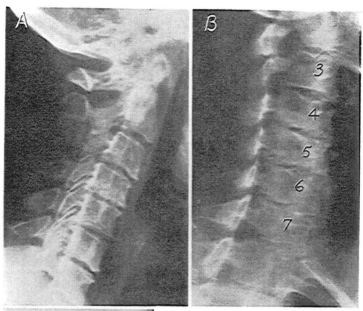

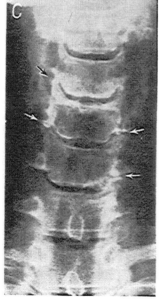

Figure 31. Spur formations which appear to be on the posterior margins of the fourth, fifth and sixth vertebrae in the lateral view are at the margins of the lateral interbody joints as shown in the oblique and anteroposterior views. Note the marked anteroposterior narrowing of the intervertebral canals in the oblique view, from the second through the fifth canals.

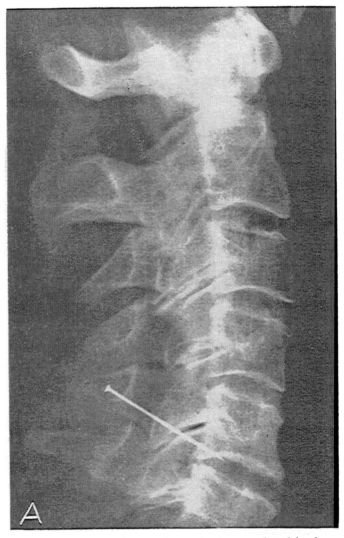

Figure 32A. Lateral x-ray of a specimen. A pin was placed in the posterior portion of the lateral interbody joint in A. Position of pin can be seen within the joint in B.

the lateral interbody joint. A semioblique view, Figure 32B, shows the lateral interbody articulation and the position of the pin within the joint. Dissection of this specimen revealed that there was marked bulging posterolaterally of this joint which caused

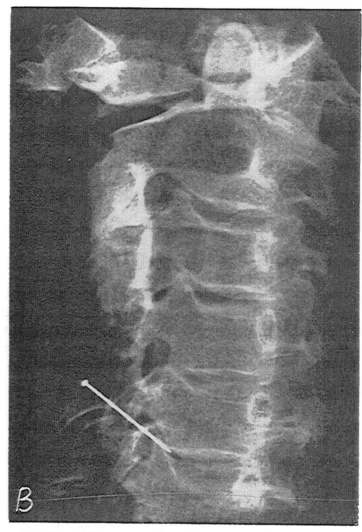

Figure 32B. Semioblique x-ray of specimen. A pin was placed in the posterior portion of the lateral interbody joint in A. Position of pin can be seen within the joint in B.

foraminal narrowing and which was not demonstrable in the radiograph. The articular surfaces of the lateral interbody joint showed marked chondromalacic changes and marginal spurs. Similar changes were found at the lateral interbody joint between the fourth and fifth vertebrae in this specimen. Certainly, the radiographs do not indicate the extent of the pathology.

The Role of the Cervical Discs

The terms "disc disease" and "cervical disc" are used as diagnoses of cervical spine disorders. These terms per se are of no diagnostic value and should be discarded. They present a question of semantics and if they are used as diagnostic terms their meaning should be properly defined. The correct terminology is "disc disorder," unless there is extrusion of disc material, in which event it should be designated as such.

The term "disc disease" should imply an infection within the fibrocartilaginous disc or discs—a rare occurrence. If such an infection does exist, encroachment of the intervertebral canals may occur to produce irritation or compression of the cervical nerve roots.

The term "cervical disc" when used as a diagnostic term conveys the idea that a disc has been ruptured and that disc material has been extruded posterolaterally, as in the lumbar area, to cause compression of the proximate cervical nerve. This is an erroneous impression which has developed because of the belief that the cervical nerve roots lie immediately posterior to the intervertebral discs. This relationship does not exist in the cervical spine. The fibers of the cervical nerve roots leave the spinal cord at the level of the corresponding vertebral body as shown in Plate 3-1. As can be seen, the uppermost fiber of each nerve root leaves the cord at the level of the inferior margin of the disc above it, and the lowermost fiber of each nerve root leaves the cord well above the margin of the disc below it. None of the nerve root fibers passes over the intervertebral disc.

The nerve root fibers converge with decreasing degrees of obliquity and make their exit from the vertebral canal at the lateral extremes of the canal. They are well protected from the intervertebral discs by a "safety zone," which is the body of the vertebra lying directly anterior to the anterior nerve root fibers (Plate 3-1). As they make their exit from the spinal canal at near right angles, they leave the "safety zone" and pass immediately into the intervertebral canals. Here they are in intimate contact with the lateral interbody joints and with the posterior joints, and by virtue of their position between a potential pincher, they are extremely vulnerable to insult on even the slightest derangement of the canals.

Disc material can be extruded posteriorly, in which instance it would cause compression of the spinal cord rather than the nerve roots (Plate 3-2). If a large amount of disc material were extruded posteriorly, it might cause compression of the upper and lower nerve root fibers of the proximate nerve roots but it would cause compression of the spinal cord as well, in which instance the symptoms might be greatly aggravated by flexion of the neck. Disc material can be extruded at the lateral extreme of the posterior portion of the disc and cause pressure on the axilla of the nerve root, but here again there should be compression of the lateral side of the spinal cord.

Disc material is rarely extruded posterolaterally or posteriorly in the cervical area. We must keep in mind that the intervertebral discs do not extend to the posterolateral margins of the vertebral bodies as they do in other areas of the spine because of the posterolateral interbody joints. These small joints are so placed that they take much of the strain off the intervertebral discs, and they are, therefore, much more vulnerable to injury and to degenerative changes than are the discs themselves. The posterolateral upward projections on the superior surfaces of the vertebral bodies extend farther posteriorly than they do anteriorly and they are cupped posteriorly so that they serve as barriers to posterolateral extrusion of disc material (Fig. 8), except at the seventh vertebra where in certain instances the upward lips are not well developed, as shown in Figure 33. In rare cases, the upward lips are not well developed on the superior surface of the sixth vertebra. These variations at the sixth and seventh vertebral bodies, in my opinion, account for the preponderance of disc extrusions at these levels as reported by most neurosurgeons.

The posterior longitudinal ligament in the cervical area is com-

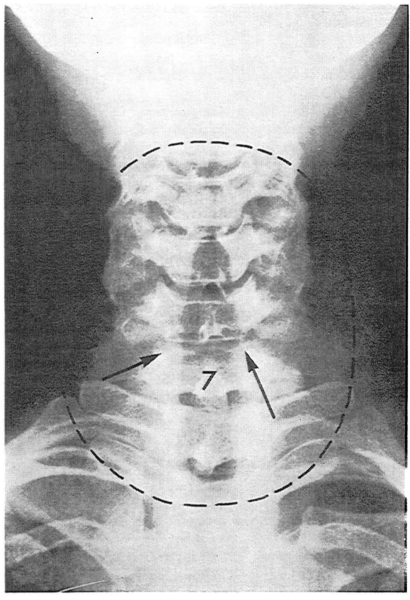

Figure 33. An anteroposterior view of a cervical spine which shows an absence of the upward lateral projections on the body of the seventh vertebra. Hence, there is no barrier to posterolateral extrusion of disc material at this level.

posed of two distinct layers and it is much denser, stronger and wider than in the other areas of the spine. It, too, acts as a barrier to posterior extrusion of disc material (Fig. 34).

In most instances, the annulus fibrosus is thicker posteriorly than it is at its anterior portion. The vertical diameter of the cervical discs is greater anteriorly than posteriorly, and the discs, therefore, have a much wider anterior exposure between the mar-

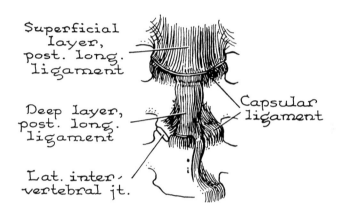

Superficial layer, post. long. ligament

Deep layer, post. long. ligament

Lat. intervertebral jt.

Capsular ligament

LUMBAR

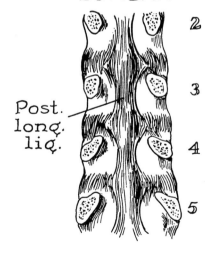

Post. long. lig.

2

3

4

5

Figure 34. The posterior longitudinal ligament. Cervical portion composed of deep and superficial layers (upper). Lumbar portion composed of one layer which is denticulated (lower).

Ligament is denticulated.

gins of the vertebral bodies than they have at their posterior portions.

The most likely exit for the nucleus pulposus of a cervical disc, or of disc material itself, is at the point of least resistance which is anteriorly or anterolaterally in most instances.

Disc material might be extruded posteriorly if there were undue relaxation, weakness or an actual tear in the posterior longitudinal ligament as well as in the annulus fibrosus. If the posterior longitudinal ligament is not torn, disc material might escape through a break or crevice in the posterior portion of the annulus fibrosus and the deep layer of the posterior longitudinal ligament. It might migrate upward or downward between the superficial and deep layers of the posterior longitudinal ligament. In this event, some of the fibers of the ventral portion of the nerve root either above or below the disc might suffer compression, but pressure should be exerted upon the spinal cord as well.

Schmorl and Junghanns have described the formation of bony nodes at the posterior vertebral margins and at various levels on the posterior aspect of the vertebral bodies anterior to the posterior longitudinal ligament. They believe that these nodes represent prolapsed disc material which has ossified and that they are potential or actual factors in spinal cord compression. They might cause pressure upon some of the fibers of the ventral portion of the adjacent nerve roots, also, depending on their location.

Hyperplasia or thickening of the capsular ligaments of the lateral interbody joints and osteophytic formations at the margins of these joints may give the appearance of extruded disc material beneath or anterior to the nerve root or roots. It is my impression that the surgeon who sees and feels a bulge anterior to the nerve root may interpret this finding as disc extrusion. Even in the dissecting room, one's first impression may be that these changes about the lateral interbody joints may represent disc extrusions until one cuts and retracts the nerve roots so that the true picture can be seen. Further dissection of these joints often reveals that similar and even more marked protrusions or bulges occur at the anterior portion of the lateral interbody joints. Complete exposure of these joints reveals chondromalacic changes as seen in other synovial joints, with the typical moth-eaten areas in the contiguous articular surfaces.

The so-called "hard discs" as described by Stookey, and which were thought to be chondromas, are in reality the result of osteophytic changes about the margins of the posterolateral interbody joints which are covered by thickened or hypertrophied capsules.

Degeneration or disintegration of cervical discs, which is the result of some traumatic experience in most instances, does not necessarily produce nerve root irritation. However, as the involved disc narrows, the annulus fibrosus bulges circumferentially and the proximate vertebra settles to cause some narrowing of the intervertebral canals, which may result in compression or irritation of the nerve roots within the canals. The discs between the fifth and sixth and between the fourth and fifth vertebrae are most frequently involved, but a disc at any level may become narrowed, as illustrated in Figure 35.

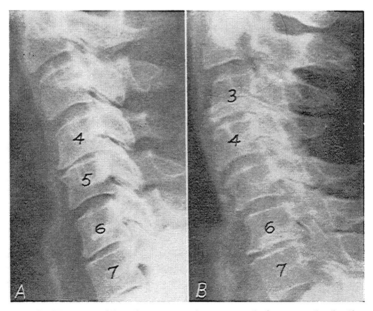

Figure 35. Hypertrophic changes and narrowed intervertebral discs at various levels.

Fractures and Dislocations

Certain fractures of the cervical vertebrae may be responsible for cervical nerve root irritation. Hemorrhage and swelling into the joints or displacement of a bone fragment may cause foraminal narrowing. Fractures of the posterior facets or of the vertebral arches cause mechanical derangements of the intervertebral canals as shown in Figure 36A and B. Such fractures may not be demonstrated in the usual post-injury radiographs. Flexion-oblique and

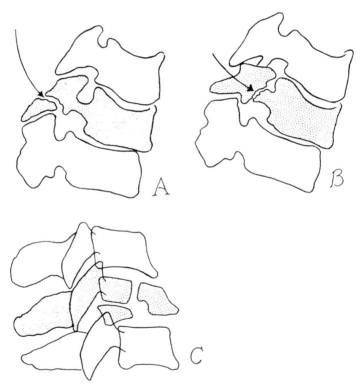

Figure 36. A fracture of a posterior facet (A) or of a vertebral arch (B) permits forward luxation of the involved vertebra and causes marked derangement of the intervertebral canals formed by that vertebra and the contiguous vertebrae. A posteriorly displaced fragment of a vertebral body causes narrowing of the intervertebral foramina and of the vertebral foramen (C).

lateral-oblique views may be necessary to show these fractures, especially if they occur unilaterally.

Compression fractures of the upward lateral projections of the vertebral bodies cause pressure upon the adjacent nerve root or roots. These fractures, too, are difficult to demonstrate in the usual radiographs, as shown in Figure 37.

Crushing fractures of the vertebral bodies may cause backward displacement of the posterior fragment or fragments to encroach upon the intervertebral foramina as well as the vertebral foramen. Such fractures may cause pressure upon the spinal cord and upon the origin of the nerve root fibers (Fig. 36C).

Fractures of the superior facets of the lateral masses of the atlas and fractures of the posterior arch of the atlas may cause irritation or compression of the first nerve root, and fractures of the facets of the atlantoaxial articulations and of the lamina of the axis may cause compression or irritation of the second nerve roots

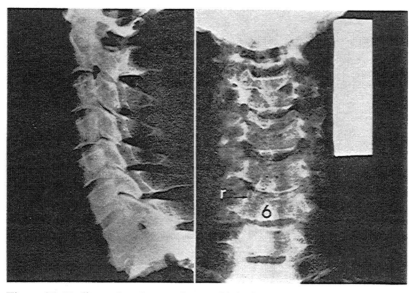

Figure 37. Radiographs of a specimen which show no evidence of any fracture. However, dissection of this specimen revealed a severe compression fracture involving the upward lateral projection and extending into the body of the vertebra on the right side of the sixth vertebra.

(Fig. 38). The close proximity of the vertebral arteries to the lateral masses of the atlas and to the superior facets of the axis renders these arteries extremely vulnerable to injury when fractures occur at these areas.

Sudden forceful flexion of the cervical spine may cause dislocation of the posterior facets without actual fracture of the facets. Displacement of the inferior facets forward over the superior facets of the adjacent vertebra may cause compression of the adjacent nerve roots, as well as compression of the spinal cord, as the dislocation occurs and narrows the vertebral foramen (Fig. 39).

Posterior dislocations may occur when the head and neck are forcibly hyperextended. However, these dislocations usually reduce themselves and there may be no x-ray evidence that such dislocations have occurred. Dislocations almost always result in cord compression as well as nerve root compression, with loss of

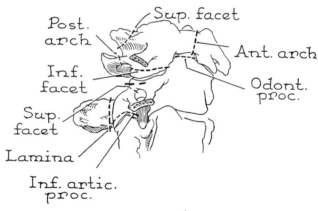

Figure 38. Fractures of the atlas and axis which may cause nerve root compression. Fracture of a superior facet of the atlas may cause pressure on C1 nerve root. Fracture of the posterior arch of the atlas may cause compression of either C1 or C2 nerve root. Fracture of the inferior facet of the atlas may cause irritation of C2 nerve root. Fracture of the superior facet of C2 may irritate C2 or nerve root. Fractures of the lamina of the axis may produce swelling and hemorrhage with irritation of C2 and 3 nerve roots. Fractures of the anterior and posterior arches of the atlas with spreading apart of the lateral masses may cause compression of C1 and C2 nerve roots.

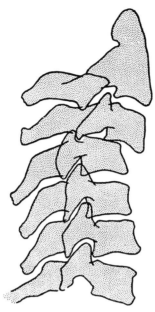

Figure 39. Tracing of a radiograph which shows dislocation of the third vertebra on the fourth. This causes impingement of the fourth nerve roots and of the spinal cord.

motor and sensory functions. The spinal cord and nerve roots may be so badly traumatized that they are reduced to pulpy masses of neural tissue and hemorrhage. If the victim of such an accident survives, the chances for complete functional recovery are extremely remote.

Sudden and forceful flexion of the neck may cause a complete disruption of the transverse ligament of the atlas resulting in complete forward dislocation of the head and atlas on the axis. This, of course, causes marked compression of the spinal cord and the victim does not usually live to tell the tale.

Congenital Anomalies

A variety of congenital anomalies occur in the cervical portion of the spine. Most of these anomalies per se are not the direct cause of cervical nerve root irritation. The nerve roots are adjusted to these anomalies, usually. However, trauma superimposed upon

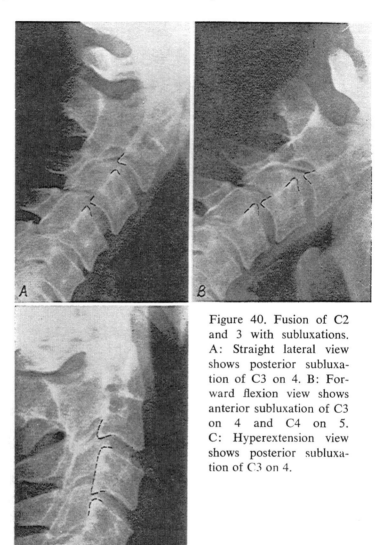

Figure 40. Fusion of C2 and 3 with subluxations. A: Straight lateral view shows posterior subluxation of C3 on 4. B: Forward flexion view shows anterior subluxation of C3 on 4 and C4 on 5. C: Hyperextension view shows posterior subluxation of C3 on 4.

such anomalies may be responsible for involvement of the nerve roots. Variations in the size and shape of the articular processes and in the angles of inclination of the articular surfaces may alter the anteroposterior diameters of the foramina. Overton called attention to the variations in the angle of inclination of the posterior articulations of the second and third vertebrae, and he believed that these changes might be causative factors in irritation of the third cervical nerves.

Congenital fusion of two or more vertebrae may be responsible for mechanical changes in the intervertebral canals above or below the fused areas because of the increased stress and strain placed upon the adjacent joints as they attempt to take over the function of the fixed vertebrae (Fig. 40).

THE VERTEBRAL ARTERIES

The vertebral arteries as they traverse the transverse foramina anterior to the nerves may be responsible for compression of the nerves when the neck is forcibly hyperextended and the arteries

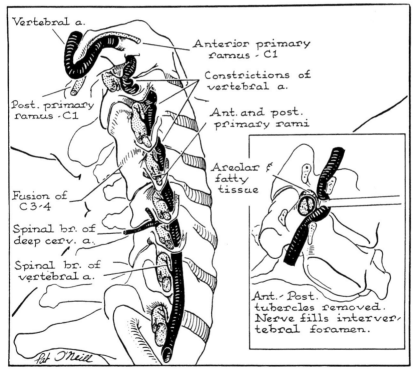

Figure 41. The vertebral artery—a sketch which shows the relationship of the adjacent structures, and actual constriction of the artery at three levels.

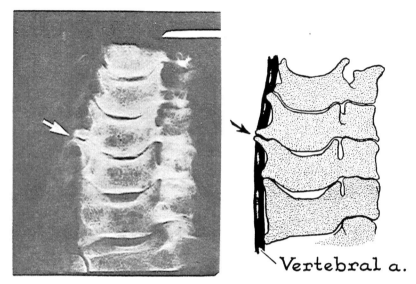

Figure 42. Radiograph of a specimen from which the posterior joints and the transverse processes have been removed to show clearly the extensive osteophytic formation at C5 and C6 lateral interbody joint. The diagram shows the relationship of the vertebral artery which was actually pushed behind the spur formations. The artery was constricted but not occluded. However, rotation of the head to that side would cause occlusion of the artery.

are drawn backward toward the superior margins of the articular processes. Compression of the nerves will be more marked if sclerosis of the arteries is present. Actual compression of the arteries themselves is not unusual in this hyperextended position, especially if there are spur formations at the lateralmost margins of the lateral interbody joints, or if there are adhesions about the arteries (Figs. 41 and 42). Actual constrictions of the vertebral arteries may occur at any level, but the most frequent sites are above the level of the third vertebra where the arteries are especially vulnerable to trauma. Many investigators have shown, by vertebral angiography, very definite obstructions in the vertebral arteries which occur with changes in the position of the head.

THE ROLE OF THE SYMPATHETIC NERVE SUPPLY

Any mechanical disturbance which gives rise to cervical nerve root irritation gives rise also to involvement of the cervical sympathetic nerve supply either by direct irritative factors or by reflex stimulation. Inasmuch as it has been shown that the fifth, sixth, seventh and eighth nerve roots do contain preganglionic sympathetic fibers, irritation of the nerve roots may give symptoms and findings of direct stimulation of the sympathetic components contained within these nerve roots. Irritation of the nerve roots may cause pain anywhere along the segmental distribution of the nerves, resulting in muscle spasm and vasomotor ischemia.

Inflammation of the ligamentous and capsular structures give rise to pain and may give rise to reflex stimulation of the postganglionic fibers of the cervical sympathetics. If the pain is not relieved, it may become a self-perpetuating pain stimulus, such as occurs in Sudeck's atrophy. Evans has called this phenomenon "reflex sympathetic dystrophy." Reflex stimulation of the postganglionic fibers or direct stimulation of the preganglionic fibers in the lower four nerve roots can give rise to many signs and symptoms which may not appear to be caused by irritation of the cervical nerve roots. Such symptoms include blurring of vision, dilatation of the pupil, loss of balance, tinnitus, auditory disturbances, headaches, swelling and stiffness of the fingers, tendinitis, and capsulitis. These symptoms were described by Barré in 1926 and they have been labeled "the posterior cervical sympathetic syndrome." Barré pointed to irritation of the sympathetic plexus surrounding the vertebral artery and to irritation of the vertebral nerve as a source of the clinical manifestations.

The recurrent spinal meningeal nerve, which is a mixture of somatic and sympathetic fibers and which passes from the short trunk of each spinal nerve back through the intervertebral canal, may be irritated or compressed by any disorder of the intervertebral canal. This nerve is sensory as well as vasomotor. It lies anterior to the nerve root and may be compressed or irritated by any alteration in the intervertebral canal.

LOCATION AND DEGREE OF IRRITATION

The symptoms and clinical findings of nerve root irritation in the cervical spine may vary somewhat in each individual, because of the localized areas of compression as well as the degree of compression. Sunderland has classified nerve injuries on the basis of the degree of changes induced in the normal structure of the nerve. He contends that some fibers in the nerves may escape involvement while others sustain variable degrees of damage. The nature of the peripheral defect, the course of recovery and the end result depend on the particular fibers involved and on the particular type or degree of injury sustained by each. Nerves may be injured by mechanical, thermal and chemical means as well as by ischemia. He believes that there are individual variations of susceptibility of nerve fibers to injury and that some nerve fibers within a nerve are much better insulated or protected than are other fibers within the same nerve.

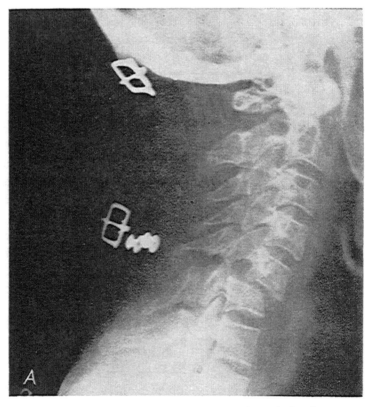

Figure 43A. Extent of mechanical derangements is no indication of severity of symptoms. A: Dislocation of C5 on 6—marked derangement with minimum symptoms.

We must keep in mind that marked derangements in the cervical spine may cause minimal symptoms, whereas apparently insignificant derangements may cause severe nerve root irritation or compression. Not infrequently, fracture-dislocations give rise to minimal symptoms and clinical findings, whereas in some cases there may be no appreciable changes, but symptoms and findings of sensory and motor deficits may be present (Fig. 43A & B).

In summary, it can be said that it is within or about the intervertebral foramina that we must expect to find irritative or compressive factors which give rise to symptoms and findings of involvement of the adjacent nerve root or roots, as well as of the structures which accompany the nerve roots within the intervertebral canals.

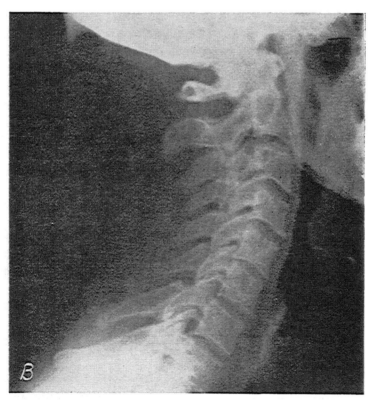

Figure 43B. Narrowed disc between C5 and 6—minimum derangement with severe symptoms.

Chapter 4

ETIOLOGY

B ETWEEN THE SKULL and the first thoracic vertebra there are eighteen true synovial joints, ten "controversial" synovial joints or the lateral interbody joints, and six secondary fibro-cartilaginous joints or the disc joints. A wide range of neck motion has been achieved by the division of the overall movement among so many serially arranged joints, each having its own limited range of motion to assure a certain amount of stability. Its position between the head, which is an eight to twelve pound weight that must be balanced and held in position on the two small facets of the atlas, and the relatively immobile thoracic spine and its great flexibility render it unusually vulnerable to injury from external forces.

An analysis of more than eight thousand patients seen by the author who have had symptoms referable to the cervical spine revealed that more than 90 percent of these patients had had one or more injuries of the cervical spine, either recent or remote. The remaining small percentage of patients had non-traumatic disorders, metastatic lesions, spinal cord tumors or primary osseous lesions.

TRAUMA

Injuries of the cervical spine have been confined to the soft tissue structures in approximately 75 percent of my cases. The remaining 25 percent suffered injuries of the skeletal structures as well as injuries of the soft tissue structures.

Injuries of the ligamentous, capsular and muscular structures are often referred to as *strains* and *sprains*. These two words are used interchangeably, but erroneously, to indicate the type of injury.

A *strain* injury indicates that joint structures have been placed under stress or tension by prolonged or by sudden force, or that they have been stretched slightly beyond their usual elastic capacity. Such injuries may be painful from a few hours to several days.

Simple *strains* leave no residual alteration in the structural efficiency of the tissues.

Sprain injuries were described in "The Edwin Smith Surgical Papyrus" (some five thousand years ago) as injuries which produced a rending, forcing or wrenching apart of articulations without actual dislocations or breaks. This indicates that the joint structures have been stretched beyond their functional capacity, resulting in tearing of various degrees or actual avulsion from their attachment to the bones, or even an avulsion of a bone fragment. *Sprains* of the ligaments and capsules heal within six to eight weeks by the formation of scar tissue, which is less elastic and less functional than normal tissue. Varying degrees of residual alteration of their functional capacity is inevitable.

Active motion under control of the patient cannot cause a *sprain* injury because the pain which results from overstretching the ligamentous and capsular structures limits injurious movements, except in neuropathic joints. Passive motion with force, either sustained or sudden, can produce injurious effects on the joint structures. Such injuries may result from sudden forceful movements of the head and neck instituted by blows on the head, face or neck, or by indirect forces applied to the body. Pulls and thrusts on the arms which cause a snapping movement of the neck may result in sprain injuries of the cervical joints. Blows on top of the head or falls from a height and landing on the feet cause compressive-avulsion type sprains. Falling from a height and landing on the neck and shoulder may produce a traction injury or a compression injury, or both.

Sudden forceful hyperextension or hyperflexion of the head and neck from any cause may result in traction and compression injuries, as well as rotational injuries. If the head and neck are rotated at the time of or during the application of the force to the side opposite the rotation, the resulting injury will be more severe.

The most frequent trauma of the neck today is caused by collisions of motor vehicles.

Automobile Accidents

The exact number of neck injuries which occur in automobile accidents can never be determined. The available statistical data relative to neck injuries are inadequate because injuries of other parts of the body which are obvious and often severe take precedence over the more obscure injuries of the cervical spine, so that a large percentage of neck injuries go unrecognized and unreported. Often times, the patient does not associate head, neck, shoulder, arm and chest pain with an injury of the neck. The pain associated with the more severe injuries may completely overshadow the symptoms referable to the neck.

The Mechanism of Neck Injuries

To describe the mechanism of neck injuries which occur in head-on collisions, Davis, in 1944, used the term *whiplash*. However, Crowe claims that he used the term in 1928, but there is no published record of this in the medical literature until 1963. Credit for the coinage of this term has been given erroneously to Gay and Abbot who published an article on the subject in 1953. Their concept of the mechanism of the whiplash was in error.

It should be understood clearly that head-on collisions cause a sudden forceful flexion of the neck followed by a recoil in extension, as described originally by Davis. Rear-end collisions produce a sudden forceful hyperextension of the neck followed by a recoil in flexion, as shown in Figure 44A. If a car is struck at the side, the passenger in the struck car is thrown toward the side of the impacting force and then to the opposite side or away from the impacting force, as shown in Figure 44B.

The mechanism can be understood better if we keep Newton's Law in mind: *a mass at rest remains at rest until acted upon by some external force and a mass in motion remains in motion until acted upon by some external force.*

Rear-end collisions produce a sudden acceleration of the portion of the body which is in contact with the seat of the struck car. The head, being a mass at rest, remains at rest until acted upon by some external force. The marked flexibility of the neck with the weight of the eight to twelve pound head resting upon its otherwise free end results in forceful hyperextension of the neck as the body is accelerated forward. The head hits the top of the back of the seat or the headrest in most cars now (but which is usually

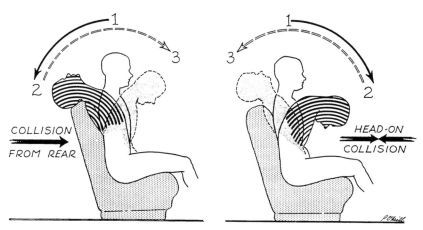

Figure 44A. The whiplash. If car is hit in the rear the neck is thrown into hyperextension and then hyperflexion. Head-on collisions cause sudden hyperflexion of the neck followed by a hyperextension recoil.

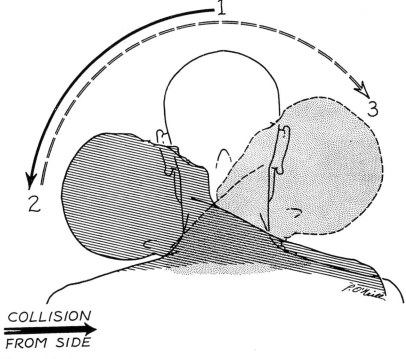

Figure 44B. The side-lash. In a side collision, the head and neck, and the body if unrestrained, are thrown to the side from which the impact occurs and then to the opposite side.

much too low and not properly designed to protect the head and neck) and this impact plus the reflex contraction of the neck muscles start the head in forward motion. The head continues forward until it is acted upon by some external force, such as contact with some stationary portion of the car and/or the restraining action of the soft tissue structures which hold the head and neck on the body.

Sudden deceleration of a moving vehicle occurs in a head-on collision with another vehicle or with a stationary object. Inasmuch as the body of the passenger in such a vehicle is unsupported from the front, it is thrown forward as it continues its momentum until it strikes some stationary part of the car such as the steering wheel, the windshield or the dashboard. The head continues forward unless it hits an immovable object, or until it is acted upon by some external force. It then recoils in extension. Usually, therefore, the lashing effect on the neck is less severe in head-on collisions than it is in rear-end collisions. This explains why the driver of the striking car in rear-end collisions rarely suffers a significant neck injury, unless his body is held in contact with the back of the seat by some restraining device or unless he is able to brace his body against the back of the seat.

The term whiplash, therefore, indicates the mechanism which can produce injuries of the cervical spine. It is not, and was never intended to be, a diagnostic term. Although the term has fallen into disrepute, it is used extensively and at least one lexicographer has defined it very well. The use of the term will continue in spite of the many attempts to squelch it, but it should be used correctly and never as a diagnosis.

The forces which must be absorbed by the neck when two vehicles collide cannot be measured accurately by mathematical formulas. McKeever attempted to measure these forces in his analysis of the mechanism of injuries of the neck, and he tried to show that the neck shortens at the point where the inert head is immediately vertical to the accelerated or decelerated body, as the case may be. He believed that because of this shortening of the neck an avulsive or compressive injury must occur somewhere in the cervical spine. By starting with a presumed set of facts he was able to show that the neck shortens one and thirty-five hundredths of an inch. He showed by his theorum that 527 pounds of kinetic energy must be absorbed by the neck as the body comes directly under the head (see Fig. 45). Cameron and Cree showed later that McKeever's concept omitted certain important factors such as lofting of the head and the element of torque, and they concluded that no known mathematical premise can explain all the forces involved in crash accidents because of the many variables which are ever present and which must be taken into consideration. Such variables include the site of impact, the direction and force of the impact and the velocity. Also, one must consider the stature, the sex and the age of the passenger(s), as shown by the "Seventeenth Stapp Car Crash Conference."

More important than the exact mechanics of acceleration and deceleration collisions is the recognition of the injuries of the neck which result. As stated previously, the greatest amount of stress

COLLISION FROM REAR

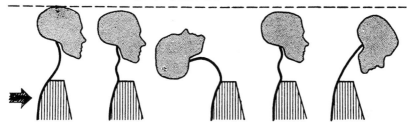

HEAD-ON COLLISION

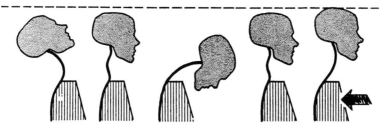

Figure 45. McKeever's concept of the mechanism of injury of the cervical spine which occurs in vehicular crash accidents.

and strain on active movement of the cervical spine in hyper-extension occurs at the C4-C5 level and in flexion it occurs at the C5-C6 level. In the absence of preexisting changes in the cervical spine from previous disorders, it is at these levels that we can anticipate the greatest amount of injury. However, injury may occur at any level. Cameron demonstrated that the element of torque plays an important role at C1 and at C7 and postulated that torque may explain the frequent midcervical injuries.

The injuries which occur may involve only the soft tissue structures which bind together the bony structures–the capsules, the ligaments, the muscles (especially those which bridge no more than two adjacent bony parts) and the intervertebral discs. Concomitant injuries of the bony structures occur often, and contusion of neural and vascular tissues are not unusual. Traction and

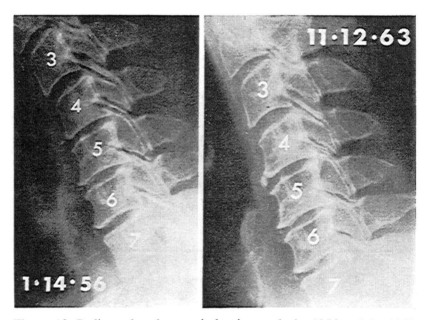

Figure 46. Radiographs of a cervical spine made in 1956 and in 1963, which illustrate avulsion of bone fragments at the anteroinferior margins of the bodies of C4, C5 and C6 and the subsequent changes. Note the swelling of the soft tissue structures anteriorly in the film made immediately following a rear-end collision in 1956.

shearing forces may cause injury of the brain stem, and in many instances concussion of the brain and injuries of the spinal cord occur. Injuries of the lower back often accompany the neck injuries, but these are usually of minor significance.

INJURIES CAUSED BY REAR-END COLLISIONS. Forceful hyperextension of the neck, which occurs when the body is accelerated forward, places traction on the anterior longitudinal ligament. The deep fibers of the ligament which are attached to the margins of the vertebral bodies and loosely to the annulus fibrosus of the intervertebral disc may be stretched, torn or avulsed. A piece of bone may be torn from the inferior margin of the vertebral body or bodies as shown in Figures 46 and 47B. An actual tear or rupture of the underlying annulus fibrosus may occur to allow escape of nuclear or disc material, or the disc may be avulsed from the cartilaginous plates of the vertebral bodies (Fig. 47C), as demonstrated by Macnab in his experiment with a monkey.

Compressive forces placed on the posterior structures results in avulsions of the capsular ligaments, an infolding or creasing of the interlaminar ligaments and contusion of the articular cartilage of the posterior joints as the joints are jammed together (Figs. 47B, C, D).

The longus capitis muscles and the intertransverse muscles may be torn from their attachments to the bones (see Fig. 47E).

Fractures of the spinous processes, of the laminae (Fig. 107) and of the portion of the bone between the articular facets (the interarticular isthmus) may occur, as shown in Figure 50. Fractures of the facets themselves or of the vertebral arches occur in some instances, and these may be unilateral or bilateral. The upward projections on the posterolateral surfaces of the vertebral bodies may be compressed on one side because of the torque effect which occurs when the neck is forced into hyperextension. Contusion of the nerve roots within the intervertebral canals may result from the pincherlike effect which occurs with forced hyperextension and with posterior subluxations (Fig. 47I).

Fractures of the odontoid process of the axis may occur as the anterior arch of the atlas is forced against it, or fractures of the

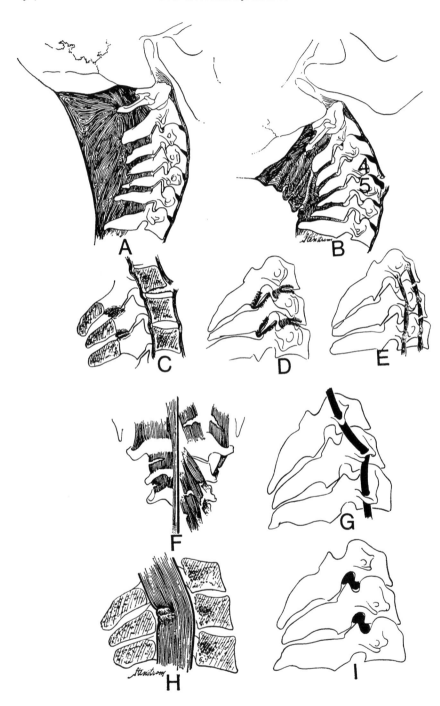

anterior arch itself may be produced. One of the transverse processes of the atlas may be fractured, as well as the facets on the lateral masses (Fig. 38).

If the head is rotated to one side and tilted to the opposite side (rotation and lateral bending occur together), the torisonal effect causes greater damage on one side than on the other side. At the atlantoaxial joints, the guy ligaments may be torn or stretched to give rise to lateral instability with lateral subluxation or slipping of the head and atlas on the axis, and/or rotation of the axis in its relationship with the atlas and skull (Figs. 11 and 12). Tears of the anterior suboccipital muscles, of the capsular ligaments of C1 and C2, the intertransverse and longus capitis muscles on the side opposite to which the head is turned may occur (Fig. 47F); also, the vertebral artery may be compressed as it passes beneath the lateral mass of the atlas (Fig. 23).

Fractures of the articular processes of the axis may occur.

Figure 47. Injuries caused by forceful hyperextension of the cervical spine: A is a side view of the cervical spine which shows the vertebrae, the nuchal ligament, the anterior longitudinal ligament, the discs, the transverse processes and their transverse foramina, the upward lateral projections on the bodies of the vertebrae from C3 through C7, the posterior apophyseal joints and the spinous processes. In B, note the creasing of the nuchal ligament and the tear of the anterior longitudinal ligament with avulsion of a fragment of bone at the anteroinferior margin of C4; in C, there has been a tear of the anterior longitudinal ligament and a separation of the disc from the cartilaginous plate on the inferior surface of the body of C4. There is creasing of the interlaminar ligament and overriding of the apophyseal joints also. In D note the tearing of the capsules of the apophyseal joints and of the anterior portion of the capsules of the lateral interbody joints. In E there is tearing of the intertransverse and the anterolateral muscles which are attached to each vertebra. The short anterior suboccipital muscles may be torn, as shown in F. The vertebral artery may be forced against the posterior wall of the transverse foramen, as shown in G. Actual compression of the posterior portion of the spinal cord may occur from infolding of the interlaminar ligament (H). The nerve roots and their accompanying structures may be compressed from subluxation by the pincherlike effect produced, as shown in I.

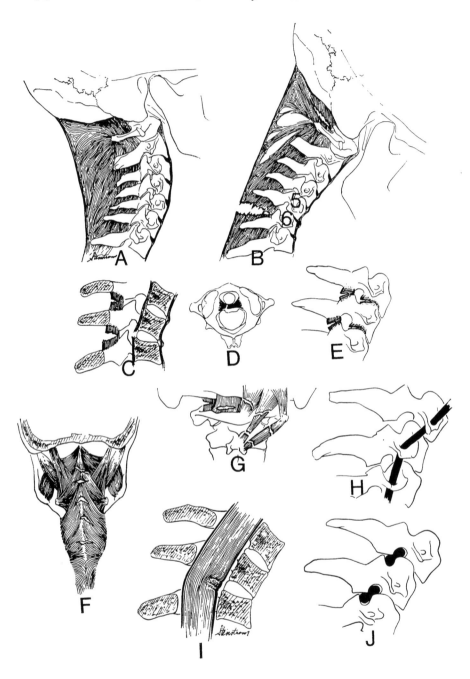

Often, these fractures are not noted in the immediate posttrauma radiographs, but are clearly visible after a period of several weeks, as shown in Figure 51.

The vertebral arteries may suffer trauma as they are pulled backward against the posterior wall of their bony rings through which they traverse, or by fracture of the adjacent bone structures or by injury to the proximate soft tissues (Fig. 47G). Injuries of the spinal branches of the arteries within the intervertebral canals may occur.

INJURIES CAUSED BY HEAD-ON COLLISIONS. Forceful hyperflexion of the neck which occurs as the body is decelerated suddenly may tear or stretch the nuchal ligament, the posterior longitudinal ligament, the interlaminar ligaments, the capsular ligaments of the lateral interbody joints and the posterior joints (see Fig. 48B, C, E). Avulsion of the margins of the articular facets and of the spinous processes may occur. Dislocations of the posterior facets, with or without cord injury, occur in some instances (Fig. 39).

Compression fractures of the vertebral bodies are not unusual, but they may not be evident in the immediate postinjury radiographs, as demonstrated in Figures 52 and 105. They can be seen in subsequent films when more compression and healing have occurred.

Figure 48. Injuries caused by forceful hyperflexion of the cervical spine: A is the side view of the cervical spine with the structures shown as described in Figure 47. In B one can see tears in the nuchal ligament and anterior extrusion of disc material at C5 and C6. In C there is a tear of the posterior longitudinal ligament and of the interlaminar ligaments. D shows a tear of the transverse ligament of the axis. In E there are tears of the capsules of the lateral interbody joints and of the posterior joints. F shows tears in the posterior pharyngeal raphe. Tears of the posterior suboccipital muscles are shown in G. In H, the vertebral artery is pulled against the anterior wall of the transverse foramen. Creasing of the anterior portion of the spinal cord may occur in acute flexion, especially if subluxation and/or bulging of the intervertebral disc posteriorly occur, as seen in I. With forward subluxations the nerve roots with their accompanying structures may be compressed, as shown in J.

If the head is rotated at the time of the accident, a vertebral arch or a posterior facet may fracture because of the shearing force. This occurs usually on the side opposite that to which the head is turned. A fracture of a transverse process may occur on the side to which the head is turned. The lateral masses of the atlas and axis may suffer compression fractures.

The transverse ligament of the atlas may be sprained or stretched as forceful hyperflexion of the neck occurs (Fig. 48D). If the head is rotated at the time of the injury, the guy ligaments may be torn, also (Fig. 49B), and allow lateral slipping of the

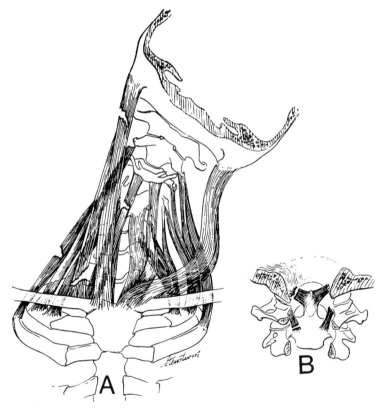

Figure 49. Injuries which may occur if the neck is rotated and bent laterally or from forces applied from the side: As shown in A, the muscles that are on stretch may be torn. The alar ligament and/or the atlantoaxial ligament may be torn, as shown in B, as well as tears of the capsules of the lateral interbody joints.

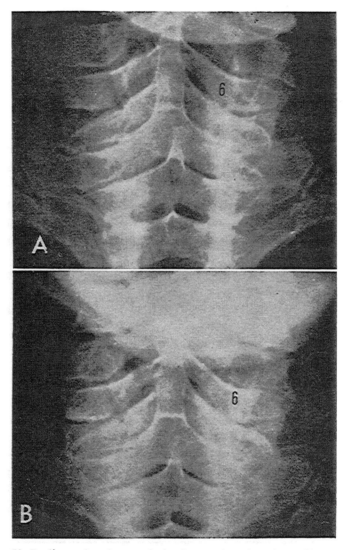

Figure 50. Radiographs of a cervical spine made a few days after an injury and six months later. There is a compression fracture of the interarticular isthmus on the right side of the sixth vertebra, as shown in A. There is some increased narrowing of the isthmus in B and the fracture appears to be healed.

head and the atlas on the axis, and/or rotation of the axis in its relationship to the head and atlas.

INJURIES CAUSED BY SIDE COLLISIONS. Collisions in which the side of one vehicle is hit by the front end of another vehicle, which occur at intersections of streets or roads usually, may result in any of the above injuries depending on the force of the impact, the position of the head and the buffering effect produced by the construction of the vehicles involved. Actual tears of the lateral neck muscles may occur, as shown in Figure 49A, and tearing of the alar and atlantoaxial ligaments and upper joint capsules may occur (Fig. 49B).

Any of the above described mechanisms may result in contusion injuries of the vertebral arteries resulting in vasoconstriction and obliteration. These findings have been demonstrated by angiographic studies of the vertebral arteries.

Ligamentous instability and the resulting structural changes which result from the above described injuries may produce irritation of the cervical nerve roots or actual compression of all the structures within the intervertebral canals.

Injuries of the Brain and Spinal Cord

Injuries of the brain may be associated with the above described injuries of the neck. Gurdjian and his coworkers at Wayne State University have shown that sudden setting into motion or acceleration of the body and the head at different rates of acceleration may cause a head injury. Sudden deceleration, which occurs when the moving body and head come in contact with a nonmoving or slower moving object, can produce the same effect. Such injuries to the brain or to the intracranial contents may result from rear-end, head-on and side collisions.

Injury to the brain and to the brain stem may be the result of pressure gradients created by pressure build-up or by shearing forces and mass movements of the intracranial contents. The increase in intracranial pressure from acceleration and deceleration of the head is directly related to the degree of these forces. Following these injuries, alterations in the cell structure within the brain stem were found, but no changes in the cortical structures resulted.

These findings are of significance in view of the work done by Torres and Shapiro at the University of Minnesota. Electroencephalographic abnormalities were found in 46 percent of "whiplash" injuries of the neck and in 44 percent of closed head injuries. The symptomatology and the clinical findings were comparable in both groups of patients. The mechanism in the production of the electrical abnormalities following whiplash injuries was explained on the basis of direct influence on the brain tissue by acceleration and deceleration forces, which was described, also, by Denny-Brown and Russell in 1941.

The brain may be injured as it hits the inner table of the skull. Vascular insufficiency to the brain is produced by constriction or occlusion of one or both vertebral arteries within the transverse foramina of the cervical vertebrae. It was concluded that marked brain dysfunction can occur as a consequence of the whiplash as well as from direct injury of the head.

Thomas has stated in his discussion of concussion in the book *Impact Injury and Crash Protection* that a brain concussion, which occurs often in crash accidents, is an immediate and transient impairment of neural function, such as alteration of consciousness, disturbance of vision and equilibrium, and disorientation resulting from mechanical forces. Injury to the reticular formation of the brain stem accounts for the loss of consciousness and is the sheer stress developed in the brain stem as a result of the elastic flow produced by pressure gradients along the brain stem axis; acceleration, both translational and angular, appears to be the most likely cause of the increased intracranial pressure.

The emotional reactions which occur sometimes following acceleration and deceleration injuries of the neck indicate that brain damage is more common and more extensive than we have realized, and that the so-called psychoneurotic-type symptomatology can be explained and determined on an organic basis. Although we do not fully understand the physiological mode of the psychodynamic processes, brain dysfunction does occur and is not restored to normal by legal procedures as some would have us believe.

The spinal cord within the vertebral foramen is vulnerable to injury by compression or laceration from fractures of any of the bony components of the foramen, by dislocations with or without fractures, by marked subluxation, by severe traction forces produced by sudden hyperflexion of the neck, by severe hyperextension forces which may produce folding anteriorly of the interlaminar ligaments to cause compression of the spinal cord. Injuries to the vertebral arteries and their spinal branches and injuries of the posterior and/or the anterior arteries may occur. Symptoms of arterial damage may be delayed as far as the spinal cord itself is concerned.

Forceful lateral bending and rotation of the cervical spine may cause injuries which involve the skeletal and soft tissue structures as well as the spinal cord. The injuries of the spinal cord may be minimal and transient, or there may be complete crushing or maceration or transection of the cord by fractures and/or dislocations, and even avulsion, of the nerve roots as shown in Plate 4.

Injuries of the Lower Back

Injuries of the spine have been studied at Wayne State University since 1953. Patrick has reported that high acceleration peaks have been recorded when an automobile hits a solid object. The experimental studies were done to determine the static and dynamic injuries to the vertebrae imposed by acceleration. It was found that end-plate fractures occurred in the lumbar area which were difficult, or impossible, to demonstrate by radiographic examination.

Many victims of automobile crash accidents present symptoms of strain injury of the lower back. The symptoms usually subside within a reasonable length of time. Sprain injuries and end plate fractures will result in disturbances of the dynamics of the adjacent intervertebral disc, resulting in some degree of permanent disability. Compression fractures of the vertebral bodies do occur, and if pain persists radiographs should be repeated at four to six week intervals.

Injuries Caused by Noncrash Accidents

Injuries may result from sudden acceleration and deceleration of motor-powered vehicles even in the absence of crash accidents. The rapid acceleration of motor vehicles, which our present high-powered engines permit, may cause a forceful hyperextension of the neck of an unsuspecting passenger.

The sudden deceleration of a moving vehicle, which the very effective power brakes make possible, may avoid a crash accident, but the unprepared passenger may keep going into the dash or the windshield, or if passenger in rear seat, into the back of the front seat or to the floor. How many times have we seen purses, boxes, suitcases, children and dogs thrown forward, to be stopped only by contact with a stationary part of the car!

A seat belt, if in proper use, will prevent the forward propulsion of the body to some extent and will lessen the possibility of serious injuries of most of the body from sudden deceleration of the vehicle, but the belt has very little, if any, deterring effect on the cervical spine as the head and neck continue in forward motion. Even the addition of a shoulder harness will not relieve, but will only increase, the forces which must be absorbed by the head and neck, although such harness may prevent contact injuries.

Comment

The statistical data concerning injuries of the cervical spine resulting from crash accidents of motor vehicles are inaccurate, inasmuch as many of these injuries are unrecognized and hence never reported. Major fractures and dislocations, internal injuries, head and face injuries take precedence over the less obvious injuries of the cervical spine, as shown in Figures 51 and 52.

Radiographs of the cervical spine made immediately or a few days after the accident may be considered to be "within normal limits," and it is presumed often that no injury to the cervical spine has occurred. Subsequent radiographs may tell a different story. Continued symptoms referable to the complex structures of the cervical spine call for repeated adequate radiographic studies even after a period of several years, if we are to understand what

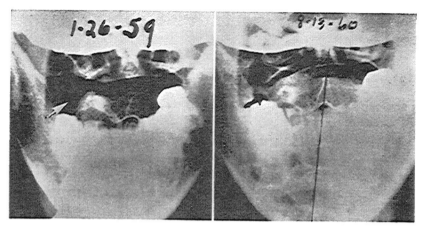

Figure 51. Open mouth views of patient who was injured on 9/14/58. The fracture of the odontoid and of the superior articular surface of the left lateral mass were not recognized initially. Subsequent films revealed the fractures as healing progressed. (This patient suffered a severe head injury and was unconscious for seven days. Concern and treatment were directed toward the head injury.)

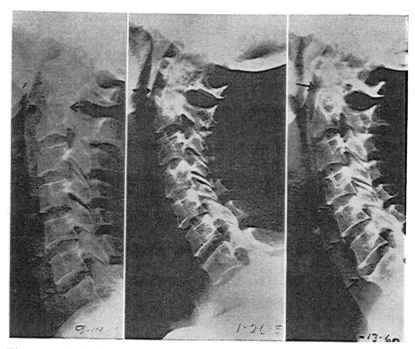

Figure 52. Initial injury occurred on 9/14/58 and radiograph made on that date shows no evidence of a compression fracture of the seventh vertebral body. (The fracture of the odontoid and the avulsion fractures of the fifth and sixth vertebrae were not recognized.) The compression fracture of the seventh vertebral body was evident in the subsequent films. (This patient suffered a severe head injury to which treatment was directed.)

happens to the neck at the time of crash accidents and the changes which occur subsequently. If we believe that injuries of the neck do not occur, or that they are of little significance, we are deluding ourselves and failing in our obligations to those so injured who consult us. The fear of legal involvement does not justify inadequate examinations and diagnoses nor the failure to institute proper therapy when indicated.

Injuries Sustained in Sports

It is not necessary to recount all the various activities known as sports which are responsible for injuries of the neck, but those which are most hazardous should be mentioned.

Football

The game of football which seems to necessitate, or at least permit, violent physical contact of the players has been responsible for many neck injuries. The greatest percentage occurs as the result of forceful hyperextension of the neck from contact of the chin or face with the ground, or from contact with some portion of the body of another player such as a flexed knee.

The unyielding plastic face-guard may be thrown or forced upward causing sudden hyperextension of the neck. In this event, the rigid back rim of the helmet may be driven against the back of the neck to cause severe injury to the ligamentous, capsular and muscular structures, and to the skeletal structures as well. Injury to the spinal cord and injury to the vertebral arteries may result in some instances.

Hyperflexion injuries may occur when a tackler's head is forced forward and downward by contact with other players.

Rotational forces may accompany hyperextension and hyperflexion injuries to add to their severity.

Trampoline

Jumping on the trampoline, especially by the novice, has caused many types and degrees of neck injuries. Hyperflexion injuries have been reported by Ellis as the result of imperfectly executed backward somersaults. If the trampolinist lands on his head or on his neck and shoulders, injuries of the cervical joints resulting in subluxations and dislocations are not unusual.

The severe injuries and the fatal injuries are usually reported, but one may postulate that many of the minor injuries are not mentioned. The acute symptoms may subside and the injuries are forgotten until years later when the inevitable joint changes have developed. Recently the trampoline has been discontinued in many schools because of serious injuries which have occurred.

Diving

Fractures and dislocations may result from improperly executed dives, especially if the head hits the bottom of the pool or some submerged object in the water. Varying degrees of injury to the spinal cord may occur from forceful hyperextension of the neck, or from hyperflexion.

Diving, even when done by professionals, may result in hyperflexion, hyperextension, compression and rotational sprains of the ligamentous and capsular structures. Repeated injuries of the ligamentous and capsular structures which may not be disabling immediately will result in the inevitable osteophytic formations which occur following such traumatic experiences, as shown by Schneider in his study of the cervical spines of the divers at Acapulco.

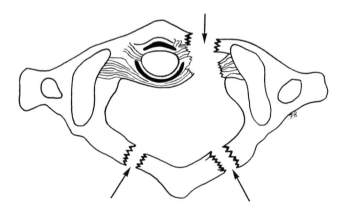

Figure 53. A diagram which illustrates a fracture of the anterior arch of the atlas at its weakest point and bilateral fractures of the posterior arch which occur when the head is forced suddenly in hyperextension.

Miscellaneous

Blows on the Head

Many injuries of the neck result from blows on the head. The extent of the injuries will depend on the amount of the force, the direction of the blow and the position of the head at the time of the impact. Sprains, disc ruptures, fractures and dislocations may occur.

Figure 53 illustrates the type of injury which may occur when the head is forced backward. The posterior arch of the atlas is forced against the lamina of the axis, causing a bilateral fracture of the posterior arch and a fracture of the anterior arch of the atlas as it is forced against the odontoid process.

A severe downward force on the head, which may be caused by a falling weight, may result in separation of the lateral masses of the atlas downward and outward when the bony ring of the atlas is fractured in at least two places (Fig. 54). The downward force may cause compression fractures of the vertebral bodies and avulsion of the capsular structures, also.

A blow on the head when the neck is in flexion may cause tearing of the posterior ligamentous and capsular structures, compression fractures of vertebral bodies, tearing of the transverse ligament of the atlas and/or rupture of one or more intervertebral discs. Dislocation of the posterior facets and varying degrees of spinal cord injuries may occur.

Falls

Any fall may produce an injury to the cervical spine. If the falling person lands on his head, neck, or shoulder, the injury is likely to be more severe than if there is no impact to these structures. The extent of the injuries is dependent upon the direction and the amount of the force or forces applied to the neck.

Sprains, subluxations, fractures and dislocations may occur in any part of the cervical spine. If the individual lands in a sitting position, we may anticipate compression type injuries. Forward falls usually produce hyperextension of the neck, causing tearing

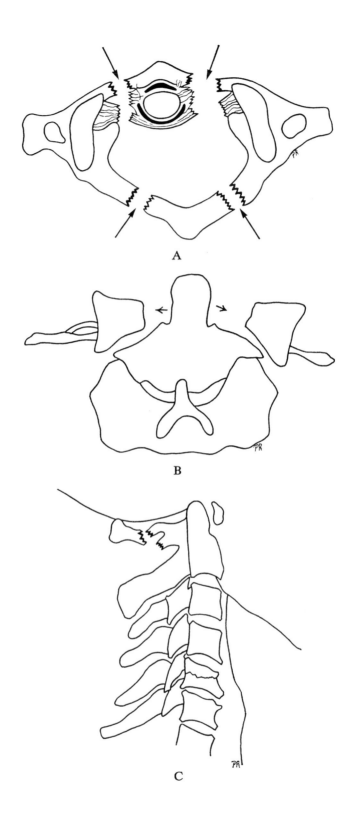

A

B

C

of the anterior longitudinal ligament, compression and avulsion of the posterior joints and possible fractures of one or more spinous processes. Compression of neural and vascular structures may occur.

If the head is forced to one side, avulsive-compression injuries occur on the side to which the head is forced and traction injuries occur on the side that makes contact with the ground or floor.

If the head is forced forward, we may anticipate traction injuries of the posterior soft tissue structures and compression injuries of the anterior structures of the cervical spine. Dislocations of the facets or fractures of the facets and/or of the vertebral bodies may occur.

Forceful Pulls or Thrusts on the Arms

Sudden forceful pulls on the arm or arms may cause a snapping of the neck with resulting sprain injuries of the soft tissue structures and either compression or traction injuries of the neural structures.

Forceful Muscular Contractions

Lifting heavy weights from a stooped position, lifting heavy objects above the head and pushing and pulling heavy loads may give rise to sprain injuries of the neck, and in some instances to fractures of a spinous process or articular facet (the effort syndrome). Forceful muscular contractions produced by electric shocks may cause similar injuries.

Unilateral Subluxations

Even in the absence of any apparent traumatic experience, unilateral subluxations may occur when the muscles of the neck are

---

←◀◀◀

Figure 54. A diagram of the atlas showing bilateral fractures of both arches, which occurred when the patient was hit on the head by a falling air conditioner, is seen in A. A tracing of the radiograph of the first two vertebrae which shows marked separation laterally of the lateral masses of the atlas is shown in B. In C a tracing of a lateral view of the cervical spine shows forward displacement of the anterior arch of the atlas and the double fracture of the posterior arch, as well as a fracture of the fifth vertebral body.

fully relaxed. This may happen when a person turns over in bed in his sleep, or when a person is under a general anesthetic if the neck is not protected as the patient is transferred to a carriage or bed.

A subluxation may occur when the head and neck are turned suddenly beyond the usual range of motion.

Some separation of the adjacent facets on one side occurs to cause elevation of the vertebra on that side and some forward displacement and rotation to the opposite side. This causes narrowing of the intervertebral foramen on the opposite side and possible nerve root impingement. The neck cannot be bent toward the side of the subluxation and the head cannot be rotated to that side.

Just what causes the facets to lock with the inferior facet elevated on the superior facet of the adjacent vertebra is debatable. Impingement of the synovial membrane or of the meniscuslike structure within the posterior joints may be the mechanism involved. The resulting inflammatory reaction may give rise to foraminal narrowing and compression of the adjacent nerve root and the other structures within the foramen.

Occupational and Postural Situations

Certain postural situations and some unusual occupational positions may result in repetitive minor traumatic insults to the joint structures and to the adjacent nerve roots. Occupations which require sudden or prolonged hyperextension of the neck, prolonged flexion of the neck and prolonged or frequently repeated rotation and lateral bending of the neck may instigate symptoms of foraminal encroachment. Some of the many postural attitudes and occupational positions are illustrated in Figures 55 and 56.

NONTRAUMATIC CONDITIONS

Inflammatory involvement of the joints of the cervical spine of nontraumatic origin comprise only a small percentage of cervical spine disorders. However, it must be remembered that many patients with cervical joint involvement are treated by the general

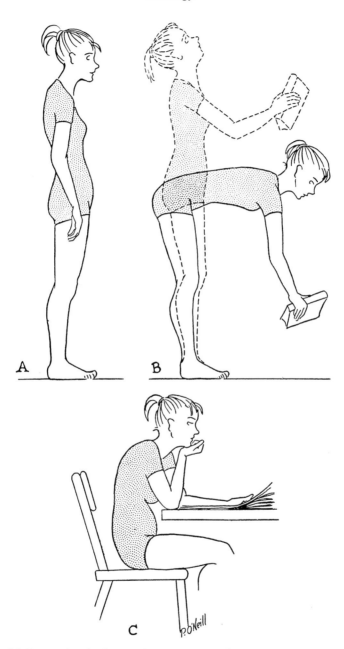

Figure 55. Postural attitudes causing hyperextension of the neck. A: Drooping shoulders. B: Stooping. C: Usual "table posture"—chin on hand.

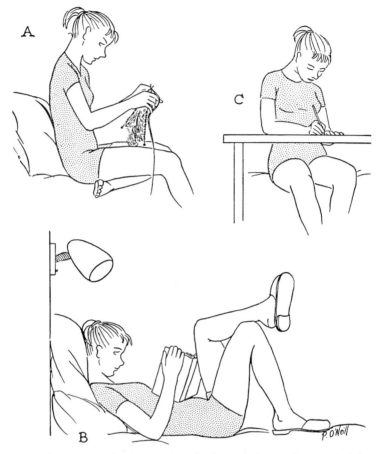

Figure 56. Postural attitudes causing flexion of the neck. A: Knitting or sewing. B: Reading in bed. C: Writing.

practitioners and the internists, so that many such conditions may not be seen by the orthopaedists.

Synovitis

An inflammatory reaction within the synovial membrane of the cervical joints may occur as a result of upper respiratory infections. Inasmuch as little is known about the innervation of the synovial membrane (it seems to be insensitive), we cannot say that inflammation of it produces pain. The pain resulting from a synovitis is, in all probability, due to the increase of synovial fluid which causes pressure on the richly innervated capsular structures and on the adjacent nerve root resulting in radicular pain. The inflammation may spread to involve the capsular structures resulting in capsulitis to produce local or reflexly referred pain.

Arthritis

Involvement of any of the structures of joints can be classified under the general term of *arthritis,* a complete discussion of which is beyond the scope of this book. A diagnosis of *arthritis* is an easy one, and who can question such a diagnosis? Certainly, any painful joint condition justifies such a diagnosis regardless of the numerous etiological factors.

Disorders of the joints adjacent to the nerve roots may give rise to radicular symptoms and findings, or pain may be reflexly referred from the capsular structures along the course of the nerve roots which supply them. Pain may be confined to the involved joint structures without radicular referral and without reflex referral. Spasm of the muscles which control joint movements occurs to provide a splinting effect on the painful joints–a protective mechanism.

Rheumatoid and Ankylosing Spondylitis

Joint disorders known as rheumatoid arthritis are the result of involvement of the connective tissue, or collagen, fibers. The exact etiology of this condition is still undetermined and it is likely that there are many causative factors. The joints of the cervical spine are not immune. The ultimate response to this disorder is ankylosis of the spine. Foraminal narrowing with irritation of the nerve roots is more likely to occur in the acute phase of this disorder when the joint structures are inflamed. As the condition progresses to ankylosis, the inflammatory reaction subsides. Local pain is relieved by cessation of joint movement and the foramina through which the nerve roots pass are found to have smooth contours with no apparent narrowing (Fig. 57). Although there may be some resulting hyperplasia of the ligamentous and capsular structures, nerve root insult is rare in the absence of motion, unless irreversible changes within the nerve roots have occurred.

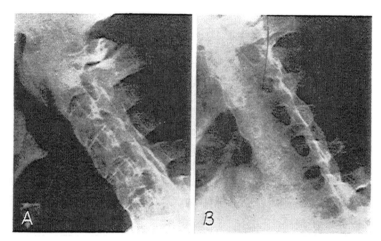

Figure 57. Radiographs of the cervical spine of a patient who has rheumatoid arthritis. Note the absence of bony encroachment of the intervertebral canals.

Rheumatoid arthritis is a generalized disorder involving many organ systems other than the synovial joints, although it is primarily a polyarthritic disorder with joint inflammation and dysfunction. The early extraarticular manifestations often help in making the diagnosis. The sedimentation rate is the most significant laboratory test, although other connective tissue disorders may give an increased sedimentation rate. Superficial rheumatoid nodules are diagnostically important findings. The rheumatoid factor as manifested in the sheep agglutination test is important but is positive in only two thirds of patients with rheumatoid arthritis. A complete discussion of all the manifestations of rheumatoid arthritis is beyond the scope of this book. A comprehensive discussion can be found in the eighth edition of Hollander's book *Arthritis.*

Decker reported that acute flexion lateral radiographs of 333 rheumatoid arthritic patients revealed that 84 had atlantoaxial subluxations exceeding the accepted normal of 2.5 mm in women and 3.0 mm in men, and that 23 showed subluxations of C3 on C4. The latter group had clinical evidence of more cord compression than did those with atlantoaxial subluxations.

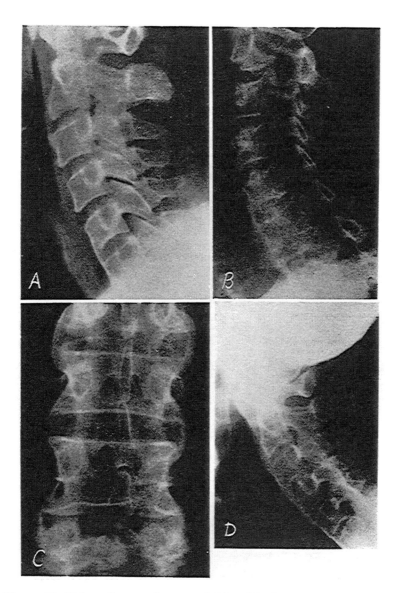

Figure 58. This patient at the age of 31, while in the Air Corps, began having pain in his sacroiliac joints with gradually increasing pain and stiffness in his lumbar and thoracic areas, and limitation of chest expansion. When examined in 1957, fifteen years after the onset of his symptoms, he was having pain and stiffness of the lower portion of his cervical spine, also. In A and C the ankylosis is evident in the cervical spine to C5 and in the lumbar spine. The radiograph D made in 1974 shows extension of the ankylosis to C2. There was motion only between the occiput and atlas and at the atlantoaxial joints. In B it can be seen that the intervertebral foramina are of normal size and contour and this was true in the oblique films made in 1974.

Rheumatoid arthritis occurs, supposedly, in the twenty to forty year age group; however, it can and does occur in other age groups.

A review of about 8000 cases of cervical spine disorders revealed only five cases who had rheumatoid arthritis. None of these had atlantoaxial subluxation but only radiographic evidence of involvement of the posterior or apophyseal joints of the cervical

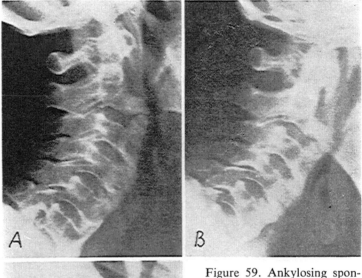

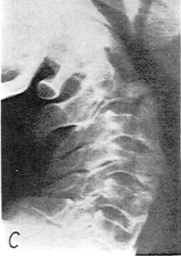

Figure 59. Ankylosing spondylitis of the anterior portions of the vertebral bodies with marked proliferative changes. This patient had difficulty in swallowing and occipital headaches. She could swallow by hyperextending her head, which caused irritation of the third nerve roots.

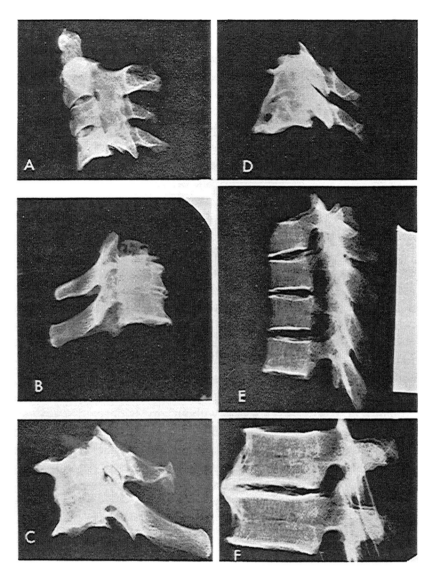

Figure 60. Radiographs of specimens showing varieties of ankylosing arthritis. In A there is fusion of the posterior joints only. In B there is fusion of the posterior portion of the vertebral bodies, and the posterior longitudinal ligament and the posterior joints are not fused. Figure C shows fusion of the vertebral bodies across the disc and of the longitudinal ligaments. In D fusion along the anterior and posterior ligaments has occurred, but the posterior joints and the disc are free. In E only the posterior joints are fused. In F there is fusion across the anterior ligament and the annulus fibrosus anteriorly is involved.

spine. Only one case diagnosed as rheumatoid arthritis, which involved initially the joints of the knees, hips, hands, elbows, shoulders and eventually the posterior synovial joints of the cervical spine, showed ankylosis of these joints, as shown in Figure 57.

Ankylosing arthritis or spondylitis is illustrated in Figure 58. The cause of this disorder is not known. It usually starts in the sacroiliac joints in young male adults and is first manifested by stiffness and pain in the lower back or, in some instances, in the hip joints as described by the patients. This disorder migrates proximally to involve almost all of the joints of the spine as well as the costovertebral joints.

Dissection of anatomical specimens has revealed several varieties of ankylosing arthritis. In some instances ossification of the anterior and posterior ligaments have been noted without involvement of the posterior joints. In other instances, the posterior joints have shown the bony ankylosis. In other specimens ankylosis has been noted between the vertebral bodies and the lateral interbody joints with the ligamentous and posterior joint structures apparently uninvolved. In still other specimens, and in some patients, marked bony proliferation bridging the anterior margins of the vertebral bodies has been found without any evidence of ankylosis of the posterior structures (Fig. 59). Some specimens have shown ankylosis of all the joints–the posterior apophyseal joints, the lateral interbody joints and the secondary disc joints (Fig. 60).

An explanation of the different varieties of ankylosing arthritis cannot be made. Each type may produce a variety of symptoms and clinical findings.

Gout

The joints of the cervical spine do not escape the arthritic process known as gout. Elevation of the uric acid content of the body fluids or hyperuricemia may be the result of excess formation of uric acid, deficient renal excretion of uric acid or diminished destruction of urates in the body. The specific lesion of gout is the deposition of monosodium urates in the articular tissues, which act as irritants to produce a proliferative reaction resulting in synovial pannus formation, cartilaginous degeneration, cystic areas in the

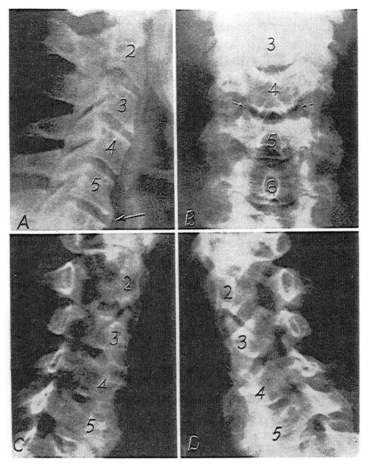

Figure 61. Radiographs of the cervical spine of a patient who has gouty arthritis. Arrows in B point to tophaceous deposits at the lateral interbody joints between 4 and 5. Note the anteroposterior narrowing of the intervertebral canals in C and D.

sub-chondral bone and proliferation of marginal osteophytes. Compression or irritation of the cervical nerve roots may occur from involvement of the adjacent joints (Fig. 61).

Disease

The author's interpretation of *disease* is a pathological process induced by an organism. Such diseases include osteomyelitis and infectious arthritis which are caused by pathogenic organisms. Encroachment on the intervertebral canals may result from involvement of the adjacent bone and joint structures. Fortunately, these conditions are relatively rare in the cervical spine.

Quillain, Barré and Strohl have described a neuroradiculitis with cerebrospinal hyperalbuminosis which they believe to be caused by a virus or some postinfectious condition, resulting in paralysis and loss of deep tendon reflexes.

Neoplasms

Primary bone tumors of the cervical spine occur rarely. Soft tissue tumors may erode the bone structure. Foraminal encroachment may occur depending on the location and extension of the neoplasm. Intramedullary neoplasms of neural origin may occur in the spinal cord. Other tumors may occur in the meninges, nerve roots and blood vessels to give rise to nerve root symptoms and clinical findings.

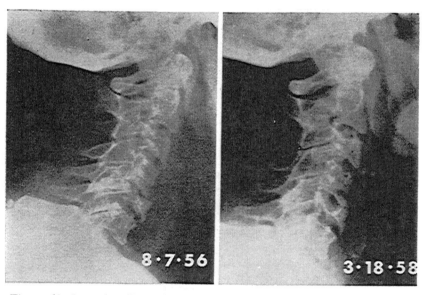

Figure 62. Lateral radiographs of the cervical spine of a patient who had metastatic carcinoma of the breast involving the fifth vertebral body. The cervical lesion was treated with x-radiation with apparent improvement, although she had continued radicular pain and paresthesias, but no motor deficit.

Metastatic Lesions

Malignant lesions of other organs may metastasize to the cervical spine. I have encountered four cases of metastatic lesions in the cervical spine from carcinoma of the breast. Such lesions may be responsible for localized cervical pain, as well as for radicular pain, paraesthesias and motor deficits (Fig. 62).

Osteoporosis

A generalized metabolic bone disorder known as osteoporosis, the cause of which is not definitely known, may involve the cervical spine. This condition is characterized by a reduction in the size and number of bone trabeculae and not infrequently results in collapse of vertebral bodies. Such collapse occurs rarely in the cervical vertebrae, but when it does happen an alteration in the intervertebral foramina results and may be responsible for irritation or compression of the nerve roots, as well as localized pain.

Degenerative Joint Disorders

Joint changes which are called degenerative in character involve the cervical joints. These disorders for the most part are the result of traumatic experiences, either single or multiple, or they may result from a mechanical imbalance of the motor units so involved (Figs. 63, 64 and 65). Traumatic insults may involve the ligamentous and capsular structures, the articular cartilage, and discs and the muscles which control the joints. The eventual picture is one of osteophytic changes at the margins of the bones to which the ligamentous structures have their attachments. In the cervical spine, these changes occur primarily at the margins of the lateral interbody joints, and to a lesser extent at the margins of the posterior joints, to cause foraminal encroachment and pressure upon the structures within the intervertebral canals. Osteophytic changes occur at the anterior margins of the vertebral bodies frequently, and somewhat less frequently at the posterior vertebral margins where they may encroach on the vertebral foramen to cause pressure on the spinal cord.

Osteophytic formations occur slowly over variable periods of time so that the nerve roots may be crowded gradually into the

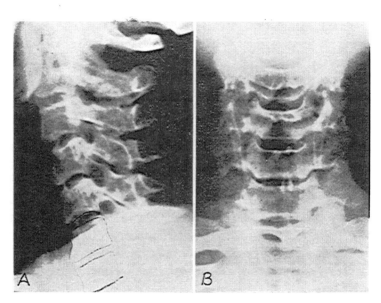

Figure 63A & B. This patient received a whiplash injury in 1937 when a heavy truck hit the rear end of the car in which she was riding. X-ray films made immediately following the injury were thought to be negative.

bottom of the canals and thus escape insult from the osteophytes until a certain stage is reached, or until some unaccustomed stress or strain is placed on the joints or on the nerve roots themselves. Some unusual movement of the neck may be the added stimulus which triggers an attack of radicular symptoms.

Injuries involving the anterior ligament of the cervical spine give rise to osteophytosis at the vertebral attachments. Bick has stated that these osteophytes form as an ossific reaction to local strain at the insertion of the longitudinal fibers into the cephalic or caudal rings of the vertebral bodies. Any structural imbalance between vertebral bodies invites their formation and they may extend along the connecting ligamentous fibers to form a bridge across the vertebral bodies to produce a fusion. The osteophytic processes per se are, in all probability, painless, but their encroach-

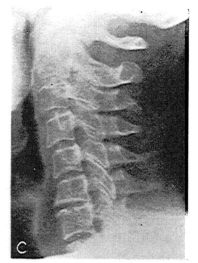

Figure 63C. The lateral view was made in 1945 following a second injury. Note the narrowing of the disc at 6 and 7 and the degenerative changes at this level. There is some narrowing of the disc between 5 and 6, also.

Figure 63D & E. In 1956, nineteen years later, this patient received another whiplash injury. Note the progressive degenerative changes which have occurred since the initial injury.

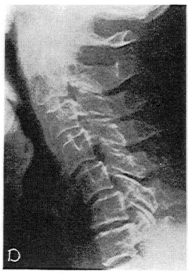
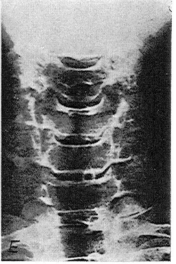

ment upon neural structures can and does produce pain and neuropathies.

The loss of disc turgosity from escape of its fluid content alters the mechanical motor unit of which it is a part and may give rise to osteophytosis at the anterior and anterolateral margins of the

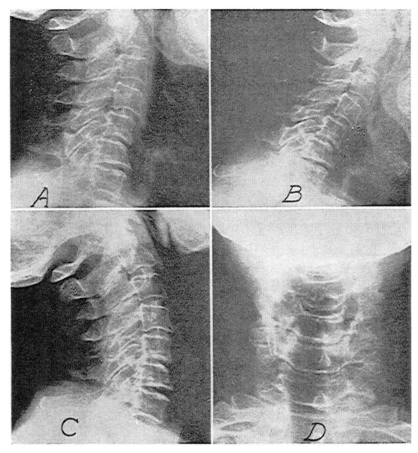

Figure 64. Radiographs of the cervical spine of the patient shown in Figure 63 which were made in 1962 following a head-on collision with a post. Note the increased changes and the increased forward subluxation of C4 on C5 and of C5 on C6.

vertebral bodies, and more rarely at the posterior margins where they may cause pressure upon the spinal cord.

The lateral interbody joints and the posterior joints may escape the ossific changes for variable periods, even for many years, in which event nerve root compression may not occur concomitantly with osteophytosis of the vertebral bodies, as shown in Figure 66.

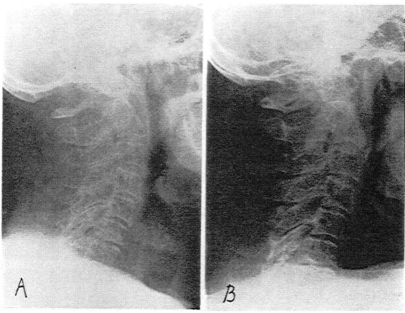

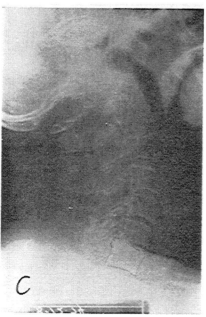

Figure 65. Films made in 1974 of the patient shown in Figures 63 and 64 show the progressive changes which have occurred during the past twelve years. In A there is no forward slipping of C4 on C5 nor of C5 on C6. There is increased narrowing of all discs below C3 and there are marked degenerative changes of the apophyseal joints. In the flexion view B there is forward slipping of C5 on C6 and forward motion is markedly limited. There is a fairly good range of hyperextension in C, but C6 slips forward on C7.

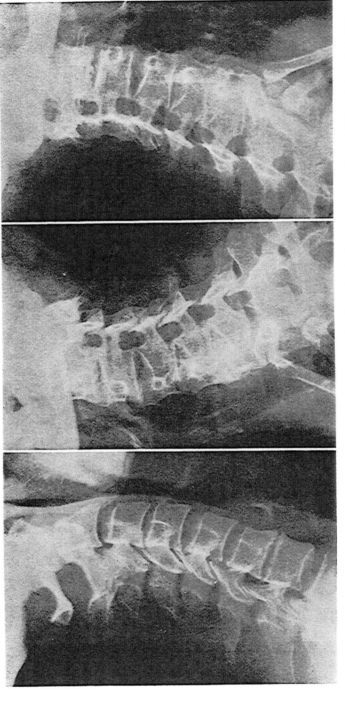

Figure 66. Lateral and oblique radiographic views of a cervical spine which show narrowed discs at C3 and 4 and at C6 and 7. Osteophytic formations are present at C6 and 7 at their adjacent anterior margins, however there is no appreciable narrowing of the proximate intervertebral canals. There are no anterior osteophytes present at C3 and 4, but there is definite encroachment on the intervertebral canals by osteophytes at the margins of the lateral interbody joints at this level.

These changes have been called osteoarthritis, hypertrophic arthritis, proliferative arthritis, spondylosis, etc. However, Bick's term *vertebral osteophytosis* is the term of choice. These changes represent the inevitable response of the spinal ligaments to traumatic experiences.

The Aging Process

If any single aging process exists, it is not known at the present time. Certain so-called degenerative changes in the spine are found more frequently in the fourth, fifth and sixth decades of life, but such changes cannot be attributed to a specific aging process. Intrinsic and extrinsic factors are involved undoubtedly.

In the spine, the water content of the fibrocartilaginous discs and of the articular cartilages decreases with age but not at the same rate in all individuals nor in all age groups. The loss of water lessens the resiliency of these structures, but they may function well within their own limited capacity, if no undue stress is placed on them.

The ligamentous and capsular structures lose some of their elasticity with age, but this does not occur in the same degree in all people. Such changes, if caused by aging, should be uniform in all the joints of one individual and not in one or two specific joints. Biomedical science has sought to define the fundamental basis of aging, but the origin of biological aging remains an enigma.

Aging per se is not responsible for nerve root irritation, but the resulting mechanical alterations which may occur can be responsible for encroachment on the foraminal structures.

Spasmodic Torticollis

Unilateral spasmodic contractions of the muscles of the neck and shoulder which may be related to a lesion of the thalamus, the globus pallidus or the basal ganglia give rise to mechanical derangement of the cervical spine from repeated overstretching of the ligamentous and capsular structures and to compressive forces upon the articular cartilages. The continuous uncontrollable and forceful contractions of the muscles may cause pain localized to

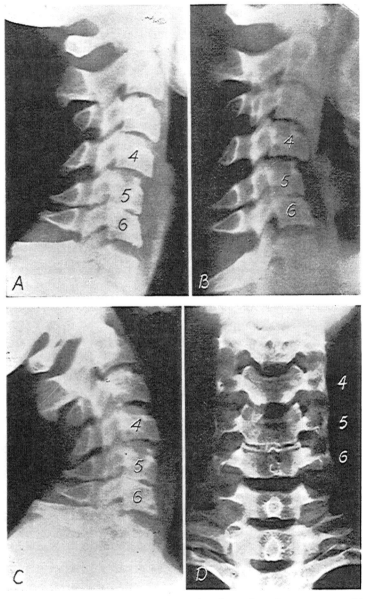

Figure 67. Radiographs of the cervical spine of a fourteen-year-old girl following a recent sprain injury of the neck. The bodies of the fifth and sixth vertebra are fused posteriorly, probably a congenital fusion, or a result of an earlier injury. Note the marked ligamentous instability between the fourth and fifth vertebrae.

the joint structures, but not infrequently radicular symptoms do occur as well as reflexly referred pains.

Anomalies

The many anomalies of the cervical spine which are considered to be of congenital or of developmental origin may or may not be directly responsible for irritation of the nerve roots. Fusion of two or more vertebrae does not usually narrow the foramina. The foramina may be smaller at the fused areas but they are always round or oval shaped and smooth in contour. However, the fixation of two or more vertebrae places an added strain on the adjacent vertebral joints as they attempt to maintain the functions of the neck, and the changes which may occur in these joints can give rise to compression of the adjacent foraminal structures (Fig. 67).

The anomaly known as *basilar impression,* which is an invagination of the atlas into the skull from elevation of the floor of the posterior fossa of the cranium, may be responsible for symptoms of nerve root involvement. However, such symptoms may not appear until the third or fourth decade of life or until some apparently trivial injury to the neck occurs. Hadley has stated that this condition may be an acquired one, secondary to increased sclerosis of the base of the skull which may occur in Padget's disease. The upward migration of the cervical spine into the skull may place traction upon the cervical nerves (Fig. 68).

Ossification of the inferolateral margin of the posterior atlanto-occipital membrane forms an arch over the vertebral artery and the first cervical nerve root as they pass through the posterior atlanto-occipital membrane as shown in Figure 69. These bony arches are found usually on both sides of the posterior arch of the atlas and they may be an actual protection to the vertebral arteries and the nerve roots. However, following injuries to the upper part of the cervical spine, adhesions may form between the artery, the first nerve root, and the bony arch or canal through which they pass.

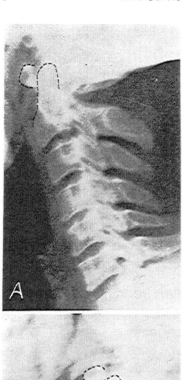

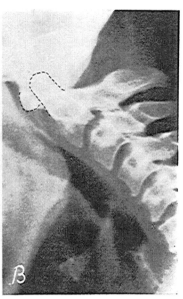

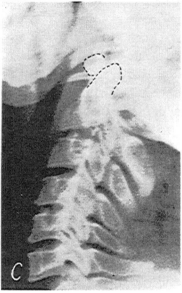

Figure 68. Basilar impression. Note that the posterior arch of the atlas remains within the posterior fossa of the skull in all positions. The flatness of the occiput is characteristic. This patient had severe occipital headaches following a whiplash injury. Symptoms were relieved by motorized intermittent traction.

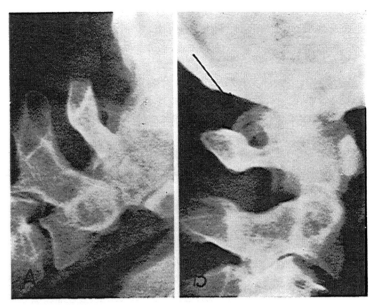

Figure 69. Congenital anomalies of the atlas. Note the bony arches over the vertebral arteries and the first cervical nerve roots. This anomaly is due to calcification of the lateral portion of the posterior atlanto-occipital ligament or membrane.

Other anomalies which may be of significance are shown in Figure 70.

Cervical ribs may, in some instances, be responsible for compression of the adjacent peripheral nerves, but they cannot cause nerve root irritation, of course.

Other Factors

There are many other factors responsible for symptoms of nerve root irritation which are worthy of mention.

Abnormal laxness of joint structures resulting from a general debilitating condition or a long illness often results in subluxations to cause foraminal narrowing. Certain somatic types, having a generalized laxness of all joint structures, may be prone to episodes of radicular symptoms.

Emotional stress, physical and mental fatigue may cause "nervous tension" and anxiety to aggravate an otherwise quiescent cervical syndrome. It has been said that fear or fright may cause the neck muscles to go into spasm. This is a far-fetched conclusion. Fear or fright cause the adrenal glands to secrete adrenalin into the blood stream where it is distributed to all parts of the body. It does not select the neck muscles only to produce spasm. The dog and cat when frightened arch their backs in preparation for *combat*.

If emotional stress does result in spasm of the muscles of the spine, once the stress has been eliminated the muscles return to their usual state. It is difficult to conceive a chronic emotional state which might produce constant and persistent muscle spasm, other than catatonia.

Patients who suffer joint disorders are reputed to be good barometers. Although this has been categorized as "an old wives tale," Hollander and his coworkers have shown that changes in weather do have a direct effect upon joint disorders, so that such changes which cause increased swelling of joint structures may be responsible for pressure upon the adjacent nerve roots to activate symptoms.

In order to complete the etiological picture, one must mention the word idiopathic, which is the term used by defeatists to signify "I don't know the cause." In many instances, there may be no immediate demonstrable etiology. However, if one searches diligently for the cause of any painful or abnormal condition, the answer can be found usually.

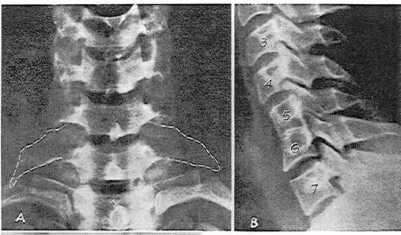

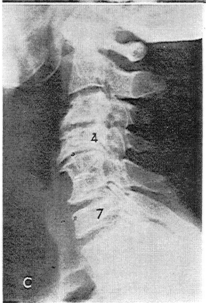

Figure 70. Other congenital anomalies in the cervical spine. A: Bilateral cervical ribs. B: Block vetebra, thought to be congenital. C: Block vertebra with marked degenerative changes above at C3 and C4.

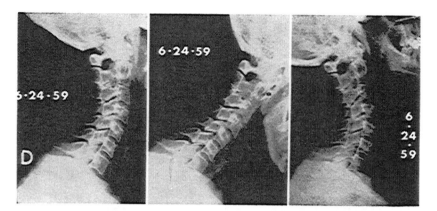

Figure 70D through H. D: Enlarged posterior tubercle of posterior arch of atlas with no motion between C2 and C3 and between C1 and C2. E and F: Block vertebra at C2 and C3 and between C7 and T1 and marked degenerative changes between C7 and C6. Note abnormalities of this patient's cervical spine in the AP view (F) and fusion of two ribs on the left side. G: Block vertebra at C2 and C3 with an unusually large intervertebral foramen. H: Underdevelopment of C5. It is interesting to note that none of these patients had any symptoms referable to their cervical spines until injuries had been imposed on them.

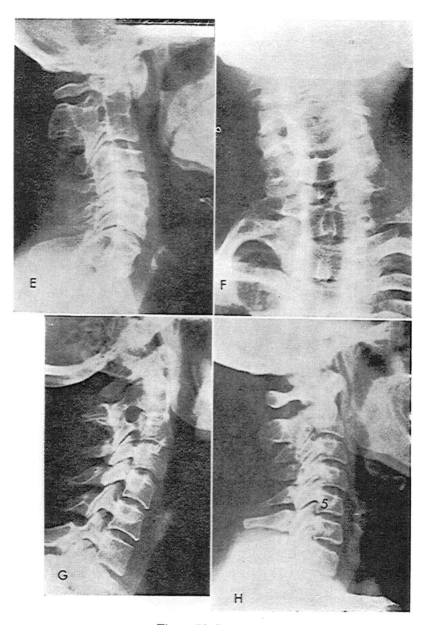

Figure 70 *Continued*

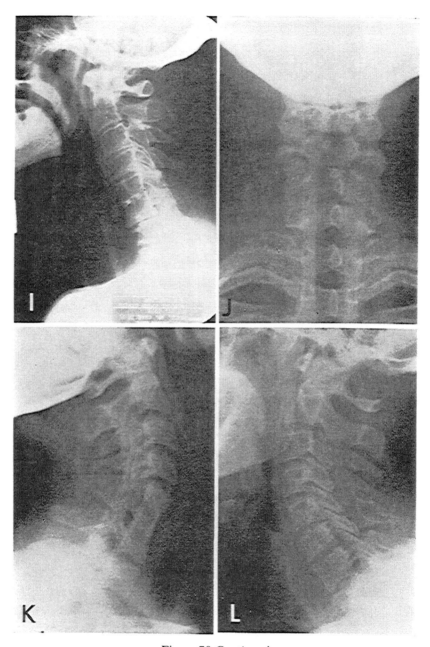

Figure 70 *Continued*

←᷂

Figure 70I. This patient, age 77, had no neck problems until his car was hit in the rear, following which he had symptoms referable to his neck. Note the narrowed discs and fusion of C5 and C6 and the forward subluxation of C6 on C7. Flexion and hyperextension views show the same amount of forward displacement. Oblique views show fusion of C5 and C6 facets on the left side and normal facets at C6 and C7. On the right side the facets at C6 and C7 are irregular and they are placed in a transverse plane. There is certainly a forward slipping of C6 on C7, but this is not the result of developmental failure of fusion of the neural arch with the pedicle. One cannot be certain that the changes at C6 and C7 are the result of congenital abnormalities. Certainly the narrowed intervertebral discs are not congenital. There are indications, however, that the forward slipping at C6 and C7 was of long standing, and in all probability the result of an unrecalled remote injury.

Figure 70J and K. Patient, age 24, had no neck symptoms until age 14 when injured in a car accident. Second injury, at age 20, occurred when a truck mat fell on her head and neck. Chief complaints were headaches and loss of balance when she put her head backward and to the left, plus numbness of the left long finger. Note marked backward subluxation of C4 on the congenitally fused C5 and C6. In the AP view note the cervical ribs. Is the fusion at C6 and C7 congenital or is it the result of the injury at age 14?

Figure 70L. Patient, age 38. Note fusion of the spinous processes of C5 and C6. This patient was involved in a severe car accident at age 22. Is this anomaly congenital or traumatic?

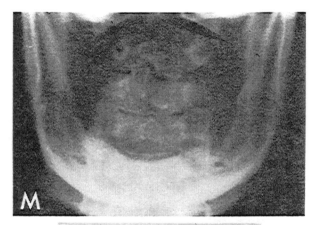

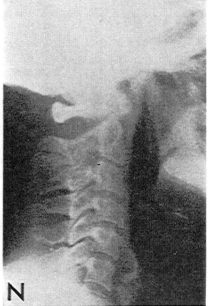

Figure 70M. Patient, age 37. Note anomalies of the spinous processes of C2 in the AP and lateral radiographs and the narrowed disc at C2 and C3 N. Patient had no symptoms until after a car accident.

Chapter 5

THE STRUCTURAL CHANGES INDUCED BY TRAUMA

TRAUMA

TRAUMA INFLICTED on the tissues of the body indicates an injury. Injury means to hurt. To hurt implies physical pain or mental pain, or both physical and mental pain. Traumatic experiences may involve local tissues with harmful effects upon the adjacent structures and upon the patient as a whole affecting his total personality. Multiple factors enter into each individual's response to injury or to trauma, and these include the physical as well as the psychic reactions. The age and sex of the individual, the nature of the injury, the circumstances of the injury, the vulnerability of the uninjured adjacent structures to the penalties of impaired function, the possible resulting disability after healing has occurred, the individual's pretraumatic personality and his tolerance for pain, the element of anxiety or emotional response to injury, the occupation of the individual, the financial and social status of the individual and the medicolegal involvement which is ever present in this era of increased insurance coverage—all of these factors are of importance in the final analysis of the eventual results of traumatic experiences.

Biochemical studies have enlightened the problems we encounter in the treatment of patients who have been injured mechanically, as well explained by Rhoads and Howard in their book *Chemistry of Trauma*. The patient has been injured and will continue to be injured until the components of the injury have been identified and resolved. Injury and the body's response to it may continue for days, weeks, months and even years.

The injury involves the entire body, not just the one or more sites of injury. The response to injury involves every system, every organ and every cell of the body. During the initial stage of healing, exudative fluid brings leukocytes, histiocytes and macrophages into the injured area which, with the assistance of proteolytic en-

139

zymes, remove or dissolve the injured tissues at the site of the injury. Two or three days later fibroblasts appear and by the sixth day fibroplasia has become extensive and later results in scar tissue which contracts and decreases the capillaries and interstitial fluid.

Mucopolysaccharides, which contain hexosamine, appear in involved tissues as early as six hours after injury. The amino acid hydroxypyroline appears in the injured tissues some four to six hours after injury and is found in the collagen, which accounts for the restoration of the tensile strength of the tissues. Tissue deficiency in ascorbic acid prevents the formation of hydroxyproline, and it has been shown that following injury there is a decrease in the plasma vitamin C and in urinary excretion. Loading the patient with vitamin C following injury results in its retention and, it is believed, aids the healing process.

The healing of bone is similar to the healing of soft tissue injury. Urist has shown that collagen develops in bone to a greater degree than in other tissues of the body and that bone repairs itself completely and flawlessly with time, which is not true of soft tissue injuries.

Rhoads and Howard have shown that every system of the body is affected by trauma and that the adrenal cortical response results in a decrease in permeability of vascular structures in the injured tissues and lessens the inflammatory reaction and produces hyperglycemia resembling a diabetic type glucose tolerance curve following injury, as well as glycosuria. It increases the breakdown of tissue protein to amino acids and provides extra energy when needed. It is provided by the response to injury, but it should not be administered unless there is a deficiency. A normal adrenal function is an essential part of traumatic defense.

Renal response to injury is the retention of water which may be due to vasoconstriction resulting in the decreased blood flow and glomerular filtration. Increased posterior pituitary function causes an increased absorption of water by the renal tubules. Sodium is retained by the kidneys, but the plasma level may drop. Renal excretion of potassium in large quantities follows injury. Calcium and magnesium metabolism may be altered. Alteration in carbohydrate and protein metabolism and also lipid metabolism occur to some extent.

Gastrointestinal, pancreatic, hepatic and thyroid functions are all affected by trauma, much of which is undoubtedly the response of the adrenal cortical system to unexpected injury, as well as by the emotional disturbances which are always present following injuries of minor or maximal magnitude in most individuals. Especially in collisions of automobiles, the passengers are usually angry and afraid; anger and fear, of course, stimulate the adrenal cortical system to give rise to various responses.

Physical characteristics influence the body's response to injury and the personality influences the emotional reaction. McLaughlin states that the body and soul are one and that the soul is reflected in a personality which responds to a traumatic experience fully as much as the physical unit. The emotional electrolytes, which he describes as fear, hope, triumph, ambitions, defeat and frustrations, must be maintained in balance for the preservation of pride, dignity and self-respect—just as physical electrolytes must be in balance for proper healing of tissue injuries. An unstable balance may be disturbed profoundly by an insignificant injury, whereas a mature and stable personality may take the consequences of a serious injury in stride.

Disturbances of emotional equilibrium following a traumatic experience are manifested often by somatic symptoms and findings which are lacking recognizable organic basis. However, emotional disturbances may give rise to physiological and symptomatic reactions which may be as consistent as those which accompany disturbances in fluid and electrolyte balance. The psychic factor is anxiety—a powerful force which may be equally as disabling as a severe physical handicap.

Injuries of the musculoskeletal system which result in pain and impaired function have an effect on the psyche of the individual and the resulting disability or impairment may be out of proportion to the severity of the injury and to the resulting physical handicap. To label any condition which cannot be explained easily as *psychoneurosis* is indicative of diagnostic poverty and infers that those symptoms and signs which cannot be explained readily do not exist.

The changes in the structures of the cervical spine which occur as a result of trauma must be understood if one is to interpret the resulting syndromes of cervical spine disorders and if one is to prognosticate concerning the eventuality of such conditions. One must be familiar with the changes which occur in synovial joints, the fibrocartilaginous disc joints and the osseous structures, as well as the ligamentous, capsular, vascular, muscular and neural structures. Pain pathways, although there is much controversy concerning them, should be studied by all who attempt to treat pain syndromes.

INFLAMMATION

Trauma imposed on living tissues results in an inflammatory reaction. For many years, the concept of tissue reaction has been that a traumatic insult or irritation of tissues causes arteriolar dilitation, which may be preceded by momentary vasoconstriction. This is followed by an increased rate of blood flow, then capillary dilitation and increased permeability, exudation of fluid, packing of red cells within the capillaries to give rise to slowing of or stasis in the blood flow, pavementing of white cells in the capillaries and exudation of these cells into the area. Certain substances are liberated at the site of injury which have the capacity to increase the permeability of blood vessels. The discovery of such mediators as serotonin, histamine and bradykinin have helped to enlighten the problem of vascular leakage which may continue for days, weeks and months. However, these substances exert their effect for only short periods of time, perhaps from thirty minutes to one hour.

The recent work of Majno, Palade and their researchers has unveiled some startling findings concerning what takes place in the fine vessels as a result of trauma. They have shown, contrary to former beliefs, that leakage does not occur in the capillaries but that it occurs on the venous side of the vascular tree. Only venules of a strictly circumscribed range of diameters are subject to leakage, and such leakage occurs through tiny gaps between contiguous endothelial cells which have been induced by the mediators of inflammation, such as serotonin prostoglandins. The duration of the leakage is not dependent on the direct response to injury or on the agent responsible for the inflammatory focus.

These changes may occur at varying rates of speed and the inflammation may be of short duration or it may persist for months or years. The eventual outcome is a reparative response. Some inflammations are resolved with relatively perfect repair, but more often injury results in scarring which is the usual residual of tissue damage. With continued chronic inflammation there is hyperplasia of the inflamed tissues. This is true of the ligamentous and capsular structures of the cervical spine, which are found to be thickened frequently at the time of surgical explorations and in anatomic dissections.

This analysis of the current knowledge of inflammatory responses explains many of the problems with which we are confronted in our study of cervical spine disorders.

THE LIGAMENTS AND THE CAPSULES

The ligamentous and capsular structures of the joints have elasticity to provide certain ranges of motion, and they have tensile strength to resist deforming forces. If they are subjected to a deforming force beyond their functional capacity, they do not regain their original length when the deforming force is removed. If the deforming force or stress is removed before the ligaments rupture, some recoil is possible, but they never regain their original size or shape. If rotary forces are applied, tautness of the ligaments is greater on the side of the applied force, and the ligaments are relaxed on the opposite side, so that the taut ligaments receive the deforming forces. The breaking load may be minimal depending on the position of the joint and the amount of rotation.

However, we must keep in mind that there is a difference between usual and maximal joint movement. Movement may be forced beyond the usual range without damage to the ligaments, but there is a greater risk of ligamentous rupture by a force applied when a joint is near its maximal range of motion than by a greater force when the joint is near its midposition.

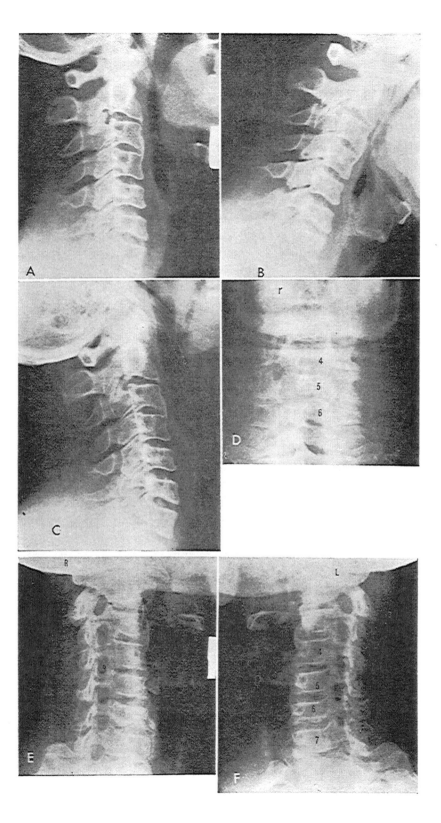

When a ligament has been sprained (torn or avulsed from its attachment to bone), an inflammatory reaction occurs. Many factors will influence the extent and duration of the inflammation and hence the resulting functional impairment. Repair of injured capsular and ligamentous tissues is slow, probably because of the meager blood supply to these structures. The usual time for repair is six to eight weeks under ideal circumstances following surgical repair or fixation, as shown by Clayton and Weir.

Healing occurs by the formation of scar tissue, which is less elastic and less functional than normal ligamentous tissue. If the inflammatory reaction persists, hyperplasia or thickening of the tissues occurs, which further decreases their elasticity and tensile properties, and, therefore, the range of joint movement.

Immobilization of joints or functional inactivity results in stasis of circulation and is a common cause of posttraumatic joint stiffness. A small amount of movement in injured joints, rather than complete immobilization, reduces the inflammation by mobilizing or dispersing the tissue breakdown products from the site of injury and prevents to some extent fibrous arthrosis.

Fibrous ankylosis may occur following trauma of the ligamentous structures and such immobilization of joints may lead to actual bony ankylosis, as shown in Figure 71.

In the cervical joints, pain may be caused by the inflammatory

---

← ◂

Figure 71. Nature's response to injury of joint structures. Lateral radiographs are shown with the neck straight in A, with forward bending in B and with backward bending in C. Note that there is no motion between C2 and C3 because of fibrous ankylosis and there is none between C3 and C4 because of bony ankylosis at the anterior margins of these vertebrae. An anteroposterior view is shown in D and on the left side there are osteophytic formations at the posterior joint margins at C4 and C5 and at C5 and C6 plus marked narrowing of the interarticular isthmus of C6 on the left side. In the right oblique view (E), the intervertebral canals are of fairly normal size and contour, whereas in the left oblique view (F) there is anteroposterior narrowing of the canals at C4 and C5 and at C6 and C7 which is the result of osteophytic formations at the margins of the posterior joints at the third canal and at the lateral interbody joint margins at the fifth canal. Date of injury 6/16/49. Films made 3/27/63.

changes within the ligaments and capsules and/or by insult to the adjacent nerve roots.

THE SYNOVIAL MEMBRANE

The synovial lining of joints, which is concerned with secretion and absorption of synovial fluid, has a very rich blood supply and a very meager nerve supply, if it has any nerves other than those which accompany the blood vessels. The fluid which it secretes is essential for normal joint function. Injury of the synovial membrane is painless, but the inflammatory reaction resulting may cause an increased secretion of fluid, which in turn causes increased intraarticular pressure. The increased pressure causes stretching of the capsular structures with resulting pain. If the inflammatory reaction is not soon resolved, pannus may extend over the articular cartilage on the margins of the zone of attachment of the synovial lining to the articular cartilage. If the pannus persists, adhesions may form to give joint stiffness. Persistent inflammatory reactions may give rise to permanent hyperplasia of the synovial lining of joints with resulting impairment of varying degrees of joint function.

Again, the tissue breakdown products are dispersed and adhesions prevented by limited joint movement, or movement within the subpain threshold.

THE ARTICULAR CARTILAGE

The articular cartilage of the synovial joints is of the hyaline variety. Chondrocytes are distributed through an intercellular matrix which is composed of 70 percent water. The mucopolysaccharide chondroitin sulphate provides resilience of the cartilage. It varies in different joints and with the age of the patient. The cartilage is somewhat compressible. It has no nerve supply and no direct blood supply but obtains nourishment from the synovial fluid. The peripheral portions, where there is a transition from the highly vascular synovial membrane to the avascular cartilage, may be better nourished than the central areas, and it has been suggested that this might possibly influence the proliferation of cartilage cells at the margins of joints.

Injuries to articular cartilage occur when sudden or sustained pressures are applied. This results in fragmentation or fibrillation of the cartilage from pressure necrosis and leads to eventual degeneration. Excessive use of joints in the absence of specific trauma or in the absence of altered dynamics of the joints does not per se result in degeneration of articular cartilage in experimental animals, as shown by Lanier. Degenerative changes in cartilage are painless and occult and are difficult to detect until alteration in other joint structures has occurred to give rise to pain and limitation of motion.

No warning signal is experienced when articular cartilage is injured because of the absence of any nerve supply. Inasmuch as it has no blood supply it does not repair itself following injury, although fibrous tissue cells may bridge a gap or crack in the cartilage or a fibrocartilage may fill the defect partially.

Once the articular cartilage has been injured, the joint is on its way to degeneration. It may function well and painlessly until the degenerative processes of the joint structures have reached a certain stage or until some other traumatic insult is imposed upon them.

THE MUSCLES

The muscles, which reinforce the ligamentous and capsular structures and which are responsible for joint movements, are rarely injured except by direct trauma. The short muscles and those with attachments to the bony processes which they span are more susceptible to tearing than are the long muscles which do not have multiple attachments as they span several joints.

The short suboccipital muscles and the intertransverse muscles are vulnerable to the traumatic effects of acceleration and deceleration forces, especially if the head and neck are rotated and bent laterally. However, any of the neck muscles may suffer injury of some degree. Over-stretching of the muscles causes pain and spasm which may subside fairly promptly or which may persist, depending on the severity of the injury and the duration of the resulting inflammatory response.

Forces which compel joint motion beyond the usual range give rise to reflex contraction of the antagonist muscles to protect the joint. The nerve supply of joints is derived from the same nerves that supply the muscles which move the joints, as shown by Hilton in 1863. Therefore, inflammation within the ligamentous and capsular structures which gives rise to pain may involve reflexly the area muscles to produce muscle spasm and splinting of the injured joints.

Irritation of the nerve roots gives rise to muscle spasm along the segmental distribution of the nerve roots. If the spasm is not resolved promptly, ischemic changes occur with resulting fibrosis and permanent impairment of variable degree. This may occur in muscles subjected to direct trauma where the vasospasm and ischemia initiated by trauma may be severe.

THE BLOOD VESSELS

Trauma is one of the most potent factors, if not the most potent factor, in the production and spread of vasospasm. The vasospasm may be transitory or it may be persistent. One cannot be certain of the exact mechanism involved. Direct trauma to an artery can and does cause vasoconstriction. On the other hand, exposure of arteries in the extremities where ischemia has developed following fractures has often revealed no evidence of actual trauma of the arteries, yet extensive vasoconstriction has been present. One can postulate that the products of the inflammatory response in the adjacent tissues may initiate the vasospasm. On the other hand, the lack of certain enzymatic products in the traumatized area may be responsible for the irritation of the sympathetic nerve supply of the vessels and for the spread of the constriction far beyond the area of trauma.

The vertebral arteries and their spinal branches are vulnerable to direct injury, especially in the upper portion of the cervical spine. The forceful movements of the joints beyond their usual range may traumatize the vertebral arteries and their sympathetic nerve supply. If the vasoconstriction persists, as it may well do, permanent narrowing and complete constriction of the arteries may result. Symptoms of vascular insufficiency of the posterior portion of the brain are not unusual following trauma to the neck.

Intimal damage may give rise to the formation of sclerotic changes within the arteries to cause luminal narrowing. Vascular insufficiency of the spinal cord may result from vasoconstriction or narrowing of the anterior and posterior spinal arteries, which are cranial branches of the vertebral arteries, or from involvement of the lateral spinal branches of the vertebral arteries.

The vertebral arteries may be compressed by osteophytic processes at the lateral and anterior margins of the lateral interbody joints. Inasmuch as these osteophytic changes occur gradually over a long period of time, the arteries may escape complete compression except during positional changes of the head and neck. Certain positions of the neck may cause complete blocking of one or both vertebral arteries, which has been demonstrated repeatedly by angiography.

Obstruction of the vertebral arteries does not usually cause fibrosis of the cervical muscles because there is a rich anastomosis of the muscular branches with the deep and ascending cervical arteries and with the descending branches of the occipital arteries.

The vertebral veins may be injured when trauma is imposed upon the cervical portion of the spine. Each vertebral vein begins between the skull and the atlas by the union of off-sets from the internal vertebral plexuses as they issue from the vertebral canal. In the transverse foramina, the vertebral arteries are surrounded by plexuses of venous channels. At the lower part of the neck, efferent branches from the venous plexuses unite to form a single trunk on either side which exists from the foramen in the transverse process of the sixth cervical vertebra and descends to end in the back of the upper part of the innominate vein. Injury of the venous plexuses within the transverse foramina may be of little significance, whereas injury to the vertebral veins between the transverse foramina of the sixth cervical vertebra and the innominate veins may give rise to serious venous congestion.

THE NERVES

A direct traumatic insult to the nerve roots gives rise to inflammation in the dural sleeves and perineural tissues. This may result in fibrosis. Adhesions may occur between the dural sleeves and the adjacent capsular structures. Normally, the nerve roots are free in the intervertebral canals and can be moved within a definite range of approximately one-quarter to one-half an inch. Frykholm, however, believes that the dural sleeves are normally attached to the proximate bones. This has not been found to be true in my dissections of anatomical specimens. Nerve roots that have been injured or that have been compressed by capsular thickening or bony encroachments cannot be moved within the intervertebral canals until they are freed by sharp dissection.

Nerve roots subjected to compressive forces by osteophytic encroachments show varying degrees of distortion and perineural fibrosis. Hadley has illustrated well the changes which occur within and about the nerve roots. His microphotographs leave no doubt concerning the fate of nerve roots whose canals have been narrowed.

THE SPINAL CORD

Concussion, contusion, compression and laceration of the spinal cord may result from trauma to the cervical spine. Functional impairment is transitory in many instances of concussion because this injury is the result of indirect injury to the neck. If contusion of the cord occurs, petechial hemorrhages are present. These may be localized or diffuse depending on the extent and the severity of the injury. Return of function may be complete but it is more likely to be incomplete.

Spinal cord injury without demonstrable bone injury does occur and should not be overlooked. Hemorrhagic necrosis usually involves the central gray matter and may extend into the proximate white matter, with paralytic and sensory changes resulting.

Compression of the cord by fracture fragments and by dislocations or by extruded disc material results in more extensive impairment of function in most cases, and one can anticipate less reparation (see Plate 4). Laceration of cord tissue may be caused by sharp fragments of bone. If there is not complete transection of the cord, the situation may not be completely hopeless. Some regeneration and return of function may be expected, but some deficit will remain.

The return of function in all cases is dependent on the severity and extent of the damage caused by the trauma, and on the reversibility of the changes imposed on the cord.

THE FIBROCARTILAGINOUS DISCS

The literature concerning the physiology and the pathology of the intervertebral disc is voluminous. Postulations about its behavior are numerous and varied. The work done by Keyes and Compere in 1932 showed that the loss of nucleus pulposus material constituted the basic cause for changes within the disc and the surrounding structures. This work has been verified by Rabinovitch and others.

Loss of nuclear substance from whatever cause starts a disc on its way to degeneration. If any of the confining structures of the nucleus is disrupted the nuclear material escapes into the adjacent tissues. Inasmuch as the mechanico-dynamic function of the disc joint suffers a disturbance, certain joint changes occur. The disc narrows in its vertical diameter as the annulus fibrosus bulges circumferentially. Continued movement produces strain or stress on the attachment of the annulus to the margins of the adjacent vertebrae. Cartilage cells are laid down at the periphery, just as they are at the margins of other joints. These cells become ossified and are demonstrable as spurs or lips.

The cervical spine is subjected to many traumatic experiences in childhood. Such injuries, minor though they may be, may be responsible for the beginning of disc degeneration. The changes may proceed very slowly or very rapidly, depending on the severity of the trauma and on the individual's inherent tissue response to injury. Some of the disc injuries which occur in childhood may lead to vertebral body fusion which may be interpreted as being of congenital origin.

Cervical discs are very vulnerable to trauma, but the incidence of disc extrusion is much less than in the lumbar portion of the spine. The presence of the lateral interbody joints in the cervical area, except in rare instances where they are not well developed, do give some protection to the proximate discs.

Rupture of the nucleus pulposus through the cartilaginous plate and into the body of the vertebra to form a Schmorl's node has

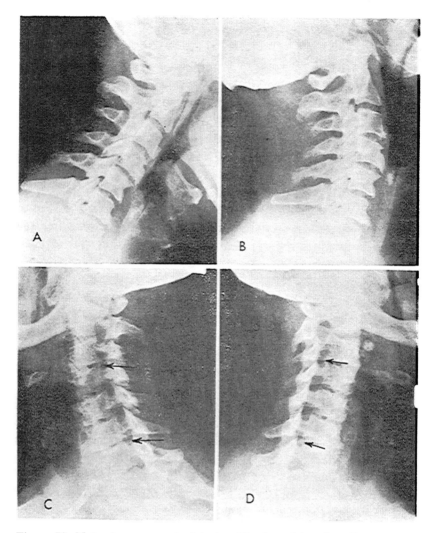

Figure 72. Nature's response to injuries. The lateral bending films (A and B) show motion at all joints. There is degeneration and narrowing of the intervertebral discs and anterior osteophytosis. However, only the intervertebral canals at C3 and C4 and at C6 and C7 are narrowed by osteophytic formations at the lateral interbody joint margins.

been noted in the cervical spine only when there has been a fracture of the vertebral body. Schmorl's nodes are found frequently in the thoracic and lumbar vertebrae. Why they are not found in the cervical vertebrae is conjecture. Perhaps the lateral interbody joints prevent fracturing forces reaching the cartilaginous plates, or perhaps the size of the discs and the fact that they do not extend to the posterolateral margins of the vertebrae may provide some protective factors for the plates.

Once a cervical disc loses its nucleus, joint function is altered and greater forces are applied to the lateral interbody joints by the usual movements of the neck. In most instances, the lateral interbody joints take the brunt of the disturbance and, if they are well developed with long upward lips on the superior surface of the vertebral bodies, narrowing of the intervening disc may be minimal, but the osteophytic changes at the margins of these joints may be extensive (Fig. 72). However, in other instances we find marked osteoproliferative changes at the anterior and anterolateral vertebral margins, with little evidence of lateral interbody joint involvement.

Although we do not know all the factors involved in disc degeneration, we can be certain that a traumatized disc will show certain changes within it which influence the adjacent structures. These changes are said to be degenerative in nature, whereas they actually represent nature's attempt to repair the disturbance in the tissues caused by trauma, and are the result of functional adaption.

OSTEOPHYTOSIS

Bick has supplied the most acceptable explanation of the changes which occur at the margins of joints or at the attachment of the ligamentous and capsular structures to bone. Ligaments and capsules are most frequently injured–sprained or avulsed–at their bony attachments. The inflammatory reaction and the disturbance in the mechanico-dynamics of the involved joint or joints give rise to the formation of cartilage cells at the periphery. The cartilage cells become ossified later to give rise to the bony spurs, as stated previously (Figs. 73 and 74). These changes, when seen

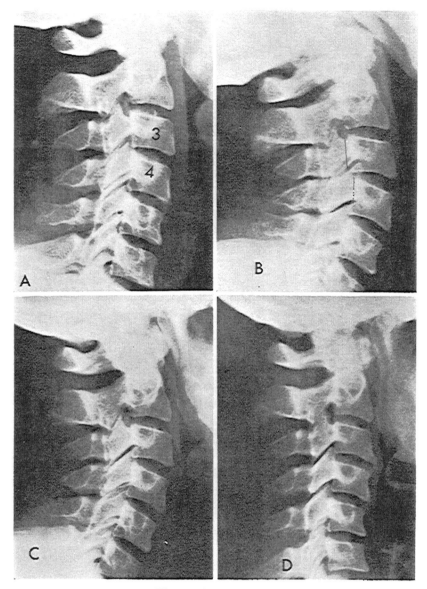

Figure 73A, B, C, & D

in radiographs, are called osteoarthritis, proliferative arthritis, de-generative arthritis or aging of joints (see Figure 104 A-D). They are, however, the result of trauma–either single or repeated–and they are indicative of joint disorder, traumatic in origin. They

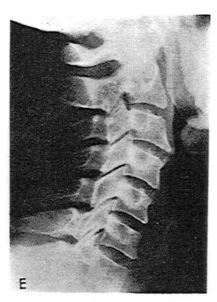

Figure 73. Nature's response to injury. This patient received a hyperextension injury of his cervical spine on 6/17/56 and the immediate post injury radiograph revealed no hint as to the location of the injury, as shown in A. Six months later the lateral view made with the neck in hyperextension showed marked instability at C3 and C4 as shown in B. Two months later the straight lateral view (C) showed restoration of the forward curve but slight posterior subluxation of C3 on C4, and beginning osteophytic changes at the adjacent anterior margins of these vertebrae. Sixteen months later a forward bending lateral film (D) showed marked limitation of flexion and increased osteophytic changes at the adjacent anterior margins of C3 and C4 and some narrowing of the intervening disc (this film is rotated to the upright position). Another straight lateral film made four years later (E) shows increased osteophytic changes.

are not the result of so-called "physiologic aging," although they are found in variable degrees in the spines of elderly people and in the spines of bulls, bears, gorillas, horses and other animals.

Nontraumatic osteoarthritis may be the result of biologic, genetic and metabolic factors. These same factors may play a part in traumatic arthritis or in joints subjected to trauma, thus making differentiation virtually impossible.

The osteophytic formations per se are usually painless, unless they encroach on adjacent neural structures or unless a traumatic

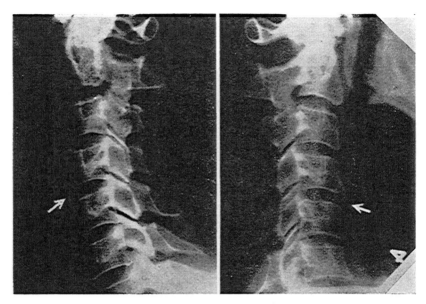

Figure 74. Nature's response to injury. Lateral view of the cervical spine of a patient who was injured in 1956 reveals no indication of the site of injury as shown in the film on the left. Four years later a lateral film shown on the right reveals that the injury involved the anterior longitudinal ligament and the development of osteophytic formation.

incident occurs to activate an inflammatory reaction within the involved ligamentous structures.

Osteophytic formations may proceed to a certain stage, and if they are not constantly activated by continued stresses and strains from excessive movement beyond the functional tolerance of the joints they may become quiescent for variable periods of time.

In the cervical spine, the most frequent site of osteophytosis is at the margins of the lateral interbody joints where the ossific formations encroach on the intervertebral canals and their contents, as well as on the vertebral arteries in many instances (Fig. 42).

These changes at the anterior margins of the secondary disc joints are next in frequency. They occur at the posterior margins of the vertebrae less often, where they may encroach on the spinal canal and cause compression of the spinal cord, depending on their extent and on the size of the spinal canal and cord.

The irregular bony nodules which are sometimes found on the

posterior aspect of the cervical vertebral bodies may be osteophytic processes which have formed at the attachment of the deep layer of the posterior longitudinal ligament following injury to the ligament, rather than extruded disc material which has migrated between the posterior longitudinal ligament and the vertebral body as suggested by Schmorl and Junghanns. The deep layer of the ligament is so firmly attached to the vertebral bodies that migration of disc tissue between it and the vertebral body is virtually impossible unless the ligament has been avulsed from the bone. However, it is possible for disc fragments to migrate between the deep layer and the superficial layer of the ligament.

The extent or size of the osteophytic process is no indication of its age nor of the severity of the traumatic experience which produced it, nor of the resulting symptoms. Each individual's response to trauma may vary. There are many factors involved and one cannot determine when, where and to what extent these changes may occur. That they will occur following trauma is inevitable as long as movement continues.

As these changes occur at the margins of the lateral interbody joints, they cause a decrease in the anteroposterior diameter of the intervertebral canals and produce pressure or compression of the structures within the canals. The nerve roots may tolerate the compressive forces inasmuch as they occur slowly over a period of time. The nerve roots, and their accompanying structures, may be forced into the bottom of the canals where they may escape from joint movements. This is especially true if there is associated narrowing of the proximate disc. As the disc narrows, the vertebral bodies approach each other to shorten the length of the cervical spine proportionately. The spinal cord does not shorten within its shortened tube–the vertebral canal–and the corresponding nerve roots may sag in proportion to the narrowing of the disc, so that they may be easily displaced into the bottom of their canals.

An acute traumatic experience superimposed on joints having marginal osteophytic changes may cause sufficient inflammatory reaction to result in increased compression of the adjacent nerve roots and so give rise to irritation of the nerve roots that had become adjusted to their already narrowed environment.

Chapter 6

SYMPTOMATOLOGY

A DETAILED ACCOUNT of the origin, duration and character of the patient's symptoms is an essential factor in the diagnosis of cervical spine disorders, of recent origin or of long standing. Obtaining an adequate history is time-consuming in many instances, but the examiner must not despair. Some seemingly insignificant symptoms are often worthwhile guideposts to diagnosis. A suggested outline for recording the historical facts is shown in Figure 75.

HISTORY

Occupation and Age of Patient

It is important to know the patient's occupation and what activities his work or his everyday living require. Work which necessitates prolonged or even intermittent hyperextension or hyperflexion or rotation of the neck may have a causal relationship in the production and prolongation of symptoms.

The age of the patient may be of some significance, inasmuch as cervical nerve root involvement with radicular symptoms is seen most frequently during the third and fourth decades of life, in spite of the fact that degenerative changes in the cervical joints may be more evident in the older age groups. One must keep in mind that disorders of the cervical spine can and do occur at any age.

Accident or Injury

Inasmuch as 90 percent of cervical spine disorders are related to injuries, it is especially important to obtain as much information as possible concerning the mechanism of the injury. Unless the patient has suffered a recent injury, it may be difficult on first interrogation to obtain a history of any traumatic experience. One must keep in mind that many types of injuries may be responsible for cervical disorders, although the patient may not associate such injuries with any symptoms referable to the cervical spine. Trauma

HISTORY OUTLINE

OCCUPATION_____AGE_____

INJURY: Date_____ Car Accident_____ Head-on_____ Rear-end_____

     Side impact_____ Other_____

     Fall_____ Where_____ How_____

     Blow_____ Head_____ Face_____ Neck_____ Back_____Other _____

     Other Mechanism_____

SYMPTOMS: Time of onset_____ Sudden_____ Gradual_____

     PAIN: Head_____ Neck_____ Shoulder_____

        Arm_____ Elbow_____ Forearm_____ Wrist_____

        Fingers_____ Chest_____ Back_____

        Character of pain: Constant_____ Intermittent_____

        Sharp_____ Dull_____ Burning_____ Other_____

        Aggravation_____. Relief_____

     STIFFNESS: Neck_____ Shoulder_____

        Elbow_____ Wrist_____ Fingers_____

     NUMBNESS: Head_____ Neck_____Face_____ Tongue_____

        Shoulder_____ Arm_____ Forearm_____ Fingers_____

        Constant_____ Intermittent_____

     WEAKNESS: Neck_____ Arm_____ Hand_____

     EYES: Blurring_____ Tearing_____ Pain_____

     EARS: Loss of balance_____ Tinnitus_____ Hearing_____

     THROAT: Dysphagia_____

     CHEST: Dyspnea_____ Pain_____

     HEART: Palpitation_____

     HEAD: Dazed_____ Unconscious_____

     OTHER:_____ Nausea_____ Vomiting_____

        Lower Back_____

        Legs_____

PROGRESS:_____ Improved_____ Worse_____

TREATMENT:_____

PAST HISTORY: All Injuries and Dates_____

_____

     Illnesses_____

     Surgery_____

     Marital_____ Children_____

     Social_____ Work Record_____

Figure 75. An outline for recording historical data.

of other parts of the body may overshadow or mask an injury of the neck. How many times have we had patients with fractures of the wrists or arms who complain of neck and suprascapular pain, for which the sling is blamed!

If the patient has had a recent injury, it is important to know when and how it occurred. A large percentage of patients has been involved in vehicular crash accidents, and one should determine the type of collision–rear-end, head-on or at the side. It is important to know the position of the patient in the car at the time of the impact. Was the patient the driver of the car or was he a passenger in the front or rear seat? Was he looking straight ahead or was his head or body turned to one side at the time of the impact? Was he thrown from the car? Did his head or any part of his body hit a stationary part of the car? The answers to these questions may give some clue concerning the severity of the injury to the neck.

Not infrequently, symptoms of injury of the cervical spine develop following a fall. It is important to know where the patient fell and how he fell. He may have fallen from a height landing on his head and neck and shoulder, or he may have fallen because his feet slipped from under him, or because he turned his ankle or because he lost his balance. He may or may not have hit his head on a stationary object as he fell. At any rate, one should determine the cause of the fall and how the patient landed.

A blow on the head, face, neck, or back from a falling object or from a swinging object, which may have been man-powered or otherwise, may have produced the injury.

There are other mechanisms of injury such as sudden pulls or thrusts on one or both arms, contact sports, diving, somersaults, or turning or jerking the head suddenly.

Symptoms

The symptoms referable to the cervical spine may have occurred immediately following an injury or the symptoms may have appeared a few hours, days or even weeks after the injury. They may have appeared suddenly or they may have come on gradually.

Pain

In most instances, the chief presenting symptom is pain of varying duration, degree, character and location. Each patient may have his own peculiar way of relating his pain image, but whatever the description it should be recorded, keeping in mind that the patient's individual constitution is therein mirrored. This may be an important clue. Well-localized areas of pain are of diagnostic significance in the diagnosis of cervical nerve root irritation, whereas generalized and ill-defined pains are not the result of nerve root irritation per se. When the patient states that he "hurts all over" a dubious attitude on the part of the examiner is justified. One must then make an attempt to have the patient localize the pain by asking specific questions.

Pain in the head, or headaches, is a frequent complaint in cervical spine disorders. The pain may be at the back of the head, the top of the head or in the temple area. The pain may be one-sided or it may involve both sides of the head.

Pain in the neck may occur at the back of the neck, at the sides of the neck or at the front of the neck. The pain may radiate into the shoulder on one or both sides or into one or both arms, from the shoulder to the fingers. The patient may complain of pain in the anterior or in the posterior portions of the chest, even in the absence of actual trauma to the chest. Pain may occur between the shoulders in the upper portion of the back, in the midportion of the back or in the lower back, which may be of radicular origin or may be the result of an actual injury to the lower back.

The character of the pain is important. It may be constant or it may be intermittent and it may be aggravated by certain movements. The pain may be sharp, a dull ache, a burning sensation or it may be described in some other manner by the patient as he relates it to some other pain experience. The patient may have found nothing which relieves his pain or he may relate that changing positions, or taking one of the usual well-advertised pain relievers or the use of heat give him some relief.

Stiffness

Following an injury, or in the absence of a recent injury, the patient may experience limitation of motion of the neck to one or both sides, or in hyperextension or flexion. Limitation of shoulder, elbow, wrist and finger motion may occur. Such limitation of motion may be the result of actual joint involvement or may be the result of nerve root irritation or of reflex dystrophy.

Tendinitis

Tendinitis of the shoulder, elbow and wrist are frequently associated with cervical spine disorders. Fibrosis of the tendon sheaths and of the palmar fascia are associated often with disorders of the cervical spine. The frequency of their occurrence leads one to postulate that there is a causal connection which may be the result of reflex dystrophy and circulatory changes or vasospasm. Swelling of the fingers is not unusual and this contributes to the stiffness of the finger joints.

Numbness

Numbness and tingling may occur anywhere along the segmental distribution of the nerve roots, without actual demonstrable hypesthesia or sensory changes. Numbness and/or tingling may be present following a recent trauma of the neck with irritation or compression of the nerve roots, or in patients who have degenerative changes in the cervical joints. The patient may awaken with numbness and tingling of one or both hands, which is often relieved by changing the position of the neck or arms. In other instances, the numbness may be constant or it may occur at any time. Numbness of the head, face and tongue indicate involvement of the posterior branches of the second and third nerve roots which make synapses with the afferent branches of the trigeminal nerves and communications with the sympathetic nerves. Numbness of the neck, shoulder, arm, forearm and fingers may be the result of irritation or compression of any of the nerve roots which supply the skin in these areas, or it may be due to circulatory embarrassment.

Weakness

Weakness of the muscles of the neck, arms, and hands may be noted by the patient. The patient may have difficulty balancing his head on his neck because of weakness of the neck muscles. He may complain of weakness of the arms and inability to work with his arms above his head. Weakness of grip is a frequent complaint and patients often drop things from one or both hands. The patient may not be cognizant of an actual weakness of the gripping muscles and he may say "things just slip from my hand"–an embarrassing situation when all the cups get broken or a skillet of hot grease lands on the floor or on the patient's feet.

Eyes

Eye symptoms are frequent following trauma to the neck and in the presence of degenerative changes about the cervical joints. Blurring of vision is a common complaint and the patient may state that he has had his eyes checked and his glasses changed without noticeable improvement. The blurring occurs intermittently and may be relieved by changing the position of the neck. Increased lacrimation may occur from time to time. Many patients describe pain in one or both eyes or pain behind the eyeballs. They may complain that the eyeballs are being pulled backward into the head or are being pushed outward. These symptoms are the result of irritation of the cervical sympathetic supply to certain eye structures via the plexuses surrounding the internal carotid arteries and their branches. The orbital muscle, which bridges the infraorbital groove and the inferior orbital fissure, contracts when the sympathetic nerves are irritated. This causes venous congestion and a sensation of protrusion of the eyeball, in all probability.

Horwick, Harry and Kasner have described eye symptoms called *asthenopia* which they believe are the result of shearing of the minute branches of the basilar artery that supply the oculomotor nucleus, to cause changes in accommodation, convergence and pupillary mechanisms.

Ears

Disturbances in equilibrium may result from irritation of the sympathetic fibers surrounding the vertebral arteries or it may be the result of vascular insufficiency. The loss of balance may be so severe that the patient is afraid to walk unassisted. There is a tendency for the patient to fall or to veer to the side of involvement. Some patients bump into door facings and others give a history of actual falls. Many times, the patients have consulted ear specialists and have been treated for Ménière's syndrome to no avail. Proper orthopaedic measures have given relief in many cases.

Ringing and roaring in the ears and transitory or partial deafness are noted by some patients. The tinnitus is the result of vascular insufficiency from the vasospasm or from actual obstruction of the vertebral or basilar supply in all probability.

Throat

Following neck trauma, it is not unusual for the patient to complain of difficulty in swallowing. This may be the result of swelling of the anterior neck structures or to cervicoglossopharyngeal irritation or to tearing of the median raphe of the pharyngeal constrictor muscles. It may be due to actual tearing of the longus colli muscles and the anterior longitudinal ligament with hemorrhage and swelling, as illustrated by Macnab in the monkey which he subjected to sudden deceleration with the head and neck free to lash backward and forward, which it did like a bouncing ball, believe me.

Other symptoms referable to the mouth and throat have been described by some patients. The craniocervical nerve connections and the sympathetic communications give us plausible explanations for some of these seemingly bizarre symptoms.

Chest

Shortness of breath, or dyspnea, may be the result of pain in some of the respiratory muscles which are supplied by the cervical nerve roots. The shortness of breath may not be accompanied by pain, and the patient simply states "I can't seem to get a deep breath."

Injuries of the chest occur often when the patient has been injured in a car accident and may be caused by the chest striking the steering wheel or steering post or by hitting some other stationary object in the car. Such complaints should be investigated thoroughly.

Heart

Palpitations of the heart, or tachycardia, may be noted by the patient when he lies down or when he assumes some unusual position or when he hyperextends his neck. Unusual heart symptoms without electrocardiographic changes do occur following acute trauma to the neck and in patients who have degenerative joint changes in the cervical spine. Irritation of the fourth nerve root which supplies the diaphragm and the pericardium, and/or irritation of the cardiac sympathetic supply, may be the cause of some of the unusual heart symptoms.

Head

Patients state often that they are dazed or addled following neck injuries, even in the absence of actual known trauma to the head. Some patients relate a short period of unconsciousness. Sometimes the head strikes a stationary portion of the car, in which event a concussion is explained easily. However, when a

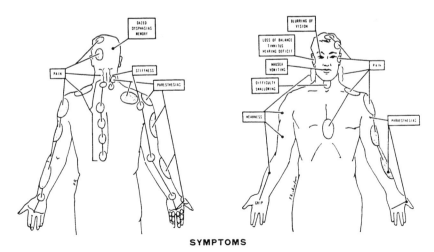

SYMPTOMS

Figure 76. Graphic illustration of the symptomatology.

neck is lashed backward and forward or forward and backward or from side to to side the brain is thrown against the inner table of the skull and a concussion may result with no evidence of external injury.

The patient may complain of dysphasias of various types. This is not unusual following acute trauma of the neck, which may be the result of an actual stretching effect on, or trauma of, the brain stem. Often the patient complains of memory disturbances. Figure 76 illustrates graphically the symptomatology.

Miscellaneous

Nausea and vomiting following acute neck injuries may occur. Pain, soreness, or stiffness of the lower back are frequent complaints. Occasionally, a patient complains of ill-defined leg pains and paresthesias. Actual injuries of the lower back of the nature of strains or sprains may occur, or the injury may involve the cartilaginous plates of the vertebral bodies. Leg pains and paresthesias in all probability are the result of irritation or compression of the spinal cord itself.

Occasionally a patient complains of "drop out" attacks, which may occur when the patient is standing or walking. These attacks come on without any warning and the patient is able to get up immediately and continue with his previous activity. The patient does not lose consciousness. Kubala and Millikan believe that the drop attack is a diagnostic symptom of intermittent vertebral-basilar arterial insufficiency. In the twenty-nine cases reported by them, they found that one-third had the attacks precipitated by certain movements of the neck, especially hyperextension. My files reveal ten patients who have had drop attacks.

Black-out sensations occur frequently following trauma and in patients who have marked osteophytic changes in the cervical spine. These sensations occur usually when the head and neck are hyperextended. Sudden, but transitory, vertebral artery insufficiency is the most plausible explanation for this symptom.

Progress

It is important to know whether or not the symptoms have improved or worsened. Some patients relate an improvement in their symptoms, following a traumatic experience, with the passage of time. Other patients, whose symptoms were mild at first, may find that the symptoms have grown worse with the passage of time.

Treatment

It is always interesting to know what treatment the patients have had. Many of them have had all the treatment modalities known to man tried upon them and many of them have had no treatment. Some have improved with treatment, some have improved without treatment and some have grown worse no matter what treatment was tried, or possibly–just possibly–because of certain treatments, as asserted by Harold Crowe, excessive ultrasound especially.

Past History

Most individuals have suffered traumatic experiences. It is very important to obtain information concerning all previous injuries, no matter what they were, as well as the approximate dates of their occurrence and the disabilities which resulted. Accidents of any type should be recorded although the patient may not recall or may not be cognizant of any injuries or symptoms following an accident.

Illnesses, surgery and hospital admissions should be a part of the past history.

Information concerning the marital status of the patient may be significant. His work record and his social and economic status may be important clues in the overall picture.

Careful interrogation of the patient may uncover valuable evidence of diagnostic significance.

Comments

When one who is not completely versed in the symptomatology of disorders of the cervical spine has completed this portion of the examination, he may have drawn the conclusion that the patient is psychoneurotic. However, to draw such a conclusion is a reflection on the examiner's diagnostic ability and not on the patient, until proven otherwise. One should not be hasty in forming an opinion at this stage, but should wait until all the data are assembled. One should never conclude that the symptoms which he cannot explain readily do not exist. Any symptom as related by the patient may be an important thread in the diagnostic pattern.

Nerve impulses in each individual pass through essentially the same relay stations to reach the cerebral cortex where they are interpreted. The individual's concept of the symptoms and his reaction to them vary tremendously, and they are dependent to a large extent on associated constitutional and emotional factors.

One must keep in mind that the symptoms of cervical nerve root irritation, or compression, and the accompanying symptoms of sympathetic and vascular involvement may present a very complex picture–a picture which requires a knowledge of the basic anatomy, kinetics, physiology and pathology of the manifold intricacies of the cervical spine in order to give it interpretive meaning.

Classification of Patients

Once the history has been taken it will be noted that the patients can be classified into one of five groups, depending upon the severity and duration of the symptoms.

In the first group will fall those patients who have had a recent neck-lash injury with no history of any previous injury or symptoms.

The second group of patients comprises those who have a so-called "crick" in the neck. The pain is excruciating and is usually localized to one side of the neck. The patient holds the head tilted away from and the chin turned toward the painful side. The neck is usually in slight flexion. A diagnosis can be made as the patient walks into the office because of the characteristic position of the head. Apparently there is unilateral subluxation, or possibly an impingement of the synovial membrane of the joint. The patient usually awakens with a "crick." He may have turned over in bed or turned his head suddenly. Sleeping in a "draft" did not cause the "crick."

The third group includes those patients who have had an injury several days, weeks or months previously. The symptoms were mild at first or were thought to be of little significance. However, as motion of the neck is continued latent symptoms develop.

The fourth group consists of patients who give a history of intermittent pain and stiffness over a period of years. These patients usually have gone from one doctor to another and have been labeled "neurotics." They have been treated for arthritis, neuritis, fibrositis, fasciitis, bursitis, migraine or pseudo-angina. Treatment has been directed to some localized area when it should have been directed to the source of the trouble–the cervical spine.

The fifth group consists of those patients who have acute exacerbations of chronic symptoms. Usually the present symptoms appear following sudden hyperextension of the neck, which may occur in the course of their usual activities, or from some unusual but apparently trivial movement of the neck. Stooping, lifting, holding the head in one position for long periods of time, reaching backward or above the head, throwing something, trying to prevent a fall or any unguarded movement of the neck may have caused the acute attack of pain and disability.

Comments

Classification of the patients according to symptomatology may be of little practical value but it is of interest from a statistical standpoint.

Inasmuch as neck injuries and liability insurance have increased markedly during the past decades and promise further increment, one might wish to categorize those patients who are covered by insurance as "medical legal" cases, and those who are not so covered as "private patients." Such grouping has little value from the standpoint of diagnosis and treatment but it may give interesting comparative data.

In some instances, a litigant may have a motive for magnifying his symptoms. However, the examiner cannot afford to conclude that the patient is mendacious because of the multiplicity of his complaints. As our knowledge of what happens to the very complex neck structures increases, we are in a better position to explain the complaints and to segregate those patients who do not have plausible injuries or symptoms from those who do have cause for concern.

Chapter 7

THE CLINICAL EXAMINATION

EXAMINATION OF THE PATIENT who has symptoms referable to the cervical spine is the second important step toward making a diagnosis. The examination should not be undertaken lightly; it should be done with consistent thoroughness, and all findings whether positive, negative or questionable should be recorded. This is true wherever the examination is done—in the hospital emergency room or in the doctor's office.

On examination it may be difficult to determine which nerve root or roots are actually irritated, inasmuch as the segmental distribution of the cervical nerves is not confined strictly to the corresponding embryologic segment.

In many instances at least one fiber of a nerve root fails to continue in that particular nerve root but descends to join the adjacent distal nerve root. For instance, one of the fourth nerve root fibers which leaves the cord at that level may actually leave the spinal canal with the fibers of the fifth nerve root (Fig. 25). If this fourth nerve root fiber is irritated within the foramen of the fifth nerve root, findings indicating involvement of the fourth nerve root may be present.

There is an overlap of the peripheral sensory distribution, also, so that no one area of skin is supplied by any one nerve root. Stimulation of the sympathetic supply adds further confusion in the exact location of the site of involvement.

In many instances more than one nerve root is irritated. If surgery is contemplated, it is important to localize the site or sites of irritation, but for conservative treatment the exact designation of a specifically irritated nerve root is not essential.

It is my belief that the fifth nerve root is irritated most frequently and that the sixth, fourth, third, second, and seventh roots are irritated in that order of frequency. Figure 77 illustrates the so-called segmental distribution of the fifth nerve root and shows that

170

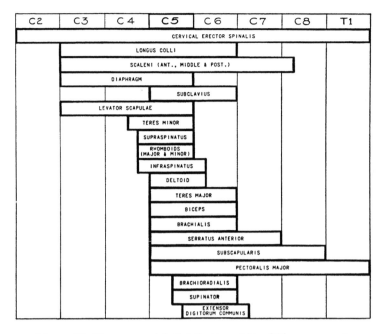

C2	C3	C4	C5	C6	C7	C8	T1

CERVICAL ERECTOR SPINALIS

LONGUS COLLI

SCALENI (ANT., MIDDLE & POST.)

DIAPHRAGM

SUBCLAVIUS

LEVATOR SCAPULAE

TERES MINOR

SUPRASPINATUS

RHOMBOIDS (MAJOR & MINOR)

INFRASPINATUS

DELTOID

TERES MAJOR

BICEPS

BRACHIALIS

SERRATUS ANTERIOR

SUBSCAPULARIS

PECTORALIS MAJOR

BRACHIORADIALIS

SUPINATOR

EXTENSOR DIGITORUM COMMUNIS

Figure 77. The segmental distribution of the fifth nerve root.

all the areas supplied by this nerve root receive innervation from at least one other nerve root.

It must be remembered that irritation or compression of a nerve root may cause pain and/or sensory changes anywhere along its distribution. Localized areas of tenderness and muscle spasm will be found at the site of the painful areas. Not infrequently, some areas of segmental tenderness are found of which the patient may not be cognizant. These myalgic areas are found by deep palpation, inasmuch as hyperalgesia or superficial tenderness is not present.

The examination form used by the author affords a simple outline of the pertinent points in the examination (Fig. 78).

POSTURE

The general posture of the patient, his movements, his facial expressions, how he sits, how he stands and how he walks should

EXAMINATION OF THE CERVICAL SPINE

Name _____ Date _____ Age _____

Posture _____ Height _____ Weight _____

Degree of Limited Motion: Right _____ Left _____

  Lateral Bending &/or Pain _____ _____

  Rotation &/or Pain _____ _____

  Flexion &/or Pain _____ _____

  Extension &/or Pain _____ _____

Shoulder Motion &/or Pain _____ _____

  Abduction _____ _____

  External Rotation _____ _____

  Internal Rotation _____ _____

  Flexion _____ _____

  Extension _____ _____

Head Compression Test:

  Lateral Bending _____ _____

  Extension _____ _____

  Flexion _____ _____

  Rotation _____ _____

Shoulder Depression Test: _____ _____

Tenderness &/or Muscle Spasm:

  Head _____ _____

  Neck _____ _____

  Scalene _____ _____

  Sternomastoid _____ _____

  Suprascapular _____ _____

  Upper Rhomboid _____ _____

  Mid Rhomboid _____ _____

  Lower Rhomboid _____ _____

  Tail of Trapezius _____ _____

  Latissimus Dorsi _____ _____

EXAMINATION (Continued)

Name _____   Date _____

Pectoral _____   _____

Tip of Shoulder _____   _____

Insertion Deltoid _____   _____

Extensors Forearm _____   _____

Other _____   _____

Radial Pulse on Elevation of Arm _____   _____

Reflexes: Biceps _____   _____

Triceps _____   _____

Brachioradialis _____   _____

Other _____   _____

Sensory Changes: Posterior Shoulder _____   _____

Outer Surface Shoulder _____   _____

Arm _____   _____

Forearm _____   _____

Hand _____   _____

Fingers _____   _____

Other _____   _____

Circumference Arms: _____   _____

Forearms _____   _____

Muscle Weakness: Shoulder _____   _____

Arms _____   _____

Forearms _____   _____

Wrist and Fingers _____   _____

Strength of Grip _____   _____

Patient Right or Left Handed _____   _____

Dilated Pupil _____   _____

Blood Pressure _____   _____

Heart _____   _____

Bruit Arteries of Neck _____   _____

Reflexes Lower Extremities _____   _____

Other Abnormal Findings _____   _____

Figure 78. A form to be used for recording the examination.

be noted. The patient who lolls in a chair and who bobs his head up and down or wags it from side to side as he talks is having little if any pain. The patient who has symptoms referable to his neck has a tendency to protect the movements of the neck. He does not loll and he does not bob or wag his head, unless, of course, he is enjoying a remission of his symptoms.

If the patient is ambulatory, the examination should be done with the patient sitting on a stool or on a straight-backed chair. The examiner should stand behind the patient to test the motion of the neck and shoulders and to palpate for painful areas and muscle spasm, and to do the head compression test and the shoulder depression test.

MOTION OF THE NECK

Motion of the cervical spine cannot be determined by simply asking the patient to move his head. The examiner should place his hands on either side of the patient's head as he stands behind him and move the head and neck passively through the ranges of motion–lateral bending, rotation, flexion and extension. The average amount of lateral bending is from the straight position to eighty degrees, although some patients may have ninety or more degrees of lateral bending. This movement can be measured with a goniometer. Limitation of lateral bending, especially if there is a difference between the two sides, is significant and should be recorded in degrees of movement or of limitation of movement.

The range of rotation in the average person is from the straight position to ninety degrees, but a few may have more rotation than that. Limitation of rotation is significant and should be recorded in degrees for accuracy. The amount of rotation can be measured by the Cervigon (Fig. 79). However, one accustomed to making these measurements can estimate the range of motion quite accurately without the aid of measuring devices.

Forward flexion and hyperextension are difficult measurements to make by any of the current devices. The average person can flex the neck forward so that the chin touches the sternum and as he does so there is a smooth backward curve of the neck which can be seen easily. If the examiner can place one finger between the chin and the sternum as the neck is flexed, flexion is limited by ten degrees; if two fingers can be placed there flexion is limited by twenty degrees; if three fingers are needed to span the distance flexion is limited by thirty degrees, and for each added finger needed add an extra ten degrees. Observation of the neck is important as these estimates are made, inasmuch as the movement in flexion may occur between the head and the upper two vertebrae and between the seventh cervical and the first thoracic vertebrae, with little or no motion occurring between the other seg-

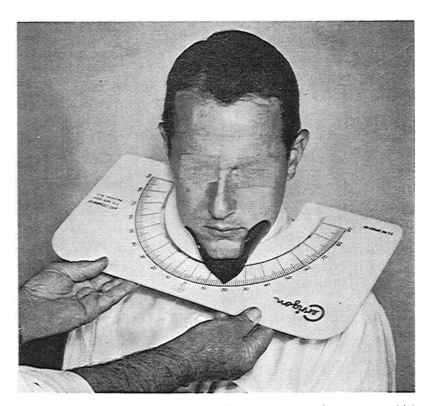

Figure 79. The Cervigon and the Cervigon MK II are instruments which are designed to measure neck motion accurately. However, it is necessary for the examiner to move the patient's head and neck through the possible range of motions in all directions rather than instruct the patient to make the movements.

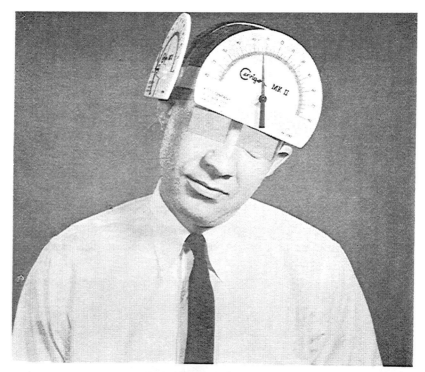

Figure 79B

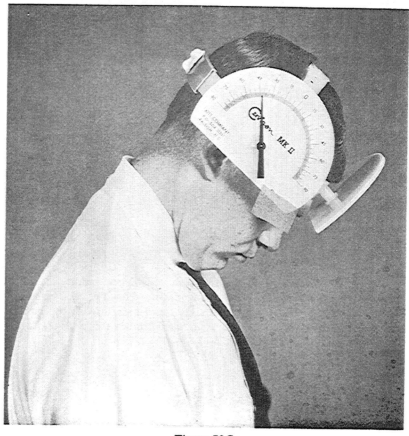

Figure 79C

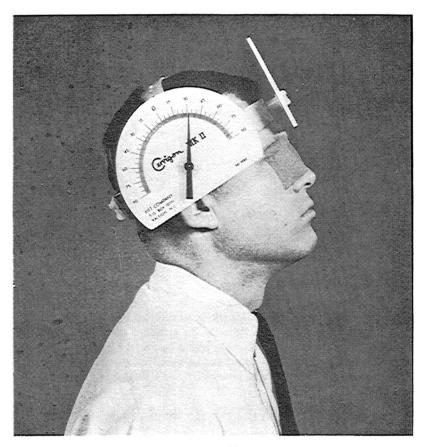

Figure 79D

ments. The location of the motion and the amount can be verified by lateral radiographs of the cervical spine made with the neck in maximum flexion.

Hyperextension of the neck is tested by placing the patient's head and neck backward. The average person can touch the base of the occiput to the spinous process of the first thoracic vertebra. Only an estimate of the range of movement is possible, unless the Cervigon MKII (Fig. 79) is used; the range should be expressed in degrees of limitation of motion as nearly as possible. The astute examiner can determine the range of hyperextension without the

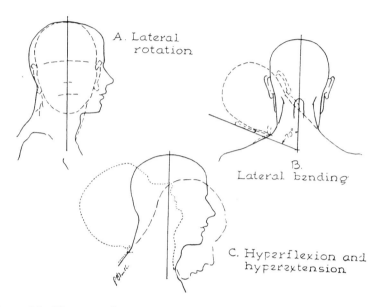

Figure 80. The normal range of neck motion. The head can be rotated laterally so that the chin is parallel with the shoulder (A). It can be bent laterally seventy to eighty degrees (B). It can be flexed forward so that the chin touches the sternal notch, and it can be bent backward so that the base of the skull touches the spinous process of C7 or T1 (C).

aid of a goniometer. If one finger can be placed between the occiput and the spinous process of T1 the limitation is ten degrees; if two fingers, twenty degrees; add ten degrees for each subsequent finger. Figure 80 shows the average range of neck motion.

All movements of the neck may be limited by pain, by muscle spasm or by a mechanical alteration in the joint and skeletal structures. If the patient is cooperative and relaxed, the motion can be ascertained easily. If he is tense and uncooperative, the testing should be repeated on several occasions. If the patient is attempting to impress the examiner with the seriousness of his injury or cervical spine disorder, he may resist movement or he may make jerking movements of the neck as the examiner attempts to move the neck.

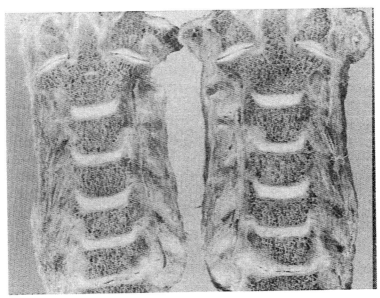

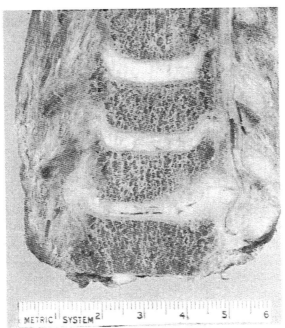

Plate 1. Median section of a cervical spine which shows no clefts in the discs except at C6-7, where the disc is definitely degenerated, is seen in the upper figure. The lower three discs are seen in the lower figure, which is an enlarged photograph of the same specimen.

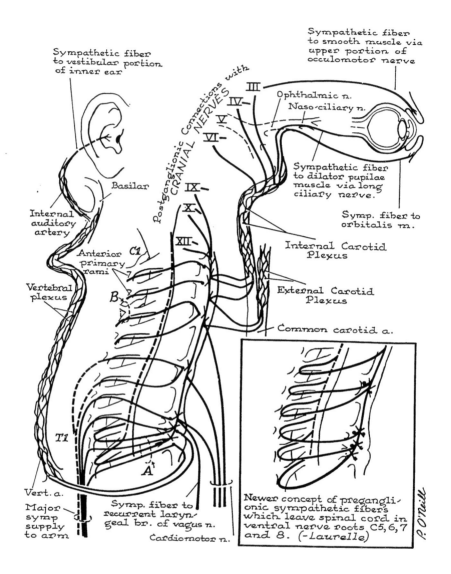

Plate 2. The cervical sympathetics. Preganglionic fibers — green. Postganglionic fibers — red. Interruption of preganglionic fibers at A will give paralysis of the cervical sympathetic supply. Irritation at B may cause reflex stimulation of the cervical sympathetics. Insert illustrates the more recent concept — that sympathetic cell bodies are present in the cervical cord from C4 through C8, and preganglionic fibers leave the cord in nerve roots C5 through T1.

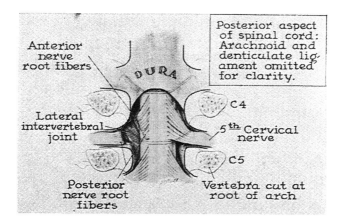

Plate 3-1. The "safety" zone for the nerve roots. The nerve roots do not pass over the intervertebral discs. The ventral fibers rest upon the lateral interbody joints, as they make their exit from the spinal canal to enter the intervertebral canals. The body of the corresponding vertebra is their protection from extruded disc material.

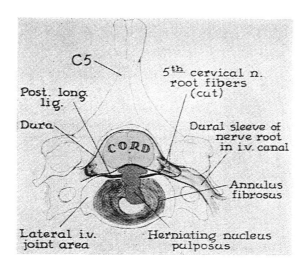

Plate 3-2. Posterior rupture of a cervical disc. The cervical nerve roots are protected by the bodies of the vertebrae, and a posterior herniation will result in cord compression rather than nerve root compression.

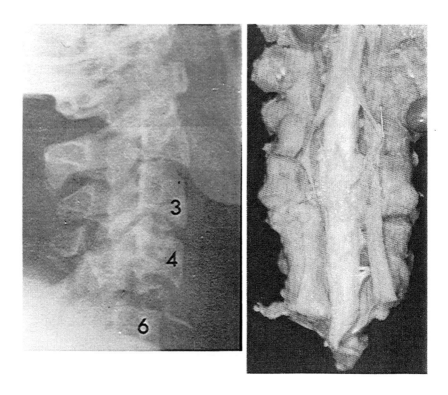

Plate 4. The lateral radiograph shows a severe fracture dislocation of C5 and multiple fractures of the posterior elements. Patient was quadraplegic but lived six months after the injury. Autopsy specimen shows marked crushing of the spinal cord and avulsion of the adjacent nerve roots.

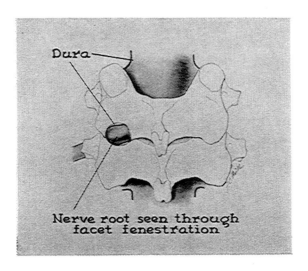

Plate 5. Facet fenestration to relieve nerve root compression. This is the simplest operation for decompression of a cervical nerve root. A laminectomy is not necessary unless there are indications of cord compression.

THE HEAD COMPRESSION TEST

This test can be done conveniently at this stage of the examination. Application of pressure to the top of the head with the head tilted to either side and with the head tilted backward and forward may cause increased pain in the neck or it may increase or cause referred pain. If the pain is confined to the neck, injury or disorder of the cervical joints is indicated. If radicular pain occurs, nerve root irritation is present.

THE SHOULDER DEPRESSION TEST

This test may be done while the examiner is standing behind the patient, as illustrated in Figure 81. With the patient's head tilted to one side, downward pressure is applied to the opposite shoulder. If this test increases the radicular pain, it indicates that there is irritation or compression of the nerve roots, that there are adhesions about the dural sleeves of the nerve roots and the adjacent joint capsules or that foraminal encroachments are present. This test places a tug on the nerve roots and if there are adhesions or osteophytic changes, radicular pain is produced.

SHOULDER MOTION

Motion of the shoulders can be tested easily while the examiner is behind the patient by raising the arms above the head of the patient, then lowering them to ninety degrees with the elbows flexed at right angles and then rotating the arms internally and externally. One should note any difference in the motion of the two shoulders and the presence of pain as expressed by the patient. If motion is tested in both shoulder joints at the same time the patient is less likely to resist the movements.

DEEP TENDERNESS AND MUSCLE SPASM

Areas of deep tenderness are well localized over the involved joints and at the sites of referred pain resulting from irritation or compression of the cervical nerve roots. The most frequent sites of deep tenderness are found over the posterior joints of the neck, over the spinous processes and the interspinous ligament, in the

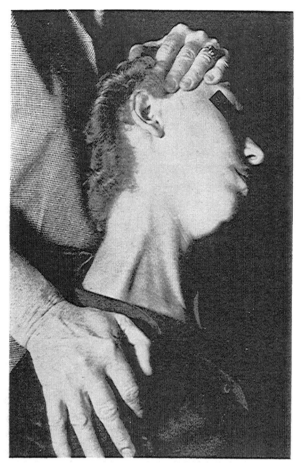

Figure 81. The shoulder depression test. If this maneuver causes a reproduction or aggravation of radicular pain, it indicates adhesions about the
dural sleeves of the nerve roots and the adjacent capsular structures, or
foraminal spurs over which the nerve root is moved or stretched.

suboccipital muscles, in the suprascapular muscles, in the rhomboid muscles between the vertebral border of the scapula and the
thoracic spine, at the superomedial angle of the scapula, in the
tail of the trapezius muscle, at the tip of the shoulder, at the insertion of the deltoid muscle and in the extensor muscles of the forearm. The areas of deep tenderness are found usually on one side,

but they may be present on both sides. Localized muscle spasm is present at the sites of deep tenderness.

Spasm or contraction of muscles, either localized or general, can be seen in some instances and can always be felt by palpation. The lateral and the anterior neck muscles, the suboccipital muscles, the suprascapular muscles, the rhomboid muscles and the lower portions of the trapezius muscles are the most likely areas where one finds muscle spasm. Muscle spasm may be the result of injury to the muscles themselves, to involuntary splinting of injured or painful joints and skeletal structures, or to irritation or compression of the cervical nerve roots or of the spinal cord.

Muscle spasm which is caused by cervical nerve root irritation may not be accompanied by pain always, but pain which is caused by irritation of the nerve roots is always accompanied by muscle spasm, which may involve an entire muscle, groups of muscles or only localized areas within the muscles.

Pain which is reflexly referred from visceral and somatic structures having cervical nerve root innervation is not accompanied by deep tenderness and muscle spasm.

REFLEX AND SENSORY CHANGES

In the presence of irritation of the cervical nerve roots, the reflexes in the upper extremities may be altered. In some instances, the reflexes may be hyperactive immediately following an injury of the neck. After a few days they become hypoactive, provided there is no involvement of the spinal cord.

The biceps is decreased or absent more frequently than the others, although the triceps and the brachioradialis reflexes may be decreased or absent, depending on the nerve roots involved or depending on the transference of impulses contralaterally or to impulses extending upward or downward within the spinal cord. The reflex changes may be transient or permanent, or they may show variations from time to time.

Sensory changes may be found anywhere along the distribution of the cervical nerve roots. Soon after an injury the changes may be manifested by hyperesthesia, but within a short time areas of hypesthesia are found. The most frequent sites of hypesthesia are

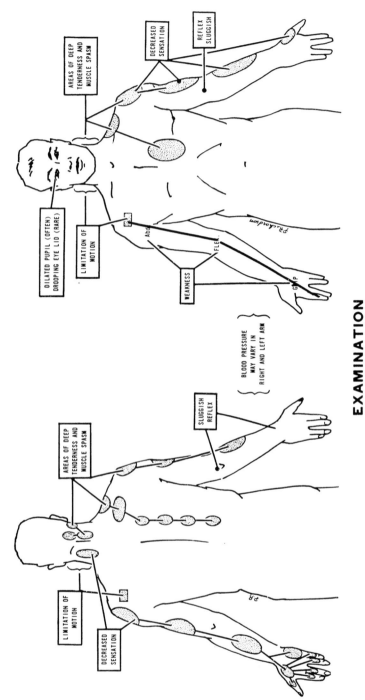

EXAMINATION

Figure 82. A graphic illustration of the clinical findings.

confined to the posterior aspect of the shoulder or the lateral aspect of the shoulder, the dorsal surface of the arm, forearm and hand, and over the thumb, index and long fingers. The little and ring fingers show decreased sensation less frequently.

The inherent overlapping of the sensory nerve supply to the skin may mask any definite sensory deficit. The sensory deficit may vary from time to time depending on the irritative factors, and the areas of sensory changes may shift from the dorsal aspect of the arm and forearm to the volar surfaces. Figure 82 illustrates the favored sites of sensory changes.

MUSCLE WEAKNESS AND ATROPHY

The routine test for muscle strength should be made. The muscles of the shoulder girdles, the arms, and the hands are supplied by two or more nerve roots which may make weakness difficult to detect in most instances. The amount of weakness may vary from day to day or from week to week, depending on the extent of nerve root irritation and on the portion of the nerve root or roots subjected to irritation.

Weakness of the gripping muscles is a frequent finding, and this weakness is best detected by the use of a dynamometer. To avoid possible error, it is wise to have the patient squeeze the instrument at least four times. The total sum of the four readings should be divided by four to obtain the average grip. The readings may be essentially the same on the four tests, but in some instances the gripping muscles fatigue easily and there may be a great discrepancy between the first and fourth readings. Patients are for the most part very cooperative in the execution of this test and it should be considered an objective finding.

The circumference of the midportion of the arms and of the forearms just distal to the elbows should be recorded at each examination. A difference in the circumference of the two arms of one-eighth to one-fourth of an inch is not unusual–the dominate extremity being the larger. In the presence of nerve root involvement, or of spinal cord involvement, confined to one side, atrophy of the muscles of the arm and/or of the forearm may develop within a period of two or three weeks. Again, the atrophy may vary from month to month, depending on the extent and duration of the nerve root involvement. Atrophy of the muscles of one extremity may result from lack of use instigated by pain or by voluntary disuse.

In some instances there may be visible atrophy of the intrinsic muscles of the hand.

THE EYES

The size of the pupils of the eyes should be checked always. It is not unusual to find dilitation of the one pupil, which indicates irritation of the sympathetic nerve supply in the neck which controls the pupillary muscles by way of the sympathetic fibers surrounding the internal carotid arteries and their branches to the eye. It may be the result of involvement of the third cranial nerve or of the midbrain. This does not represent a Horner's syndrome which results from complete interruption or paralysis of the sympathetic fibers and which causes constriction of the pupil on the side of involvement and a visible drooping of the upper eyelid as well as vasomotor changes.

A complete examination of the eyes may be indicated in many instances. The pupillary changes come and go usually and are seldom constant. Therefore, changing the lenses in the patient's spectacles does not solve the visual disturbances unless there is asthenopia, in which event plus adds and prisms are helpful.

THE EARS

Loss of balance resulting from trauma or disorders of the cervical spine is a frequent and distressing complaint. Sellers in 1952 defined equilibrium as a process of muscle tonus with or without conscious perception by which the body, its limbs, and the eyes maintain normal positions in space; by which these positions are regained when disturbed; and by which purposeful motions are consummated. The eyes, the muscles and joints with their visceral and proprioceptive senses are important components and will act under the ultimate control of widely distributed but closely interconnected areas of the central nervous system. There is one process above all others that accounts for stimulation or depression of either labyrinth in the inner ear–abnormal vasospasm or vaso-dilation and edema.

The clinical problem is to determine if the lesion is central or peripheral.

Rubin states that nystagmus always accompanies balance system abnormalities and is the one objective manifestation of equilibrium dysfunction.

Improper information supplied by the inner ear, eyes and/or the proprioceptive system leads to deficiencies or disturbances of information supplied to the central nervous system and results in dizziness, giddiness, unsteadiness or lightheadedness.

Electronystagmography has been developed as an aid in the diagnosis and to differentiate between peripheral and central causes or disturbances and it provides an objective, repeatable, permanent record of the patient's vestibular responses. Its use has supplied knowledge of the role of the connections from the reticular formation, the thalamus and hypothalamus to the vestibulo-ocular reflex pathways. Recordings of the vestibular function are important in making a diagnosis of cervical spine trauma or disorders, fractures of the temporal bone and brain concussion.

We must keep in mind, however, that patients complaining of loss of balance, lightheadedness and transitory hearing deficits following an injury of the cervical spine often respond well to traction therapy and cervical immobilization. If they do not experience relief after adequate treatment, the electronystagmographer should be consulted.

Thus far there are no tests to prove or disprove the symptoms of transitory hearing deficits of which the patients complain following trauma. The audiometer is of little value, as stated by Chrisman and Gervais, but should be utilized if symptoms persist.

BLOOD PRESSURE

Irritation of the cervical sympathetic nerve supply may give rise to vasoconstriction of the arteries which are supplied by the sympathetic fibers. It has been interesting to note that the blood pressure in the two arms varies as much as ten to twenty points in the presence of cervical spine disorders. The presence of muscle spasm in one arm may be responsible also for the variation. This is an objective finding over which the patient has no control and it should be utilized in every examination of the neck. Figure 82 illustrates graphically the usual findings.

MODIFIED ADSON TEST

Elevation of the arm may cause diminution or obliteration of the radial pulse at the wrist if there is spasm of the anterior scalene muscle behind which the subclavian artery lies on the first rib, and the head need not be tilted or rotated to the opposite side, as claimed by Adson, and certainly the test is much more frequently positive in patients who do not have cervical ribs than in those who do have. The scalene muscles elevate the first rib. Elevation of the arm produces a slight depression of the first rib, which puts the scalene on tension or causes further spasm of it to compress the subclavian artery. The radial pulse may be obliterated on one side or on both sides and may vary from time to time.

OTHER ROUTINE TESTS

At this point of the examination and with the stethoscope still at hand it is well to check the heart. If irregularities are found, an electrocardiogram should be done. Trauma to the chest is not unusual and there may be cardiac involvement.

The lungs should be checked carefully, also, especially in the event of chest trauma. Pneumothorax or hemothorax may be present. There may be costochondral separations which can be localized by palpation usually.

If the patient complains of vertigo or loss of balance or of other symptoms of vascular insufficiency such as blurring of vision, auscultation of the major arteries of the neck should be done to detect the presence or absence of bruits.

COMMENTS

One should keep in mind that adhesive capsulitis of the shoulder and calcareous deposits in the tendons of the shoulder cuff are often associated with cervical spine disorders. Pain in or about the shoulder joint from irritation of the cervical nerve roots may give rise to reflex sympathetic dystrophy with resulting changes in the capsule and tendons. Similar changes may occur at the elbow, wrist and in the fingers. Finger motion may be limited as the result of swelling caused by circulatory changes from involvement of the sympathetic nerves, or limitation of motion may be the result of fibrotic changes in the palmar fascia from ischemia. I have seen many patients develop fibrotic nodules and contractures of the palmar fascia following injuries of the cervical spine. Similar findings are well documented in the German literature.

If the symptoms as related by the patient in any way suggest the possibility of spinal cord involvement, other standard neurological tests should be made. In any event the reflexes in the lower extremities should be tested in every routine examination of the cervical spine.

OTHER DIAGNOSTIC AIDS

Certain other diagnostic tests may be helpful in differential diagnosis.

Electromyography

Electromyographic examinations are done frequently by some examiners, especially neurologists, neurosurgeons and those engaged in the practice of physical medicine. Certainly, such examinations should be done by those physicians who are trained well in the application and interpretation of such examinations. As pointed out by Norris, the electromyograph is not a simple tool and it may provide ambiguous answers to clinical problems. He states also that no EMG abnormality is pathognomic of any specific condition. Differentiation between myogenic and neurogenic disorders is usually possible.

The orthopaedist should not rush a patient to the electromyographer immediately following trauma of the cervical spine, inasmuch as no electrical changes will be found for approximately three weeks following the injury, or until Wallerian degeneration has occurred. The limitations and the advantages of electromyography should be understood well by all who rely on it as a diagnostic tool.

Electroencephalography

The electroencephalogram may be of diagnostic aid in the differentiation of brain and cervical nerve root lesions, and it should be utilized when there is a problem of differential diagnosis. One should keep in mind the work done by several investigators who have shown that the electrical abnormalities following closed head injuries and injuries of the cervical spine are comparable in approximately 50 percent of the cases, as shown by Torres and Shapiro.

SUMMARY

In summary, one can say that the clinical findings in cervical spine disorders are fairly constant, but that they may vary to some extent in each individual and at each examination. Radicular pain and tenderness and sensory changes follow fairly definite patterns corresponding to the distribution of the nerve roots involved. Involvement of more than one nerve root is the rule rather than the exception. The role of the sympathetic nerves must be considered in all cases.

Inasmuch as involvement of the spinal cord may be present, we must never conclude that it has escaped injury (until proved otherwise) or that there are no compressive or irritative factors from causes other than trauma.

Chapter 8

THE RADIOGRAPHIC EXAMINATION

Emphasis must be placed on the importance of obtaining adequate radiographic examination in all cervical spine disorders. The usual anteroposterior and lateral views may show gross pathology, but the less obvious or the obscure abnormalities may be missed entirely in these views. The clinician should not depend upon the radiologist's interpretation of "essentially negative" films. The clinical findings must be correlated with the radiographs. Inasmuch as the radiologist has little, if any, opportunity to examine the patient, the clinician must be prepared to evaluate the clinical and radiographic picture as a whole. He must keep in mind that gross derangements sometimes give rise to minimal symptoms and clinical findings, whereas minimal derangements may cause severe symptoms and marked clinical findings.

If the patient is seen in the emergency room of a hospital following a cervical spine injury, he should not be moved from the carriage until one is certain that there are no major neurological deficits. It is always safer to have lateral and, if possible, anteroposterior radiographs made before moving the patient from the carriage to the x-ray table. These views should show any major fractures or dislocations; if there are none, it is usually safe to make the routine views. If the patient is ambulatory, one may order routine views in most instances without fear of causing further injury.

ROUTINE VIEWS

The following radiographic views should be made routinely: (1) an anteroposterior view of the upper two vertebrae made through the opened mouth and with the x-ray tube tilted toward the head by five to ten degrees; (2) an anteroposterior view of the lower five vertebrae made with the x-ray tube tilted fifteen to twenty degrees toward the head; (3) an anteroposterior view made with the x-ray tube angled thirty to thirty-five degrees to-

189

ward the feet–called the caudad-angled view, as described by Abel; (4) a lateral view made with the patient sitting upright, looking straight ahead and with a sand bag in each hand to pull the shoulders downward so that the C7-T1 vertebrae can be brought into view; (5) a similar lateral view but made with the patient's head placed forward as far as possible; (6) a third lateral view made with the patient's neck in backward flexion or in hyperextension; (7) a left oblique view made with the patient sitting upright and turned at a forty-five degree angle away from the film and toward the x-ray tube, the head tilted slightly backward to avoid overlapping of the upper vertebrae by the mandible, the x-ray tube angled upward by five to ten degrees; (8) a right oblique view made with the patient facing in the opposite direction at a forty-five degree angle to the film and to the x-ray tube.

In some instances, other views may be necessary. The submental view which shows the transverse processes of the atlas should be made following trauma, especially if there are symptoms of vertebral artery involvement.

As suggested by Abel, it is important to make the caudad-angled view with the neck in right and left lateral bending positions, to localize capsular disruption or instability.

Gehweiler has recommended posteroanterior views with the patient's head turned to the right and to the left and with the patient's cheek resting on the table to show the vertebral arches. The x-ray tube is angled cephalad thirty-five degrees. We have been unable to get satisfactory radiographic views with this technique, certainly not ones that give us adequate information concerning the pillars, or articular processes, because the patients often cannot rotate their neck so that their cheeks make contact with the table. Certainly an obese or very large patient presents problems and distorted radiographs. We much prefer Abel's technique.

Stratigrams or scanigrams may be needed to show questionable fractures and anomalies (Figs. 117, 118, and 119).

Myelograms may be indicated if there are symptoms and clinical findings compatible with a space-occupying lesion.

The making of discograms has become very popular in certain sections of the country for determining the normal or degenerative status of the intervertebral disc, but their diagnostic value is questionable inasmuch as clefts may extend through a cervical disc into the lateral interbody joints without causing symptoms.

The Open-mouth View

When properly made, the open-mouth view shows the relationship of the atlas and the axis. Trauma to the neck may result in tearing or stretching of the atlantoaxial guy ligaments with resulting lateral subluxation of the head and atlas on the axis, as evidenced by the odontoid-atlas lateral mass ratio (Figs. 11, 12 and 83). If there is subluxation of the head and axis to one side, other views should be made through the open-mouth with the head tilted to the right side and then to the left side. These views will give a clue to the extent of the ligamentous damage (Fig. 84). If the subluxation is fixed and the relationship of the odontoid process to the lateral masses of the atlas is unchanged by tilting the

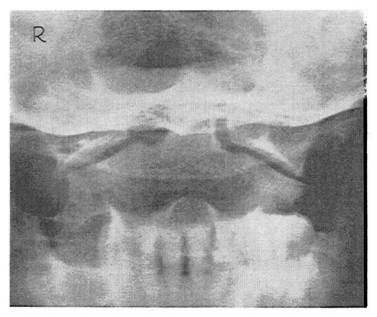

Figure 83. A radiograph of the first two cervical vertebrae which demonstrates a marked subluxation of the atlas on the axis to the right side.

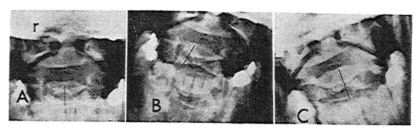

Figure 84. Radiographs made through the open mouth of a patient who had been in an automobile collision two days previously. There is narrowing of the lateral joint space on the left side, as shown in A. Lateral bending films (B and C) show relaxation of the alar ligaments bilaterally and of the accessory atlantoaxial ligament on the left side.

head to the opposite side, it is likely that this condition existed prior to a recent trauma or that some mechanical derangement is present. If the relationship shifts as the head is tilted from one side to the other, one is safe in concluding that the relaxation of the guy ligaments is of recent origin.

It is not unusual to find rotation of the axis as evidenced by the position of the spinous process away from the midline and by clear view of the transverse foramen of the axis on one side and obliteration or narrowing of the foramen on the opposite side (Fig. 85). The amount of rotation of the axis will be dependent on the integrity of the guy ligaments and to some extent on the plane of the joints between the second and third vertebrae.

An irregular line of decreased density at the base of the odontoid process indicates a fracture line usually, even in the absence of any displacement of the odontoid process (Fig. 86). A smooth line of decreased density may indicate the presence of a rudimentary disc between the odontoid and the body of the axis, or an old fracture of the odontoid process, as shown in Figure 87. Tilting of the odontoid away from the midline indicates the presence of a fracture or separation, either recent or remote (Fig. 51).

A fracture line may be seen extending through a lateral mass of the atlas or axis (Fig. 38). A compression fracture of a lateral mass may be seen in the open-mouth view; although such a fracture may not be found in the immediate postinjury radiograph it

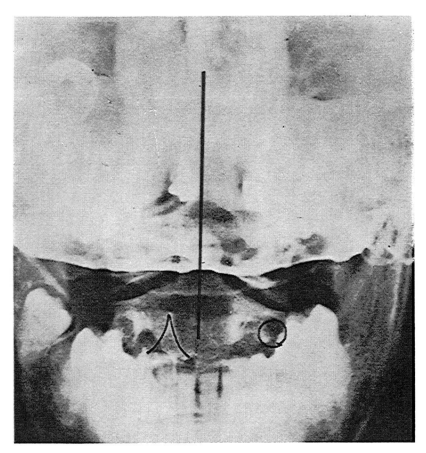

Figure 85. An open mouth view which shows rotation of the axis to the right side indicating tearing or relaxation of the accessory atlantoaxial ligament on the left side.

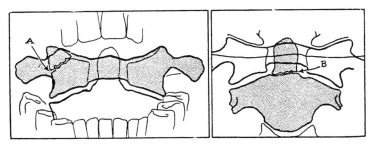

Figure 86. Sketch of x-ray films of C1 and 2 showing fracture of a superior articular facet of C1 (A), and fracture of the odontoid process of C2 (B).

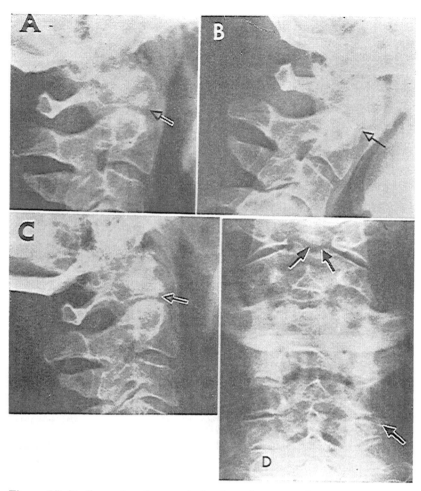

Figure 87. Radiographs of a cervical spine of a man who was injured in a head-on truck collision with a train and who had a severe head injury. The injury of the neck was considered unimportant and the neck was never immobilized. There is separation of the odontoid from the body of the axis with definite instability. In the caudad-angled view, there is narrowing of the interarticular isthmus of the sixth vertebra on the left side, and the separation of the odontoid is well visualized in this view also.

Figure 88. Open mouth radiographic view of the atlas and the axis which was made soon after an eight foot steel beam fell and struck the patient on the left side of his head. Note that there is narrowing of the joint space on the right side (arrow) and the lateral mass of the axis appears to be compressed. The film made thirteen months later shows the usual bony reaction at the site of the fracture with increased depression of the lateral mass and subluxation of the atlas on the axis to the left side.

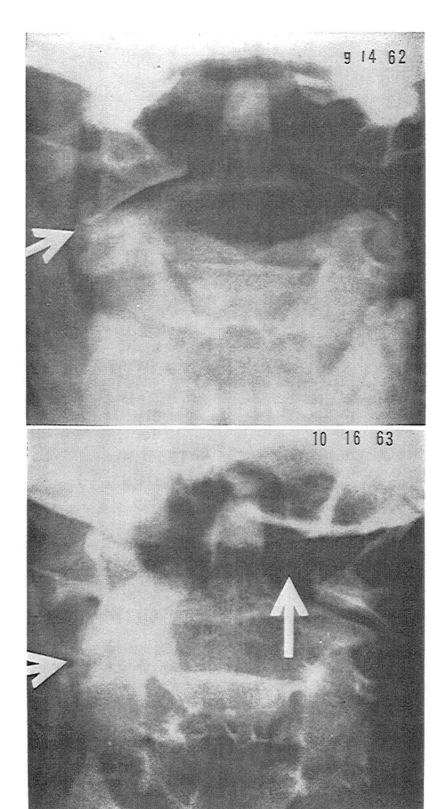

can be seen as a depressed area with increased density in subsequent films as shown in Figure 88.

A fracture of a transverse process of the atlas may be visualized in this view sometimes, although the submental view may be necessary to confirm it.

If there is wide separation of both lateral masses of the atlas from the odontoid process, one must conclude that there are fractures of the posterior arch and of the anterior arch of the atlas, inasmuch as it is impossible to break the solid ring of bone at one point only and have the lateral masses separated–there must be at least two fractures, one of the anterior arch and one of the posterior arch (Figs. 53 and 54).

Congenital abnormalities of the atlas and axis may be demonstrated in the open-mouth view. Agenesis, or failure of development of the odontoid, has been noted. An ossicle at the tip of the odontoid may be found. If the odontoid process cannot be demonstrated because of the overlying skull structures, one must suspect the presence of basilar impression or occipital invagination of the atlas, which can be verified in the lateral views. Failure of fusion of the posterior arch of the atlas may be seen in the open-mouth view, which should not be mistaken for a fracture.

The Anteroposterior View of the Lower Cervical Vertebrae

The anteroposterior view of the lower cervical vertebrae gives valuable information concerning the lateral interbody joints, the disc spaces, the vertebral bodies and in some instances the posterior facets.

Compression fractures of the upward lateral projections of the vertebral bodies may sometimes be demonstrated in this view. Dissection of anatomic specimens has revealed healing fractures of these projections which could not be demonstrated by radiographs. Flattening or sclerosis of these projections should make one suspicious of fracture, unless, of course, there is an actual absence of the projection on one or both sides (Figs. 89-92). In some instances, these projections are not well developed on the bodies of the seventh and sixth vertebrae, as stated previously.

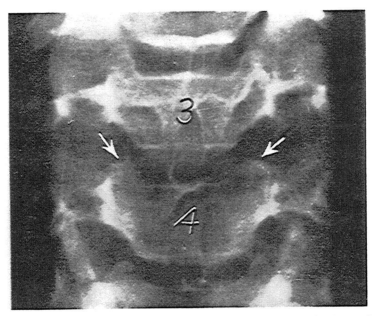

Figure 89. Compression fractures of the upward lateral projections of the body of the fourth vertebra, resulting from a side-lash injury.

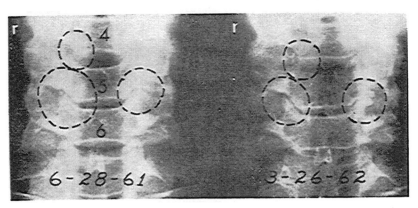

Figure 90. Anteroposterior radiographs of a patient who was injured in a rear-end collision on 6/23/61. The film made three days later shows widening of the lateral interbody joint space between the fourth and fifth vertebrae on the right side and osteophytic changes at the margins of the lateral interbody joints between the fifth and sixth vertebrae. A film made nine months later shows depression of the upward lateral projection of the body of the fifth vertebra on the right side which represents a compression fracture. There are increased osteophytic changes at the margins of the lateral interbody joints between the fifth and sixth vertebrae.

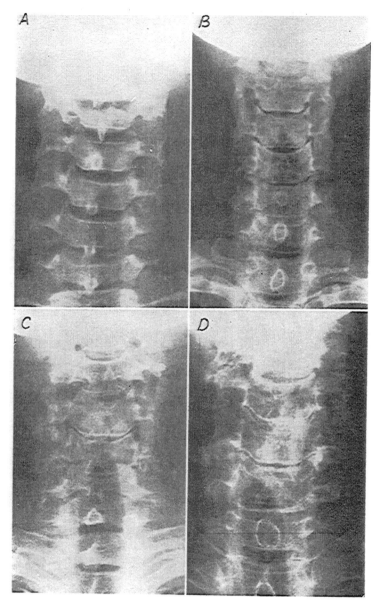

Figure 91. Anteroposterior views of cervical spines. Relatively normal appearing disc spaces and lateral intervertebral joints can be seen in A. Note marked degenerative and hypertrophic changes in B, C and D.

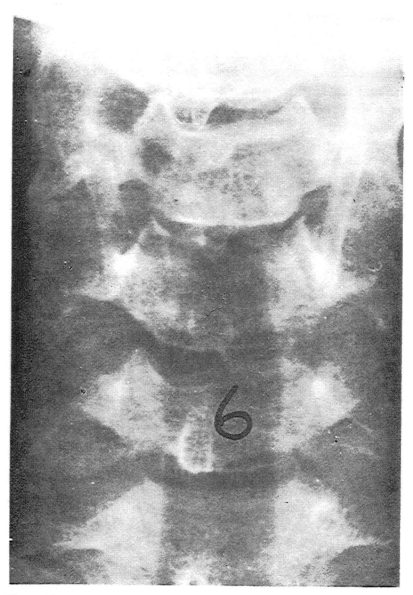

Figure 92. An anteroposterior view of the neck of a man who was injured in a rear-end collision six months previously. There is no upward lateral projection on the left side of the sixth vertebral body. The contour of the inferior portion of the vertebral body of the fifth vertebra on the left side leads one to believe that this represents a developmental anomaly.

Osteophytic changes at the margins of the lateral interbody joints are usually well demonstrated in this view (Figs. 90 and 91).

If a lateral interbody space is wider on one side than on the other side, one may suspect hemorrhage into the expanded space, a unilateral subluxation of the proximate posterior joint, a compression of the upward lateral projection, or a fracture of the vertebral arch or of the inferior facet of the proximal vertebra on the side opposite the widened interbody joint space. When there is expansion of one interbody joint space there should be a corresponding narrowing on the opposite side usually.

If there is narrowing of both lateral interbody joint spaces, the proximate disc space must be narrowed. Complete obliteration of the lateral interbody joint spaces indicates fusion of the two vertebrae. If the intervertebral disc space is obliterated, fusion of the two vertebrae is present.

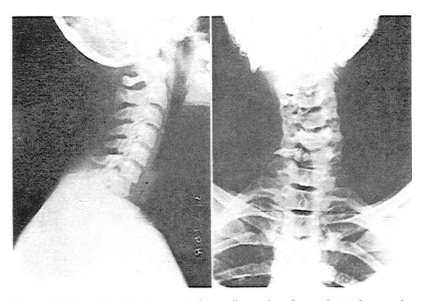

Figure 93. Lateral and anteroposterior radiographs of a patient who was injured in an automobile accident. The fracture of the articular process of the sixth vertebra on the right side can be well visualized in the anteroposterior view. Displacement of the sixth vertebra on the seventh is evident in the lateral view.

In some instances, fractures of the articular processes of the apophyseal, or posterior joints, can be seen in this view, as shown in Figure 93.

Fractures of vertebral bodies may be suspected in this view, although the extent of such fractures cannot be determined.

Hemivertebrae and other developmental anomalies of the cervical vertebrae may be noted in the anteroposterior view (Fig. 70F).

The Caudad-angled View

The anteroposterior view made with the x-ray tube tilted toward the feet of the patient is of significant value, as pointed out by Abel. It reveals the condition of the interarticular isthmuses of the sixth, fifth, and fourth vertebrae; and if the teeth are absent one can see the isthmuses of the third, second and first vertebrae. Compression and avulsion fractures of the articular processes may be noted. Immediate postinjury films may not show the fractures, but they may be demonstrated on subsequent films after narrowing of the isthmuses has occurred or there is evidence of healing of the fractures (Fig. 94).

Abel has suggested that the caudad-angled view should be made with the head tilted to each side to demonstrate relaxation or tearing of the capsular structures, which will be shown by

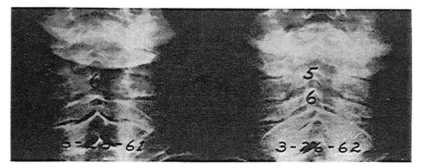

Figure 94. Caudad-angled views made three days and nine months following injury of the neck in a rear-end collision. There is slight narrowing of the interarticular isthmus of the sixth vertebra on the left side as shown in the initial film and there is increased narrowing as shown in the subsequent film, indicating beyond any doubt a compression injury or fracture.

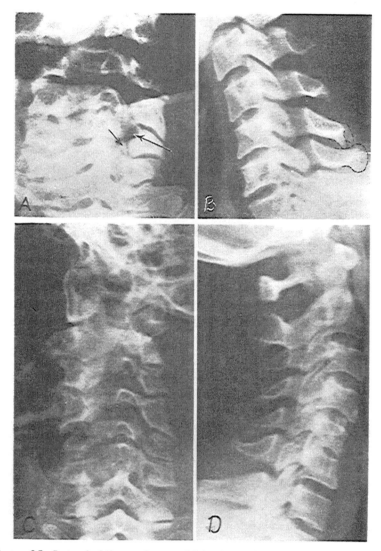

Figure 95. Lateral-oblique views, which show the posterior articulations. The patient shown in A has had a partial facetectomy at C5 and 6. The short arrow points to a fragment of bone which was not removed. This patient's symptoms were not relieved by the operation. B shows a narrowed disc between C5 and 6. Radiographs C and D are those of a patient who had received a neck injury in childhood. There is bony fusion between the posterior portions of the bodies of C5 and 6, and an avulsion of the spinous process of C5, as shown in D. The lateral oblique (C) shows that there is no bony fusion of the facets.

widening of the joint space or spaces on the side of involvement, the widening occurring on the side away from the tilt. The lateral tilt, caudad-angled views are made routinely by my technicians and are called pillar views.

This view has replaced the need for the lateral-oblique view which is shown in Figure 95. However, in some instances, the lateral-oblique may give added information.

These so-called occult fractures of the articular processes and of the interarticular isthmuses are the result of compression injuries which occur as the posterior articulations are jammed together in hyperextension injuries and/or as a shearing force is applied to the facets. Such fractures of the isthmuses result in slight but definite realignment of the vertebrae. As motion in the joints continues, osteophytic changes develop at the margins of the joints within a period of several months. These changes can be demonstrated also in this view, as shown in Figure 71D.

The Lateral Views

The three lateral views made with the patient sitting in the upright position, as suggested by Davis, are of diagnostic significance (Figs. 96 and 97).

The Straight View

A loss of the forward curve which can be noted in the lateral view made with the patient looking straight ahead is indicative of some disorder of the cervical spine. It is possible for one to straighten the forward curve by voluntary contraction of the deep lateral and the prevertebral muscle of the neck. Voluntary contraction of these muscles causes some flexion of the neck and the chin assumes a "tucked-in" position, which can be detected by the position of the mandible as it approximates or overlies the bodies of the upper cervical vertebrae.

Involuntary contraction of the muscles which straighten the cervical spine occurs to prevent painful movements of the joints of the neck, which in turn enlarges the vertical diameter of the intervertebral canals to give some relief of compressive forces on the nerve roots. Irritation of the nerve roots may be responsible

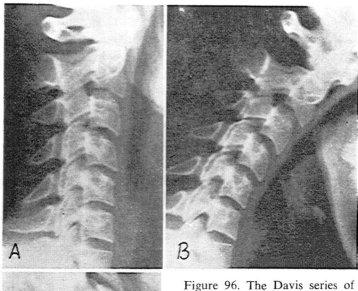

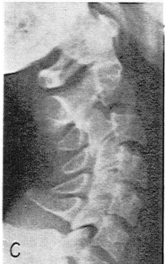

Figure 96. The Davis series of lateral radiographs. Note the loss of the forward curve in A, and the forward subluxation of the third on the fourth and of the fourth on the fifth. In the forward flexion view (B) there is marked forward subluxation of the second on the third and of the fourth on the fifth, as well as the third on the fourth. In the hyperextension view (C) there is posterior subluxation of the third on the fourth and of the second on the third. These subluxations are due to ligamentous and capsular instability resulting from a sprain injury of the neck.

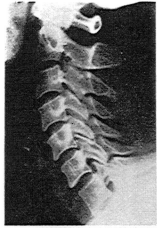

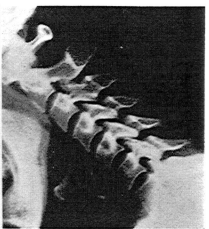

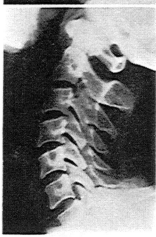

Figure 97. The Davis series of lateral radiographs of a fifty-three-year-old woman who has had no known injury to her neck. There are no subluxations and no radiographically visible degenerative changes; there is not a smooth backward curve as the head is placed forward, however, indicating some tightness of the posterior neck structures.

for the contraction of the muscles and is nature's way of attempting to relieve the irritative factor.

There are those who contend that a loss of the forward curve may be of no diagnostic significance and, therefore, omit this view. Also, there are those who contend that the loss of the forward curve may be caused by emotional tension or by fright. This is no more true of the cervical spine than it is of other parts of the spine. If fright can cause straightening of the cervical spine and if emotional tension can do it, once these conditions have been

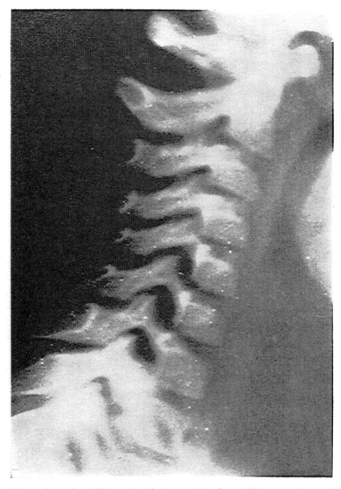

Figure 98. A lateral radiograph of the neck of a child, age three, who had had a sprain injury of the cervical spine. Note the reversal of the curve at level of the second and third vertebrae. This is a frequent finding in sprain injuries of the neck in children.

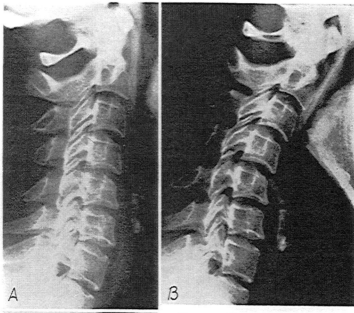

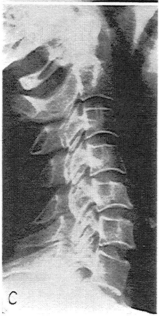

Figure 99-1. Radiographs made immediately after a whiplash injury. Note the reversal of the forward curve with posterior angulation between the fourth and fifth vertebrae. There is unusual separation of the fourth and fifth spinous processes in A with the neck straight and in B with the neck in flexion. The posterior angulation persists with the neck in hyperextension, as shown in C.

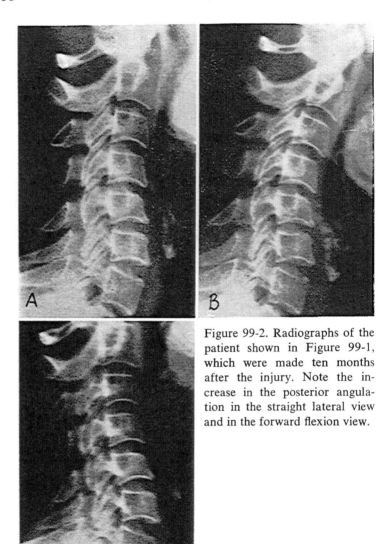

Figure 99-2. Radiographs of the patient shown in Figure 99-1, which were made ten months after the injury. Note the increase in the posterior angulation in the straight lateral view and in the forward flexion view.

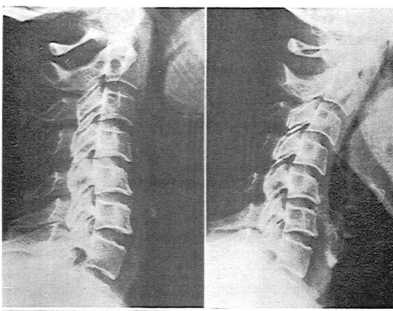

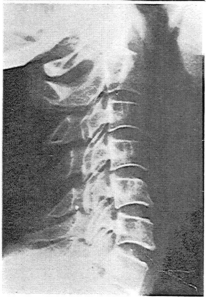

Figure 99-3. Subsequent films made six years later show continued backward angulation in all views. There are minimal osteophytic changes but there are definite irregularities of the posterior facets at the fifth and sixth and at the sixth and seventh levels. This patient received adequate treatment and was taught how to protect her neck in her everyday activities.

dissipated the forward curve should return. Only sudden fright or sudden emotional tension could possibly be of significance.

Loss of the forward curve occurs in 78 percent of all cases of cervical spine involvement and a reversal of the forward curve, which is localized usually to three or four segments, will be found in 20 percent of these cases. The apex of the reversed curve indicates usually the site of maximum involvement. In children the reversed curve may be in the upper portion of the cervical spine, as shown in Figure 98.

The reversed curve may present a sharp angulation at one specific level as seen in Figure 99. This indicates a tearing of the posterior ligamentous structures or a rupture of the intervertebral disc anteriorly at that level. Subluxation of the posterior joints upward and forward with widening of the posterior joint spaces and separation of the corresponding spinous processes may be responsible, also, for the posterior angulation.

Backward subluxations may be noted in the straight lateral

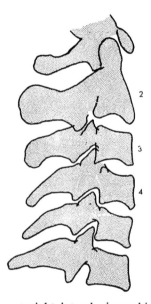

Figure 100. Tracing of a straight lateral view which shows posterior subluxation of the third vertebra on the fourth and slight subluxation of the second vertebra on the third.

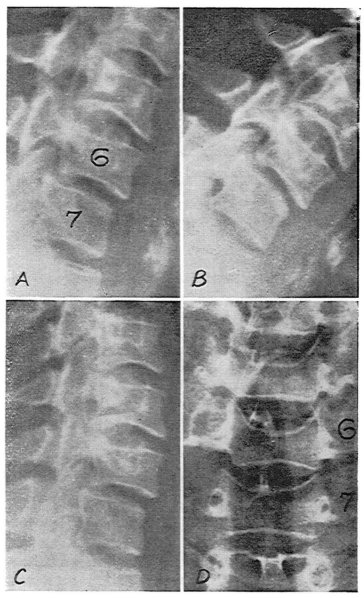

Figure 101. Persistent anterior subluxation in all lateral views, and widening of the lateral interbody joint space on the right side in the antero-posterior view indicating a unilateral facet fracture.

view. The posterior margin of the vertebral body which is displaced posteriorly is seen to lie behind the posterior margin of the adjacent distal vertebral body. The superior facets of the lower vertebra are displaced forward and encroach on the intervertebral foramina (Fig. 100).

Forward displacement of one vertebral body on the vertebral body beneath it, if present in the straight lateral view, indicates rupture of the posterior ligamentous and capsular structures, a fracture of one or both vertebral arches or of one or both posterior facets (Fig. 101A).

An increase in the interpedicular ratio may indicate the presence of a space-occupying lesion which is causing separation of the vertebrae.

The Flexion View

On clinical examination, the neck may appear to have a full range of motion in flexion. However, the lateral view made with the neck placed in maximum forward flexion may reveal that what appeared to be a normal or average range of flexion was actually taking place between the atlantoaxial and the atlanto-occipital joints and at the cervicothoracic joints with little or no motion occurring in the other joints. When there is no disorder of the cervical spine, forward flexion results in a smooth backward curve as the vertebrae maintain their alignment. If there is no backward curve, some disorder is present. Contraction of the posterior neck muscles or of the posterior intervertebral ligaments prevent forward flexion. If flexion of the neck occurs between the upper and lower joints, there will be little if any separation of the spinous processes of the intervening vertebrae in the lateral flexion view. Posterior angulation may occur at any level, but the usual angulation occurs at the fourth and fifth or the fifth and sixth vertebrae, in which event there is an increase in the interspinous ratio at these levels. Such backward angulation signifies ligamentous injury or instability at that level.

Forward subluxation of one vertebral body on the adjacent distal vertebral body as noted in the lateral flexion view represents instability of the posterior ligamentous structures, disruption of an intervertebral disc or a fracture of one or both posterior facets or of one or both vertebral arches at that level. Forward subluxations may occur at more than one level as a result of ligamentous instability (Fig. 96). Even in the absence of a known injury, a demonstrable forward slipping of one vertebral body on its proximate distal vertebra indicates ligamentous instability or skeletal instability.

When the so-called normal neck is placed in flexion, the anterior vertical diameter of the intervertebral disc spaces decreases very slightly and the posterior vertical diameter increases very slightly. If there is a marked decrease or increase of these diameters, one must conclude that the intervertebral disc has been disrupted.

If a tear of the transverse ligament of the atlas is present, or if this ligament is unduly relaxed from some involvement of its collagen fibers such as occurs in certain arthritic processes, the anterior arch of the atlas will be separated from the odontoid process in the flexion view, as illustrated in Figure 10. Any forward displacement of the anterior arch of the atlas in its relationship to the odontoid process should be considered abnormal regardless of the causative factor.

The Hyperextension View

The range and the location of backward motion can be demonstrated in the lateral view made with the neck in hyperextension. In the so-called normal cervical spine, backward motion produces a smooth forward curve as the vertebrae maintain their alignment. The spinous processes of the vertebrae approach each other with the same degree at each segmental level. The persistence of a reversed forward curve or the persistence of backward angulation indicates some disorder of the cervical spine, and may be the result of protective contraction of the muscles, or the result of permanent ligamentous and/or joint damage or the result of skeletal injury or disorder.

Persistent forwarded subluxation of one vertebral body on the

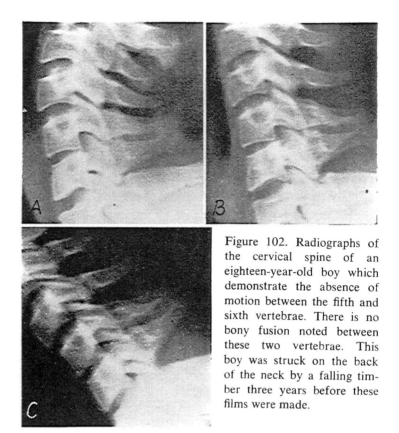

Figure 102. Radiographs of the cervical spine of an eighteen-year-old boy which demonstrate the absence of motion between the fifth and sixth vertebrae. There is no bony fusion noted between these two vertebrae. This boy was struck on the back of the neck by a falling timber three years before these films were made.

adjacent distal body as shown in the lateral hyperextension view signifies a fracture of the vertebral arch or of one or both inferior facets of the displaced vertebra (Fig. 101C).

The interspinous ratio and the interpedicular ratio of two adjacent vertebrae may be increased when the neck is placed in hyperextension, indicating that the interspinous and interlaminar ligaments have been disrupted and that the anterior longitudinal ligament is intact and probably contracted at that level, or that there is interposition of intervening joint structures.

An unusual increase in the anterior vertical diameter of an intervertebral space indicates a tear of the anterior longitudinal ligament and of the annulus fibrosus from the vertebral margins and from the vertebral plate or plates.

All lateral views may show abnormalities of the vertebral structures and the bending views may show segmental limitation of motion which may be due to bony ankylosis, or to fibrous fixation, as shown in Figure 102. If there is no separation of the spinous processes in the bending views, some abnormal condition is present.

In all lateral views, the odontoid process is well visualized usually. Fractures of the odontoid may not be seen in these views unless there is displacement. If there is invagination of the atlas into the posterior fossa of the skull, the odontoid cannot be visualized because of the overlying occipital structures (Fig. 68).

An unusually long styloid process of the temporal bone can be seen in the lateral views. The stylohyoid ligament, which may be calcified or ossified, can be seen best in the lateral flexion and oblique views (Fig. 103).

Compression fractures of the vertebral bodies can be seen in all lateral views (Fig. 104). Such fractures may not be visible in the immediate postinjury films unless there is definite distortion of the contour of the body or bodies involved. However, subsequent lateral radiographs made a few weeks or a few months after the

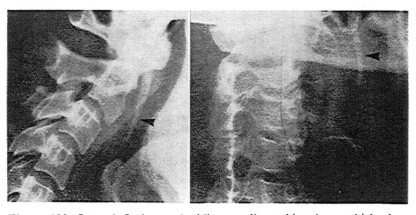

Figure 103. Lateral flexion and oblique radiographic views which show calcification of the stylohyoid ligament.

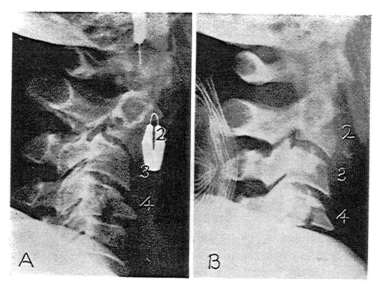

Figure 104A & B. Fracture of the body of the fourth vertebra and forward luxation of the second on the third, caused by tearing of the posterior ligamentous and capsular structures at this level, can be seen in A. Reduction accomplished by skeletal traction is shown in B.

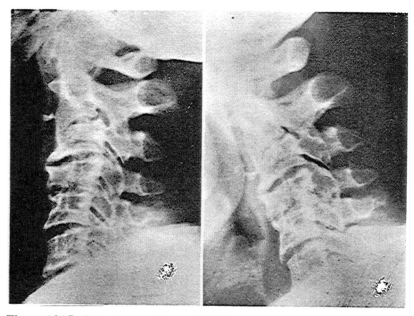

Figure 104C. Lateral extension and flexion views which were made two years postinjury show that there is complete fusion of the second and third vertebrae with forward subluxation of the second on the third and marked degeneration of the intervening disc. Note the marked osteophytic formations and apparent lack of motion at the fourth and fifth vertebrae. If the initial films were unavailable, one might conclude after viewing the subsequent films that this patient was a victim of osteoarthritis rather than traumatic arthritis.

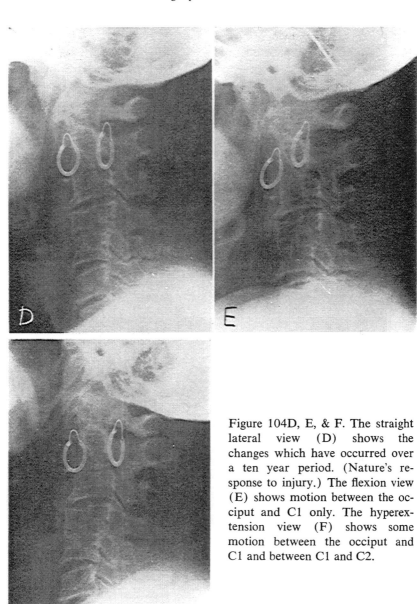

Figure 104D, E, & F. The straight lateral view (D) shows the changes which have occurred over a ten year period. (Nature's response to injury.) The flexion view (E) shows motion between the occiput and C1 only. The hyperextension view (F) shows some motion between the occiput and C1 and between C1 and C2.

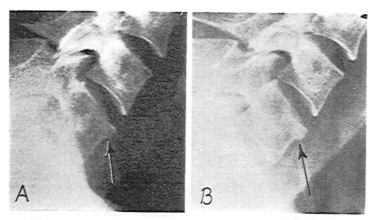

Figure 105A & B. A compression fracture of the anterosuperior portion of the seventh cervical vertebra was not noted in the initial postinjury film (A), but it was definitely evident in the film made two months later as shown in B.

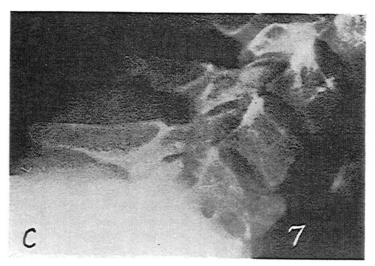

Figure 105C. Compression fracture of the body of C7 which was not discovered until two months postinjury. The shoulders prevented adequate visualization of the seventh vertebral body.

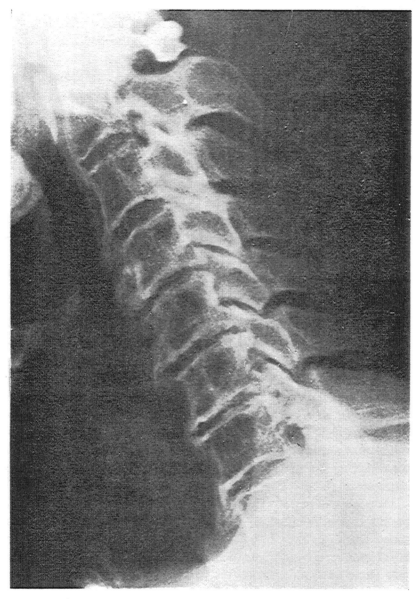

Figure 106. A lateral radiograph which shows complete fixation of all vertebral bodies at their anterior margins.

injury will establish the presence of the compression fractures beyond any doubt (Fig. 105), and subsequent films will show the
changes resulting from trauma, as shown in Figure 104D, E, F.

Avulsion fractures of the anteroinferior margins of the vertebral
bodies are revealed in the lateral views. These may be confused
with calcification within the anterior longitudinal ligament, within
the annulus fibrosus or with a detached osteophytic spur.

One may find complete calcification of the anterior longitudinal
ligament bridging the disc space or spaces. This may be the result
of trauma or of some disorder of the collagen fibers associated
with certain spondylitic conditions involving the ligamentous structures (Fig. 106). In some instances, there may be a similar process in the posterior longitudinal ligament and/or in the capsular
structures, producing complete immobilization of the areas involved. In other instances, one may find solid fusion of the vertebral bodies with complete obliteration of the intervening disc or
discs.

Narrowed disc spaces, with and without marginal osteophytosis,
may be noted in the lateral views. A decrease in the vertical diameter of a disc indicates degeneration of the disc, unless the narrowing is associated with a developmental anomaly of the adjacent
vertebrae. If a narrowed disc space is noted in the immediate
postinjury films, one may conclude that the narrowing existed
prior to the injury. However, if narrowing is seen in subsequent
films several months later, one can conclude with reasonable certainty that the known traumatic experience was the causative factor which incited the changes within the disc, which resulted in the
narrowing.

Osteophytosis of the vertebral margins may or may not be apparent in the presence of narrowing of the intervening disc, as
stated above. This will depend to a great extent on the buffering
effect produced by the lateral interbody joints. These small joints
may show marginal osteophytes which are indicative of injury or
of the stress and strain imposed on them by the disturbance of the
mechanico-dynamics of the disc following disruption of one of its
confining structures. These changes at the margins of the lateral
interbody joints are better demonstrated in the oblique views than

in the lateral views. In the lateral views, these changes may appear to be at the posterior margins of the vertebral bodies, inasmuch as the upward lateral projections on the superior surfaces of the vertebral bodies are not visible in the lateral views. In some instances, osteophytic spurs may be present on the posterior margins of the bodies, but usually these changes which appear to involve the posterior margins are at the margins of the lateral interbody joints.

The lateral views may show fractures of the spinous processes and of the laminae if there is some separation at the fracture sites (Fig. 107). Dislocation of the posterior facets without fracture of the posterior elements may be seen. Irregularities of the posterior facets and osteophytic formations at their margins may be visible in the lateral views. Overriding or subluxations, or abnormal excursions of the facets, indicate ligamentous and capsular instability.

Destructive lesions of the vertebral bodies resulting from metabolic disorders, infections, metastatic lesions and primary bone tumors are seen best in the lateral views.

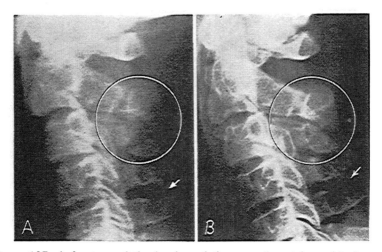

Figure 107. A fracture of the lamina of the second vertebra with forward luxation of this vertebra, and a fracture of the spinous process of the third vertebra can be seen in A. There is an avulsion of the spinous process of the fourth vertebra, also. In B the fractures are healed.

The extent of the mechanical derangements as noted in the lateral views is no indication of the extent of nerve root irritation or involvement of the spinal cord or of sympathetic and vascular involvement. In some instances, there may be clinical evidence of implication of these structures without demonstrable mechanical alterations.

Lateral views made immediately following a traumatic incident may show no abnormalities, whereas films made a few weeks later may show evidence of injury (Fig. 108). On the other hand, films made three to six months postinjury may show restoration of the forward curve and adequate realignment of the vertebrae in flexion and in extension, indicating radiographic evidence of ligamentous and capsular injury followed by some recovery. If the curves are not restored within six months, one can anticipate that the condition is permanent and recovery (restoration to the preinjury status, if known) will not occur.

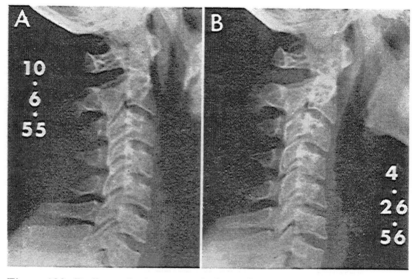

Figure 108. Radiograph A was made immediately following a truck accident. Patient had evidence of cord compression. Film B was made six-and-one-half months later. Note the reversal of the forward curve. The cord symptoms had cleared but the patient had continued radicular symptoms.

The Oblique Views

The right and left oblique views, which should be made with the patient in the upright position, show well the intervertebral canals through which the nerve roots and their accompanying structures pass. These canals, which are somewhat ovoid in shape and which decrease in size from above downward, may show alterations in their contours. Changes in the size and shape of the canals may be the result of ligamentous and capsular instability, the presence of osteophytic spurs at the margins of the lateral interbody joints and the posterior joints, fractures of the posterior facets or of the vertebral arches with some displacement, fractures of the upward lateral projections of the vertebral bodies or splayed fractures of the vertebral bodies and dislocations.

Ligamentous and capsular instability is manifested by overriding of the posterior facets, either backward and downward or forward and upward. In backward and downward slipping, the superior facet of the distal vertebra rides into the vertebral notch

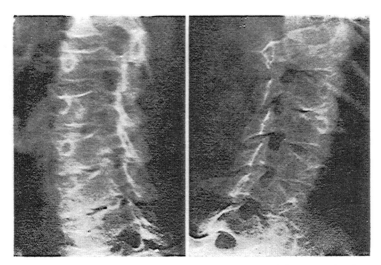

Figure 109. Oblique views which illustrate narrowed intervertebral canals by the spur formations at the margins of the lateral interbody joints. These changes occur over a period of years, but such joints and the adjacent nerve roots are much more susceptible to injury than are normal structures.

The Cervical Syndrome

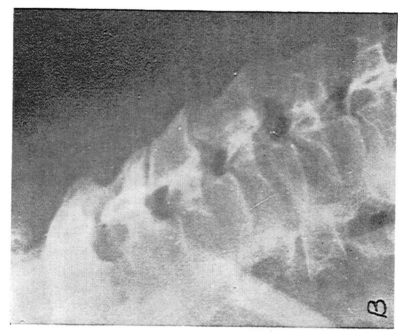

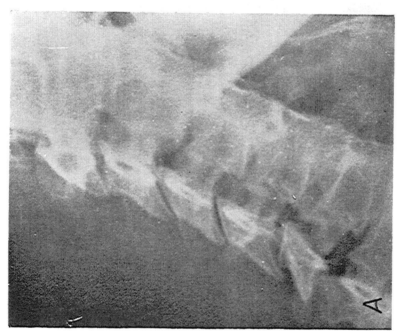

Figure 110. *Left* (A) and *right* (B) oblique-flexion views to show cause for persistent subluxations of 6 on 7 in Figure 101. Note fracture of vertebral arch of C6 in A.

to narrow the canal in its anteroposterior diameter as well as the vertical diameter. Forward and upward slipping of the facets causes an increase in the vertical diameter of the canal and widening of the anteroposterior diameter of the upper part of the canal. These conditions may be evident in one or both oblique views.

Osteophytic spurs at the margins of the lateral interbody joints project into the canals and give them the shape of dumb-bells or of boots (Fig. 109). Variations in the shape of the canals between the second and third vertebrae may be caused by spur formations or by rotation and subluxation of the second on the third vertebra.

Persistent forward subluxation of one vertebra on the adjacent distal vertebra, as revealed in the lateral views, indicates a fracture of one or both vertebral arches or of one or both posterior facets of the vertebra which is subluxated forward. These fractures can be demonstrated in the oblique views usually (Figs. 110 and 111). However, flexion and/or extension-oblique views may be necessary, as described by Boylston.

Narrowing of an intervertebral disc space results in some narrowing of the vertical and the anteroposterior diameters of the

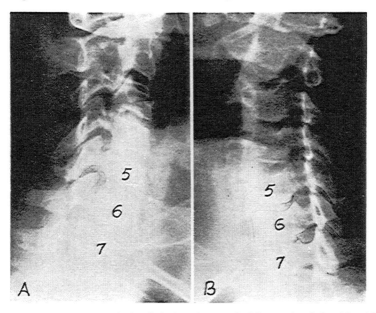

Figure 111. Fracture of the inferior facet of C6 on the left side. Note changes in intervertebral canals between C5 and 6 and between C6 and 7, and the forward subluxation of C6 and C7 on the left side only.

canals. However, the lateral interbody articulations may prevent any appreciable narrowing in either direction, especially if the upward lateral projections on the body of the distal vertebra are unusually long. If there is a loss of the forward curve of the cervical spine or a reversal of the curve, there may be no narrowing of the canals visible.

Where there is radiographic evidence of marked encroachment of the intervertebral canals, one can assume with confidence that the proximate nerve roots are compressed into ribbonlike shapes or that they have been forced into the bottom of the canals where they are found as small firm cords. No marked neurological deficit may be present in many instances.

Semioblique views, as shown in Figure 112, may demonstrate best the extent of the changes about the lateral interbody joints. The lateral oblique view and the caudad-angled view may be

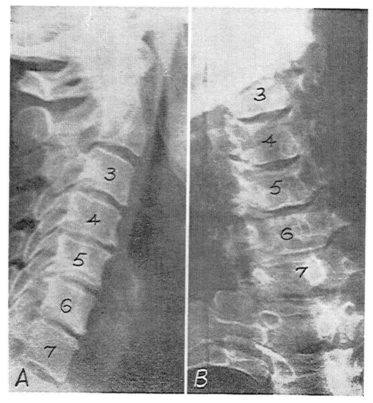

Figure 112. Hypertrophic changes—lateral and semioblique views. Note appearance of spur formation at posterior portion of C4, 5 and 6 in A. Note marked spur formation about the margins of the lateral intervertebral joints at C4, 5 and 6 in B. Spur formations do not usually occur at the posterior margins of the vertebral bodies, although the lateral film gives that appearance.

necessary to demonstrate adequately the extent of the involvement of the posterior joints, as shown in Figures 95 and 71D.

Congenital or acquired anomalies of the posterior facets can be demonstrated in the oblique views usually (Fig. 113).

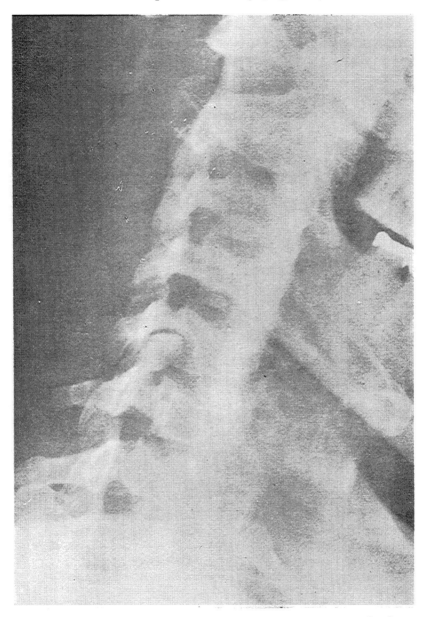

Figure 113. An oblique radiographic view which shows an unusual enlargement of the superior facet of the sixth cervical vertebra. Patient had no symptoms until he received a neck injury in a rear-end collision. The facet on the opposite side was not enlarged. What caused the enlargement is probably conjecture.

RADIOGRAPHS OF ASSOCIATED STRUCTURES

Inasmuch as I, along with other investigators, have noted the frequent association of shoulder and elbow implication in cervical spine disorders, one should not overlook this possibility. Calcareous deposits in the tendons of the shoulder cuff and in the tendinous origin of the extensor, and at times the flexor, muscles of the forearm have been found. Such disorders of the shoulder

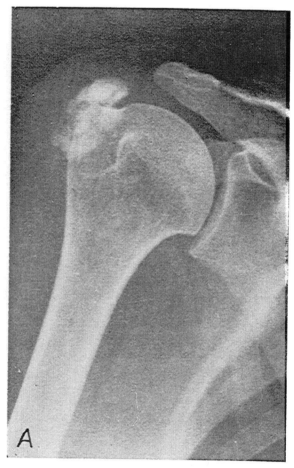

Figure 114A. Film of a shoulder showing a calcereous deposit.

and elbow may have some other etiology, but one should be cognizant of the causal relationship between these conditions and disorders of the cervical spine (Figs. 114, 115 and 116).

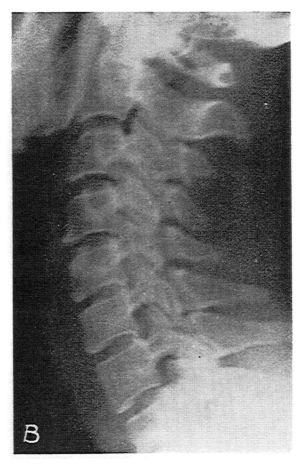

Figure 114B. Film of the cervical spine of patient in 114A, showing a narrowed disc at C5 and 6.

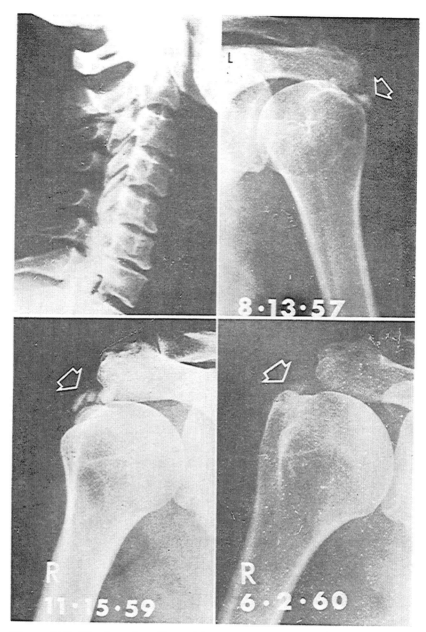

Figure 115. The lateral radiographic view of this patient's cervical spine shows narrowing of the discs at the fifth and sixth and the sixth and seventh interspaces. The film of the left shoulder shows a calcium deposit. She was having symptoms referable to her neck and left shoulder which had been present for four weeks. The calcium was removed by aspiration and irrigation.

In 1959, she fell and soon thereafter she developed neck symptoms and pain and limitation of motion in the right shoulder. Shoulder films revealed calcium deposits, which were removed. In 1960 she had a recurrence.

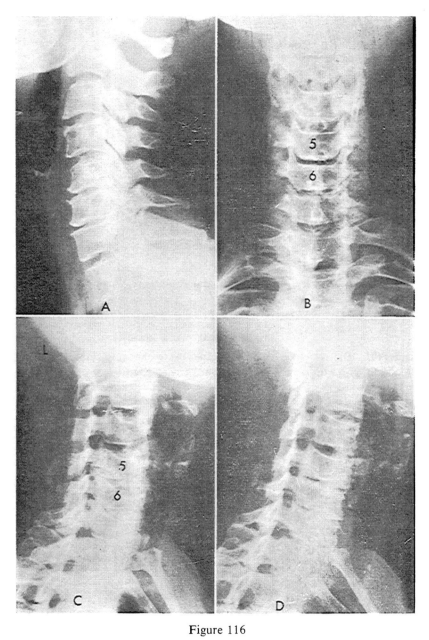

Figure 116

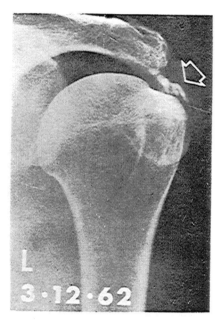

Figure 116. The patient whose radiographs were shown in Figure 115 returned in 1962 with neck symptoms and pain and limitation of motion in
the left shoulder. Radiographs of the cervical spine were made and revealed
increased osteophytic changes. Note the changes about the lateral interbody
joints at the fifth and sixth and at the sixth and seventh vertebrae, which are
more marked on the left side. The film of the left shoulder shows another
calcium deposit.

SCANIGRAMS

Obscure fractures and anomalies may require scanigrams or stratigrams for adequate visualization and diagnosis. They may be necessary for differentiation of fractures and anomalies and should be made, if possible, for proper diagnosis (Figs. 117, 118 and 119).

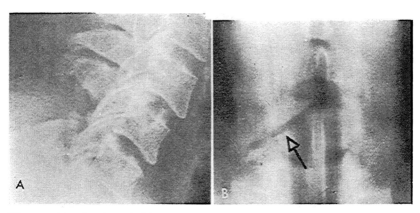

Figure 117. The lateral film (A) shows what appears to be a fracture of the lamina of the sixth vertebra. The scanigram (B) reveals a fracture of the lamina on the right side. (Courtesy of Dr. Jerry Miller.)

Next page ⟶

Figure 118. Radiographs A and B were made of this patient's cervical spine immediately following an injury: A shows some widening of the lateral interbody joint between the fifth and sixth vertebrae on the right side; B shows flattening of the anterosuperior portion of the fifth vertebral body and a narrowed disc space at C5-6. Because of continued severe symptoms scanigrams were made about two months later, one of which is shown in C, and a lateral view was made at that time (D). There was no question about an injury to the sixth vertebra on the right side and somewhat anteriorly. Other films made six months later show increased changes at C5 and C6. This case demonstrates well the need for serial radiographs. (Courtesy of Dr. Jerry Miller.)

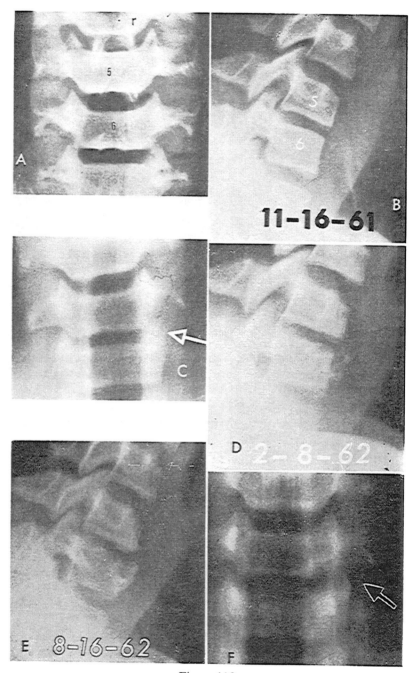

Figure 118

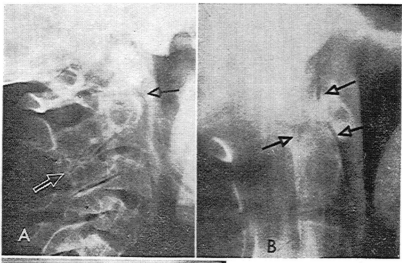

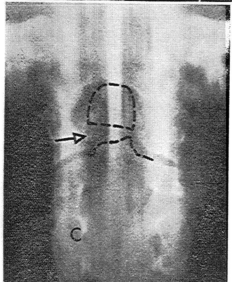

Figure 119. A lateral radiograph of the cervical spine of a seaman who had been injured some ten months previously. This film shows an abnormality of the axis and osteophytic changes at the posterior joints between the third and second vertebrae. It was impossible to obtain visualization of the odontoid process in the anteroposterior projection. Scanigrams revealed a developmental anomaly of the axis with separation of the odontoid process and an unusually large anterior arch of the atlas which articulates with the odontoid process and with the body of the axis. Whenever this man lay down or put his head backward, he experienced severe loss of equilibrium. Cinéradiography revealed definite instability of the odontoid process in flexion and extension. In all reasonable probability, the loss of equilibrium was the result of vertebral artery constriction as the head and first vertebra slipped backward with hyperextension of the head and neck.

MYELOGRAMS

Myelographic studies for diagnostic information in cervical spine disorders are done more or less routinely in many centers. As I have stated previously, and repeat now, myelograms should be reserved for those patients who present symptoms and clinical findings of cord compression or for those patients who have persistent nerve root irritation and who do not respond to *adequate* therapy. Only water soluble contrast material is recommended, i.e. metrazamide (amipaque).

In the cervical area, even a small space-occupying lesion in the vertebral canal may give findings of cord compression, inasmuch as the spinal cord more nearly fills the cervical vertebral canal than in any other part of the spine. Myelography for localization and the extent of the lesion is necessary (Figs. 120-123).

Proper interpretation of the myelograms is of upmost importance. A defect in the column of radiopaque material does not signify a space-occupying lesion necessarily. The effect of head and neck position on the spinal fluid manometrics and on the column of radiopaque material was demonstrated by Kaplan and Kennedy in 1947 when myelography was in its adolescent stage. They showed conclusively that the position of the head and neck during myelography caused blockage of the subarachnoid space, and that such blockage might be interpreted as a space-occupying lesion.

Osteophytic spurs at the posterior margins of the vertebral bodies may produce a defect in the contrast medium which cannot be distinguished from extruded disc material. The clinical findings and the symptoms may be identical. However, the routine radiographs as recommended above should give a clue to the differential diagnosis.

The presence of osteophytic formations at the margins of the lateral interbody joints may give the impression of posterolateral disc extrusions, but it should be noted that the defects in the radiopaque material lie directly over the proximate lateral interbody joints (Fig. 120).

A large unilateral defect may represent extruded disc material just lateral to the midline (Fig. 121), but such a defect may be caused by osteophytic formations at the posterior margins of the lateral interbody joints.

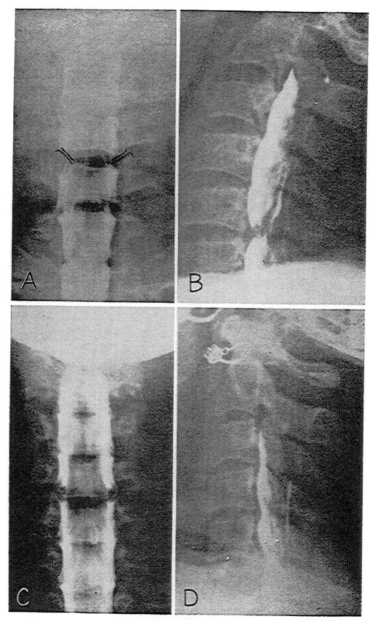

Figure 120. Myelographs of two patients reported as demonstrating a "ruptured disc" at C5 and 6 level bilaterally. The defects are caused by osteophytic spurs at the margins of the lateral interbody joints.

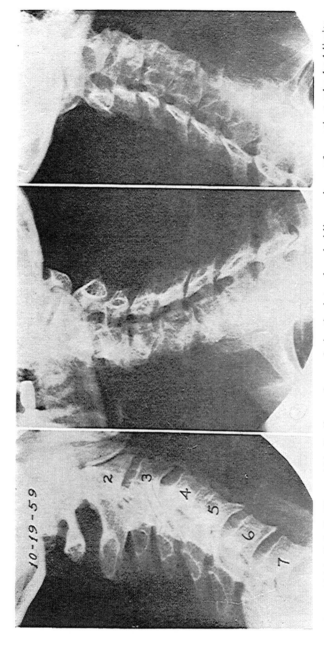

Figure 121A, B & C. Figure 121. Radiographs made in the lateral and oblique views of a patient who had limitation of all neck motion and paresthesias or radicular symptoms which were somewhat disabling. Note narrowed intervertebral canals at various levels and fusion at the fourth and fifth vertebrae.

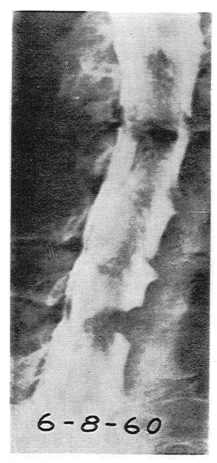

Figure 121D. A myelogram made some six months later revealed a space-occupying lesion at the level of the sixth and seventh interspace, which was on the side of the nerve root irritation.

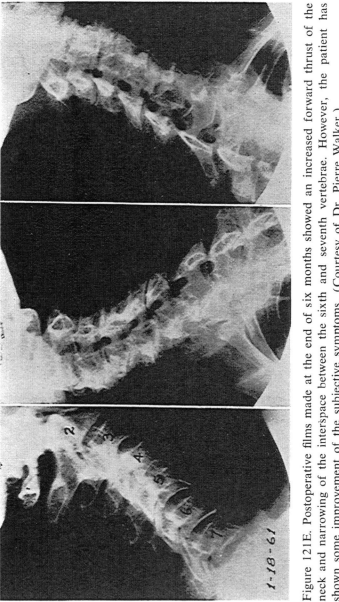

Figure 121E. Postoperative films made at the end of six months showed an increased forward thrust of the neck and narrowing of the interspace between the sixth and seventh vertebrae. However, the patient has shown some improvement of the subjective symptoms. (Courtesy of Dr. Pierre Walker.)

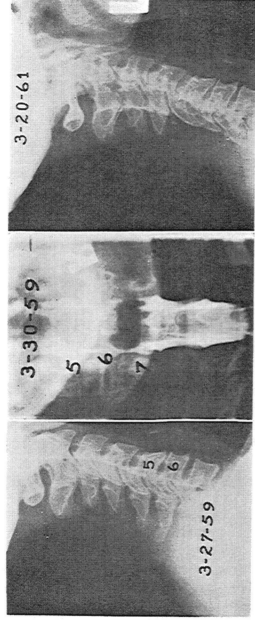

Figure 122. Myelography. The lateral view of the cervical spine shows a loss of the forward curve with some reversal at the fifth to seventh vertebrae and narrowing of the disc between five and six. The myelograph shows a space-occupying lesion at the level of the sixth and seventh vertebrae. Complete laminectomies were done at the fifth, sixth and seventh vertebrae. Two years later, a lateral view reveals the changes which occur following this type surgery when fusion of the vertebrae is not done. The patient was having continued symptoms two years postoperatively.

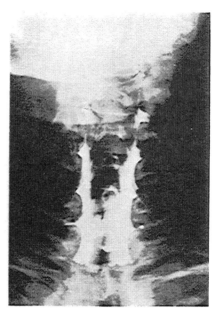

Figure 123. Myelography. The large defect in the column of radiopaque material is indicative of a tumor of the spinal cord. (See Chapter 9, third case.)

A midline defect in the radiopaque column which seems to extend over more than one segment of the spinal canal indicates a tumor of the cord usually (Fig. 123). Multiple defects as seen in the lateral views represent osteophytosis at the vertebral margins or in some instances on the posterior surfaces of the vertebral bodies.

Shapiro states in his book *Myelography* that it is important to appreciate the limitations and pitfalls of myelography if one is to use it intelligently and interpret its results properly. The myelographic finding must be correlated intelligently with the clinical findings for diagnostic accuracy.

The indications for myelography are (1) clinical evidence of a space-occupying lesion producing spinal cord compression, (2) clinical evidence of nerve root and spinal cord compression, (3) radicular or nerve root involvement which is not relieved by *adequate* nonsurgical treatment and which seems to be progressing. Many times myelography is done to ease the doctor's symptoms of impatience and the frustration of not knowing what to do for the patient whose symptoms do not abate with a few so-called conservative measures. However, one should hesitate to inject a contrast medium into the subarachnoid space unless it is absolutely necessary for diagnosis. Myelography is not risk-proof, and it should not be done unless there is definite clinical evidence of a space-occupying lesion. It will be necessary in that event for proper localization of the lesion prior to contemplated surgery. Accurate clinical localization is difficult in many instances.

Myelography is not an absolute answer to diagnostic problems in the cervical area, but it should not be omitted when the indications for it are definite.

It is almost impossible to prevent the radiopaque material from flowing into the recesses of the brain where it remains. It is assumed that this material causes no ill effects if left in the cerebral fluid or in the subarachnoid space. We cannot say that it is innocuous.

DISCOGRAMS

Discography was first done by Lindbolm in Stockholm by injecting a radiopaque material (Diodrast®) into lumbar discs to visualize their internal structures. In this way he was able to correlate the discograms with the clinical symptoms and signs.

Smith, here, and Cloward, in Hawaii, have been responsible for popularizing cervical discography. However, this procedure has not gained wide acceptance and has been condemned by many doctors–some who have used it and some who have not used it.

A normal disc with an intact nucleus pulposus will accept approximately ½ cc of the contrast medium and a radiograph made immediately following the injection will show that the radiopaque material remains within the area of the nucleus pulposus. A degenerated disc will accept more than ½ cc of contrast medium and the radiograph will show that the fluid extends through cracks or crevices within the disc and, if the annulus fibrosus is torn or ruptured, the radiopaque material escapes through the opening or openings, as the case may be, to be visualized in the vertebral canal or extending laterally into the lateral interbody joints or even into the intervertebral canals. These findings indicate disorders of the disc or discs, but they do not prove that disc material has been extruded.

The presence of a degenerated disc as shown by discography does not prove the locus which may be responsible for the symptoms. The reproduction of the pain syndrome as the needle enters the annulus fibrosus and as the injection is done is not a true indication of the location of the lesion causing the symptoms and clinical findings, as claimed by Cloward, who has outlined the pattern of what he calls "discogenic pain." Cloward presumes that the annulus fibrosus is supplied by the recurrent spinal meningeal nerves and that injecting this structure causes pain to be produced along the vertebral border of the scapula. However, as yet we do not know the correct innervation of the anterior longitudinal ligament and of the annulus fibrosus beneath it. In all probability, the nerve supply is derived from the nerves which supply the longus colli and the intertransverse muscles (the third to the eighth cervical nerve roots) following the law of Hilton which states "the nerve supply to joint structures is derived from the nerve supply to the adjacent muscles."

One cannot say that even a small needle placed in an intervertebral disc does no harm to the disc. Inasmuch as several discs are usually injected, the normal disc as well as the degenerated disc, prior to anterior interbody fusion, we may have the answer to the necessity for subsequent fusions above or below the initial area of fusion. Markolf and Morris made openings in the annulus fibrosus of fresh autopsy lumbar discs and subjected them to compressive forces allowing escape of the nuclear material, after which the openings were apparently "sealed off" by the nuclear material to form a "watertight" annulus. Does this occur *in vivo*? As yet, no one can say! Certainly, the value of this procedure is questionable.

The 1964 work of Holt has been very revealing. He performed discography on 148 discs of fifty convicts at the Missouri State Prison. None of the subjects *recalled* a neck injury or had ever had any neck, shoulder or arm pain. Therefore, these men were considered to have *normal* cervical spines. It was found that injection of as little as 0.2 cc of Hypaque® sodium produced great pain in every subject at each space injected. No definite pattern of pain foci could be established with minimal or maximal injections. Extravasation of the material was noted in all but ten of the discs. He concluded that extravasation of contrast media was of no diagnostic value. The claim of so-called discogenic pain reproduction by injecting a "responsible" disc is fallacious.

Needless to say this work has called forth numerous cheers and jeers. One can take it or leave it. I believe that this is an unnecessary so-called diagnostic test to which patients need not be subjected–especially since there may be clefts or crevices extending through some cervical discs and into the lateral interbody joints which cause no symptoms.

The wave of discography will reach its crest and then wane.

ANGIOGRAPHY

The susceptibility of the vertebral arteries to trauma at the time of neck injuries is well known. Encroachment on the arteries by osteophytic formations at the margins of the lateral interbody joints has been found. Certain postural positions of the head and neck may occlude the arteries. Muscle spasm of the suboccipital muscles may cause narrowing or occlusion of these arteries.

The symptoms of the posterior cervical sympathetic syndrome (the Barré syndrome) are due in part at least to occlusion, constant or intermittent, of one or both vertebral arteries.

Patients who do not respond to conservative therapy directed to the neck may require vertebral artery angiography (Figs. 124 and 128).

Roth has been doing cervical analgesic discography for chronic neck pain without disc extrusion, nerve root compression or neurological deficit. He injects 1 cc of lidocaine into the center of the disc and produces relief of pain. This is interesting inasmuch as there are no nerve endings in the intervertebral disc–certainly not in the center of the disc. Many cervical discs have clefts and crevices, and the most logical explanation of the relief, he claims, is that the lidocaine spreads to the posterior and the posterolateral structures, including the posterior joint capsules which are so richly supplied with nerve endings and which are often the source of neck pain.

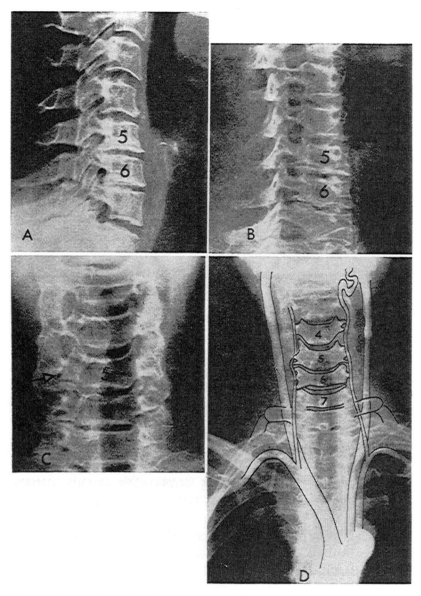

Figure 124. Angiography. Lateral, right oblique and anteroposterior radiographs of the cervical spine of a patient whose main symptoms were pain in the neck and right suprascapular area and intermittent severe loss of balance. Note the narrowed discs at the fifth and sixth and the sixth and seventh vertebrae and the marked osteophytic formations at the margins of the lateral interbody joints. Angiography was done by the consulting neurosurgeon. Constriction of the vertebral artery was found at the third vertebra rather than at the suspected fifth vertebral level. However, there was a constricting effect with positional changes especially at the level of the fifth vertebra.

OTHER RADIOGRAPHIC EXAMINATIONS

Cinéradiography when available may give additional information concerning the movements of the cervical spine and the areas of limited and/or unstable levels of motion resulting from ligamentous and capsular injuries.

Gustafson did cinéradiography on patients who had had injuries of the cervical spine in automobile accidents, and in most instances more than one study was done—one to four. He concluded from his studies that cinéradiography is of value in the diagnosis and prognosis of cervical spine injuries with or without ligamentous instability. The equipment he used reduced the amount of radiation exposure.

Okubo, in an effort to establish the cause of vertigo following cervical spine injuries, has made special studies of the upper cervical spine by means of panoramic tomography or orthopantomography. The advantage of this technique is that two identical parts, right and left, can be photographed on the same plane to give a comparative study of the two sides. Panoramic tomography moves in an orbit which is close to a circle and enables a comparison of the contrasting parts if the sagittal plane of the patient is placed on the x-ray beam axis to the curved circle. This makes it possible to observe thoroughly the joint surfaces and any variation in the intervertebral foramina which he believes cannot be visualized by routine forty-five degree angled oblique views. This, of course, entails special x-ray equipment which is not available usually to most orthopaedists.

Frequently, however, computed myelography may be necessary for accurate diagnosis.

In my experience the routine radiographic examinations which I have suggested gives me reliable information for diagnostic purposes and does not necessitate time-consuming procedures nor undue exposure of the patients to roentgen rays. If the clinical findings and the symptoms do not correspond with, nor can they be explained by, the radiographic findings, then and then only do I recommend other radiographic studies.

Chapter 9

DIFFERENTIAL DIAGNOSIS

IN MOST INSTANCES, pain of some variety is the symptom which prompts the patient to seek medical attention. It is most important that the physician understands the types of pain pathways and the changes induced by their presence. Behan said many years ago—

> Pain has its origin in the violation of nervous habitude and is a beneficent reaction through the nervous system of altered structures or disordered function against threatening forces. Intellect without objective causes may produce pain, which is called subjective pain. Pressure on pain conducting fibers may cause pain, although it is possible that severe pressure, when it is equal and constant, does not cause pain. The more variable the pressure, the greater severity of pain. Shock, anxiety, apprehension lower the pain threshold by causing a disturbance of molecular equilibrium.

Many conditions may appear to mimic the neurologic patterns of cervical nerve root irritation. It is important always to locate the primary source of the symptoms and to correlate them with the objective findings. Differentiation is difficult in many instances, but it is essential for the proper management of the disorder.

A complete discussion of differential diagnosis is not within the scope of this small treatise. However, certain neurologic premises are invaluable aids in diagnosis.

First of all, irritation of nerve root fibers or of the nerve trunk before it divides into anterior and posterior primary rami gives rise to pain and/or sensory deficits and/or decreased reflexes in the upper extremities and/or muscle atrophy or weakness anywhere along the segmental distribution of the nerve root. Sensory nerves of muscles belong to the same segment as the motor nerves. The joint structures derive their nerve supply from the muscles which control the joints. The symptoms and findings are, therefore radicular in distribution. The areas of referred pain are accompanied by *deep tenderness* and localized *muscle spasm* which are determined easily by deep palpation. The pain is deep and boring

248

in character and it is constant usually, although it may be intermittent depending on the variability of the irritation and often on certain movements of the neck. Injection of the painful areas with a local anesthetic will reproduce the pain or intensify it momentarily, and the pain may be referred along the distribution of the nerves to other areas. The pain is relieved immediately and such relief lasts well beyond the period of anesthesia–days, weeks or months. If the injection does not relieve the pain, it has been done incorrectly or there is no nerve root involvement.

Second, disorders of somatic and visceral structures which have cervical nerve root innervation may give rise to pain which is felt or expressed in other areas having the same segmental cervical nerve root supply. However, such areas of pain are not tender on deep palpation, although superficial tenderness may be present. These areas of pain represent *reflexly referred pain* along the segmental distribution of the nerve roots. It is likely that the areas of superficial tenderness represent reflex or direct sympathetic irritation with a resulting expression of peripheral tenderness caused by vasomotor changes, or they may represent irritation of the afferent pain-conducting fibers which accompany the sympathetic fibers. The painful areas are not accompanied by muscle spasm. The pain may vary from a burning sensation to actual cramping, and it is often accompanied by nausea and vomiting, sweating and pallor. The patient has an urge to move and often assumes some unusual or odd position. Sensory and reflex changes do not occur, nor is there any evidence of muscular weakness or atrophy. Injection of a local anesthetic into the painful area does not reproduce the pain nor intensify it, and if any relief of the pain is obtained it is for the duration of the anesthesia only.

Reflexly referred pain and pain of cervical nerve root origin may occur at the same time, which, of course, may confuse the picture. An inflammatory involvement of the capsular structures of the cervical joints, which are supplied by the posterior divisions of the cervical nerves, may give rise to reflexly referred pain along the distribution of the cervical nerve roots. However, involvement of the joints may cause nerve root pressure or irritation because of the close approximation of these structures.

Third, irritation of peripheral nerves or their branches may give rise to pain which may be proximal or distal to the site of the irritation. The painful areas are not tender to deep palpation, except perhaps at the very site of the irritation. Sensory changes may occur distal to the location of the irritation, as is found in the carpal tunnel syndrome and in lesions involving the ulnar nerve at the elbow for instance. There may be motor deficits distal to the site of involvement. Muscle spasm per se is unusual; however, actual contractions of muscles may occur if there is weakness of the opposing muscles.

These three premises should enable one to differentiate between irritation of cervical nerve roots and involvement of their primary anterior and posterior rami or of their branches. For instance, irritation or compression of variable degree of the branches as they leave the cervical foramina to enter the thoracic area should present no real problem, although we hear much about the *thoracic outlet syndrome* as well as the *scalenus anticus syndrome*. Many patients are having their first ribs removed or are having scalenotomies when the real problem actually involves the cervical nerve roots rather than their branches which form the brachial plexus.

The many terms used to describe what may be neurovascular compression resulting from constriction at this area are confusing, whereas a clinical differentiation may be, but should not be, difficult. Conservative treatment without surgical intervention will, in my opinion, give relief.

The fourth consideration for differentiation is involvement of the spinal cord. Pain resulting from lesions of the spinal cord is ill defined and poorly demarcated. It follows no definite nerve root pattern of distribution. Hyperreflexia and hypertonia or spasticity of the muscles are usually found. Pain is increased by coughing, sneezing or straining. Immobilization of the cervical spine does not give relief. Deep tenderness and localized muscle spasm at the painful areas does not occur. Injection of a local anesthetic into the painful areas gives only fleeting relief of pain, if any, which is associated with spinal cord involvement. Paralysis or weakness of muscles which have innervation below the lesion of the spinal cord

DIFFERENTIAL DIAGNOSIS

CLINICAL FINDINGS	IRRITATION OF: NERVE ROOTS (Referred pain)	SOMATIC & VISCERAL STRUCTURES HAVING CNR INNERVATION (Reflexly referred pain)	CERVICAL SPINAL CORD	PERIPHERAL NERVES (Neuritis)
SENSATION	Decreased	No changes or hyperalgesia	Follows no nerve root pattern	Decreased distal to lesion
TENDERNESS (Pain) and MUSCLE SPASM		Superficial, if present	Superficial, if present	Superficial, may be severe
	Deep with M.S.	No M.S.	No M.S. but may be spastic	No M.S. but there may be jt. contract. late
	Relieved by inj. with local anes.	Local inj. relieves temporarily	Local inj. relieves temporarily	Temporary relief
	Cough, sneeze strain does not increase pain	CSS does not incr. pain	CSS increases pain	Pain may be ↑ or ↓ to irritation / No effect
MOTOR CHANGES	Weakness may be present in muscles supplied by CNR	No weakness / No atrophy	Weakness or paralysis may be present & atrophy of arms & legs	Weakness & atrophy present distal to lesion
DEEP REFLEXES	Normal, decreased or absent in arms	No change	Hyperreflexia may be + Babinski	Decreased ⟶ absent distal to lesion
SYMPATHETIC CHANGES	Dilated pupil 30-40% Increased B/P in one arm	No changes	No changes usually- but may be depending on site of lesion	Causalgia distal to lesion at times

Figure 125. Differential diagnosis.

may occur, and usually does. A positive Babinski sign may be present.

The fifth consideration with which the orthopaedist is confronted on occasions is concerned with lesions of the brain, which may give rise to findings similar to those of cervical nerve root irritation, especially if recent trauma has been experienced by the patient. The clinical examination may give few if any clues. The electroencephalogram may be helpful, and angiography may be necessary. Certainly, immobilization, cervical traction and injections of a local anesthetic do not relieve the symptoms.

Comments

A complete physical examination of the patient is imperative. A cursory examination is of no value, may result in a wrong diagnosis or may cause the patient to be subjected to unnecessary and expensive tests which could have been avoided if a thorough physical examination had been done. One should not forget that

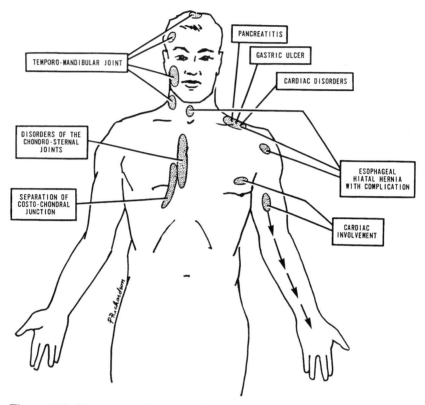

PATTERN OF REFLEXLY REFERRED PAIN
FROM VISCERAL & SOMATIC STRUCTURES

Figure 126. Sites of reflexly referred pain from somatic and visceral structures having cervical nerve root innervation.   ⟶⟶⟶

the simple *procaine test,* as described by Behan in 1914, is of invaluable diagnostic significance.

Figure 125 illustrates in chart form the principal differential diagnostic points for quick reference. Figure 126 illustrates some of the conditions involving the visceral structures which are supplied by the cervical nerve roots and which give rise to reflexly referred pain to areas supplied by the cervical nerve roots.

A few case histories may help to clarify some of the differential diagnostic points.

Case Number One: White male, age sixty-seven, had had excruciat-

PATTERN OF REFLEXLY REFERRED PAIN
FROM VISCERAL & SOMATIC STRUCTURES

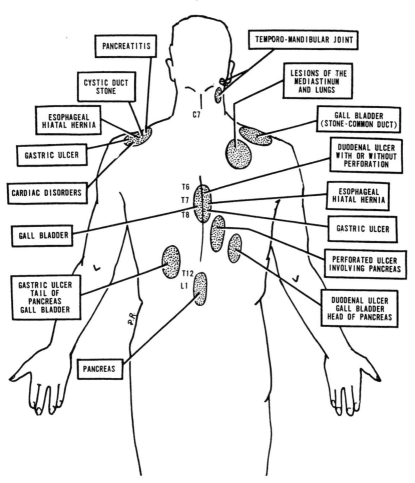

ing pain in the right shoulder and arm of several months duration. He had a marked kyphosis and scoliosis of the upper dorsal vertebrae with marked compensatory hyperextension of the neck and narrowing of the right intervertebral foramen between C4 and 5— an excellent candidate for cervical nerve root irritation. Treatment was directed toward the cervical spine without proper differential diagnosis. Procaine injections gave only temporary relief. Traction gave no appreciable relief. It was then necessary to look for a lesion of a viscera with the same segmental nerve supply. X-ray films of the chest revealed a bronchogenic carcinoma.

Case Number Two: White male, age sixty-five, complained of pain in the left arm which had been present since a fall on the elbow three months previously. He consulted his family physician who made a diagnosis of "muscular soreness." The pain became worse and he consulted a surgeon who sent him to my clinic.

His presenting symptoms were pain in the left elbow and shoulder, pain behind the shoulder and in the left chest anteriorly. Examination revealed evidence of an old abrasion over the tip of the elbow. There was a full range of elbow and shoulder motion. All neck motion was markedly limited. There was marked deep tenderness in the posterior neck muscles on the left side and in the upper rhomboid area. Tenderness over the left sixth rib anteriorly was present. The compression sign was positive on the left side. The reflexes were normal and there were no sensory changes.

X-ray films of the shoulder and elbow were negative. A single lateral view of the cervical spine revealed narrowing of the intervertebral disc between C6 and 7 and calcification of the anterior longitudinal ligament at this level.

There was some irregularity of the posterior articulations of C6 and 7. An anteroposterior view showed definite spur formation at the margins of the lateral interbody joints between C5 and 6 and C6 and 7.

A diagnosis of cervical nerve root irritation, resulting from the thrusting force of the body weight on the elbow at the time of the fall, was made.

Monocaine was injected into the tender rhomboid area. This gave him complete relief of pain in his shoulder and arm. However, the pain in his chest persisted and was always aggravated by hyperextension of the neck.

Two weeks later it was noted that this patient had some difficulty in breathing. An x-ray film of his chest revealed an inoperable bronchogenic carcinoma of the left lung with pleural effusion and pathologic fractures of the fifth and sixth ribs in the anterior axillary line.

This man had pain due to cervical nerve root irritation as well as localized pain at the site of the pathologic fractures and reflexly referred pain from the lung (C3-4-5 nerve roots).

Case Number Three: White male, age thirty-one, had had pain in his neck, shoulders, arms and hands with numbness and tingling of the third and fourth fingers of both hands for four weeks. He had had two injuries to his neck ten and fifteen years previously. He had had one attack of neck, shoulder and arm pain several months previously which had responded to bed rest and traction. His presenting symptoms had come on suddenly as he was going down some steps. They had grown increasingly more severe and were worse at night so that three or four hypos were necessary for him to get any rest. Coughing, sneezing and straining at stool caused aggravation of his pain. He had been hospitalized for cervical traction and had then been fitted with a cervical brace without relief.

Examination revealed that there was marked limitation of all neck motion and that any attempt to move the neck caused severe pain. The posterior neck muscles were somewhat spastic but there were no localized areas of muscle spasm. The biceps reflexes were slightly hyperactive. All other reflexes were normal and there were no definite sensory changes. There was no muscular weakness or atrophy.

X-ray films revealed that there was very little motion in his cervical spine. There was an anterior subluxation of C3 on C4 and a posterior subluxation of C4 on C5.

The severe symptoms and the minimal clinical findings were not indicative of cervical nerve root irritation per se. Procaine injections gave temporary relief.

Myelographic studies revealed an almost complete block at the C4 and 5 level. The spinal fluid examination revealed a protein content of 128 mg.

Neurological consultation was obtained, but due to the absence of positive clinical findings surgery was not recommended at that time.

With further bed rest and traction he improved a great deal and was allowed to return to his home. Two weeks later his pain became so severe that he was hospitalized in his home town and further neurological consultation was obtained there. A laminectomy of C3 to C6 was done and it was found that there was a fusiform enlargement of the cervical cord at C4 and 5. The neurosurgeon stated that he believed this enlargement represented an intramedullary neoplasm, but inasmuch as there were so few neurological findings he did not believe he was justified in opening the dura.

X-radiation therapy was given following the decompression operation and he was allowed to return to work after about two months. He was unable to continue his work, however, and he was then given another series of x-radiation therapy. This man continued to have pain and numbness in his arms and hands. He developed some muscular weakness which was worse following his second series of x-ray treatments. However, within eight months he was able to return to work and twelve years later was having very little difficulty.

Case Number Four: A white male, age sixty-five, complained of pain in his neck and pain in the middorsal area which radiated around his chest wall and abdomen. Complete chest, liver, gallbladder, heart and spine studies had been done six months previously. Apparently nothing abnormal was found, and no treatment was given.

Examination revealed limitation of neck motion in flexion and in lateral bending and rotation. The patient's general posture was poor at that time inasmuch as he was beginning to "slump" with resulting marked hyperextension of his neck. There was pain and superficial and ill-defined tenderness over the spinous processes of the seventh, eighth and ninth dorsal vertebrae. This finding is significant inasmuch as it is characteristic of duodenal ulcer pain. (Sir William Bennett made this observation in 1904.) There was no definite evidence of cervical nerve root irritation at that time.

The straight lateral x-ray film revealed a marked increase in the forward curve of the cervical spine with some posterior subluxation of C4 on C5. The forward flexion view revealed definite anterior subluxation of C4 on C5, C5 on C6 and C6 on C7. The hyperextension view revealed posterior subluxation of C3 on C4 and of C4 on C5.

This patient's pain was not localized but was diffuse over the middorsal area, posterior chest wall and upper abdomen.

A monocaine injection at the level of the seventh, eighth and ninth dorsal vertebrae gave him temporary relief only, as was anticipated. Inasmuch as this patient had had a previous duodenal ulcer, had been on a strict diet and had taken Banthine® he was advised to return to his diet and to the Banthine. At the end of two weeks the pain in his middorsal area, chest and abdomen had disappeared but he was still complaining of some pain in his neck. He was fitted with a shoulder brace to improve his posture. Wearing the brace gave him some relief of his pain. He was advised to get away from the pressure of his business for a vacation. He returned six weeks later at which time he was completely free of pain.

He was not seen again for another six weeks. At that time he returned complaining of pain in his left arm at the insertion of the deltoid and of pain in both wrists. The pain was always worse at night. He was given intermittent cervical traction. He continued to improve over a period of three weeks. He then had severe neck, shoulder and arm pain on the left side which required a narcotic for relief.

On examination it was noted that pressure on the left side of the neck at C5 and 6 caused a reproduction of his pain in his shoulder, arm and hand. A monocaine injection into the posterior muscles of the neck on the left side gave complete relief of pain. However, there was something about the clinical picture which was suggestive of other pathology. He was sent to a cardiologist who found that this man had had a mild cardiac infarction which was believed to have occurred six or eight months previously. Mild congestive heart failure was present and the patient was hospitalized for three weeks. Two weeks later he was rehospitalized and operated on for a perforated duodenal ulcer. Five days later he died, apparently of cardiac failure.

This case well illustrates the importance of differential diagnosis. The patient did have evidence of irritation of the fifth and sixth cervical nerve roots, but this condition was much less significant than his other lesions.

Case Number Five: White male, age thirty-four, was referred by an internist because of persistent and uncontrolled headaches of three years duration. His headache came on very suddenly as he stooped over to pick up something. Several weeks after the onset he consulted his family physician who gave him some medication for the pain. The pain was always aggravated by certain positions or movements of the head and could be relieved by tilting his head forward. The pain was located in the back of his neck and at the base of his skull with radiation behind the ears. Over a period of three years he saw an ophthalmologist, otolaryngologist, an orthopaedist and a neurosurgeon. None of these found any cause for his headaches and he was sent then to a psychiatrist who sent him to a state institution for electroshock therapy. He received seven shock treatments and was then sent home with his headache and with new symptoms of "blackouts" and loss of balance. Later his family doctor sent him to another neurologist with the suggestion that the patient might have a brain tumor. The neurologist told him that "he was crazy" and that he should be sent to an institution. He returned to the hospital for further shock treatment which gave him no relief. Later he consulted an internist who gave him histamine injections. These gave him some relief of his headaches. The internist referred him to my clinic because he thought there might be something wrong with his spine.

The presenting complaints were (1) headaches at the back of head and neck which were worse whenever he attempted to lie down—it was necessary for him to sleep propped up with two or three pillows; (2) loss of balance and inability to walk without assistance; (3) difficulty in swallowing which was more pronounced in the late afternoon; (4) stiffness of his neck; (5) numbness and tingling of the fingers of the right hand especially the little and ring fingers.

This young man was a most pathetic individual. As he sat in the examining room it was noted that his posture was very poor. He sat in a markedly "slumped" position with his neck in marked hyperextension. His face was almost expressionless. He seemed afraid to move.

Examination revealed marked limitation of all neck motion except in hyperextension. However, hyperextension caused pain in his neck and at the back of his head. There was definite tenderness on both sides of the neck posteriorly. All his reflexes were hyperactive except the abdominals which were absent. There was definite hypesthesia along the cutaneous distribution of both axillary nerves and of the fourth and fifth fingers on the right hand. When he stood up he could not walk for a few seconds because he had a sensation of "blacking out" and of loss of balance. As he walked with assistance it was noted that he walked with a wide base or with his feet some distance apart and with each step it looked as if he might fall.

X-ray films of his cervical spine revealed changes which might account for some of his symptoms. It was obvious that this patient needed treatment and encouragement. He was fitted with a shoulder brace in an effort to correct his poor posture. He was given intermittent traction and a felt collar was applied. After the sixth treatment he was greatly improved and his poor posture was corrected. Two weeks after his treatment was started he was able to go to his place of business for two hours each day. He then came in at weekly intervals for intermittent traction and for observation. He and his whole family were greatly encouraged.

At times he continued to complain of difficulty in swallowing and of occasional dizziness when he got up suddenly from a sitting position. Sneezing and coughing seemed to aggravate his pain at all times. His walking improved somewhat. However, inasmuch as his symptoms and clinical findings were suggestive of some other lesion he was hospitalized for myelographic studies, the only clinical test that had not been done. He had been told that he had two compression fractures in his lower back following the shock treatments. However, the x-ray films of his lower back and the myelographic studies were entirely negative for fracture and for any space-occupying lesion in the cervical spine.

He had a stormy time following the myelographic studies with more difficulty in swallowing and more dizziness. After a few days his symptoms subsided somewhat and he was able to return to his place of business for a few hours each day and was able to drive his car for short distances. He was last seen on December 10, 1953 at which time he was feeling much better and was in very good spirits. Three days later his wife called to report that he had a cold and that he was having some difficulty in swallowing. That night he slept very little and was unable to swallow or to take any fluids by mouth.

Early the next morning he sneezed, became cyanotic and expired befor medical aid could be obtained.

An autopsy was done which revealed the following conditions: (1) acute suppurative bronchiolitis, bilateral, with spreading and rapidly developing bronchopneumonia and with resulting generalized acute toxemia and acute myocardial degeneration; (2) persistent lymphoid tissue state, possibly being responsible for generalized lower resistance. The persistence of lymphoid tissue in an abnormal amount was found in the thymus, the thyroid, the spleen and all lymph nodes; (3) cyst of the cerebellar vermis extending into the subarachnoid space and separating the cerebellar hemispheres. The cyst was not recognizable as a specific histologic lesion. There was no evidence of inflammation or of neoplastic disease; (4) constriction of the esophagus immediately below the larynx apparently of congenital origin.

The following symptoms which this patient had could have been explained on the basis of cervical nerve root irritation: headaches, difficulty in swallowing, loss of balance, pain in the neck, numbness and tingling of the fingers, and aggravation of symptoms by hyperextension of the neck. The persistent hyperactive reflexes and staggering gait could not be explained on the basis of irritation of the cervical nerve roots. The encouragement which this patient received rather than the treatment may have been responsible for his improvement until he developed a severe and overwhelming bronchopneumonia against which he lacked the usual resistive forces.

Case Number Six: A female, age forty-one, gave a history of a fall down some stairs one month prior to examination. She could not recall hitting her head. Following the fall, she had difficulty remembering and she had experienced loss of balance. She complained of severe pain at the back of her neck and a feeling of pressure when she coughed. The pain and pressure sensation could be relieved by tilting her head forward and supporting it in this position with her hand. She complained of loss of sensation over the left side of her face and scalp.

The past history revealed that this patient had had no other injuries, the removal of one tube and ovary, no serious illnesses and that she had one child and had had one miscarriage.

Examination revealed that there was ten degrees limitation of lateral bending of the neck to the right side. Rotation to the left was painful. Flexion was limited by ten degrees. Extension was limited and very painful and with the head tilted backward the compression test produced severe pain in the neck. There was tenderness in the right suboccipital area, over the lower joints on the right side and

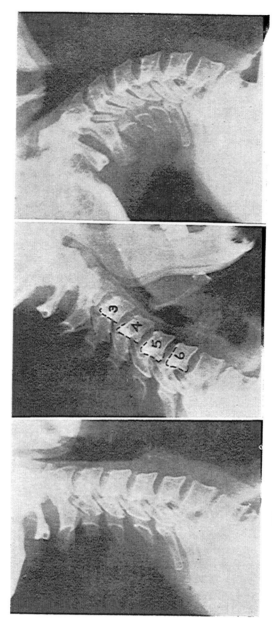

Figure 127A. Radiographs of the cervical spine of the patient described as Case Number Six. There is rather marked ligamentous and capsular instability noted in the forward flexion view.

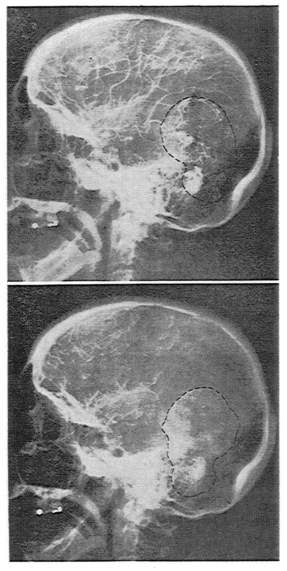

Figure 127B. Angiography revealed a large tumor of the brain as outlined in the skull films.

tenderness and muscle spasm in the suprascapular areas and at the upper and lower rhomboid areas on the left side. There was weakness of grip of the right hand. The reflexes were active and equal. There was decreased sensation over the outer surface of both shoulders, the lateral surface of both arms and the dorsal surface of the left forearm. The circumference of the arms and forearms showed no variation. The blood pressure in the right arm was 136/78 and in the left arm it was 120/78. The left pupil was dilated.

Radiographs of the cervical spine made in the routine lateral projections showed definite ligamentous and capsular instability in the forward flexion view, as noted in Figure 127A.

This patient was hospitalized for cervical traction. A spinal fluid examination was normal. She developed a nonspecific bronchitis. Coughing aggravated the pain in her neck, but this was controlled by medication. An electroencephalogram was done on the fifth day which was suggestive of focal slow activity in the right temporal region while the patient was awake, pointing to focal change in the cerebral cortex. It was recommended that this test be repeated. However, the patient was feeling greatly improved and insisted on going home. One week later she had had no severe pain in her neck or head. However, the patient did not keep her next appointment and the next communication was from Dr. Jack Woolf, neurosurgeon, some five weeks later. He had hospitalized her and had done carotid angiography as shown in Figure 127B. At operation a large meningioma was found to be growing from the tentorium, extending to the undersurface of the temporal and occipital areas and into the cerebellum. The tumor was removed and the patient had an uneventful postoperative course.

This patient did have clinical evidence of cervical nerve root irritation which occurred following a fall. However, the clue to involvement of the central nervous system was the increased pain and sensation of pressure on coughing.

Case Number Seven: Inasmuch as loss of balance or dizziness and nystagmus are frequent symptoms encountered in patients with cervical spine disorders the following case history is of significance in differential diagnosis. A 50-year-old woman was reading in bed with her neck in acute flexion. She noted a stretching discomfort in her neck but continued to read for another hour or so, and when she got to her feet she was extremely dizzy and there was a tendency to fall to one side, as well as marked nystagmus even with her eyes closed, which necessitated prompt reclining. As long as she remained quiet the symptoms subsided (after a few hours) but with movement of her neck nausea occurred, as well as a sense of dizziness. During the next month she wore a collar to prevent movements of her neck during the day and slept in a soft collar at night, which helped curtail her symptoms somewhat.

Because of continued symptoms with movement she consulted a vascular surgeon who made angiograms as shown in Figure 128. Narrowing of the left vertebral artery is clearly visible in Figure C of this series. At the time of the angiography, passive flexion of the head demonstrated suboccipital occlusion of the left vertebral artery.

The patient has had continued symptoms of varying degrees, depending on her activities and the avoidance of undue flexion and sudden movements of the neck. She has had, also, a sensation of "stickiness" in the right eye, some blurring of vision and a tingling sensation in the right cheek which are more prominent with certain activities. Through self-discipline she has learned to control movements of her neck which cause her symptoms. She takes niacin Spansules® and cyclandelate (Cyclospasmol®)—both vasodilators which help control the symptoms, also. She has been able to live a productive life, although her activities have been greatly curtailed.

The past history reveals that this patient did have Mèniére's syndrome some fifteen years prior to the onset of the above related symptoms, which lasted for nine months, but which was relieved with medication, a salt-free diet and rest. With certain activities she did have some momentary dizziness and some suboccipital discomfort. The only injury she recalled was landing on her head when she was doing tumbling. At one time she had had a temporary bilateral compression of the sixth cervical nerve roots which subsided after a few minutes.

This patient does have evidence of cervical nerve root irritation clinically six years after the sudden onset of vascular insufficiency, and one wonders if the fall on the head many years ago might have been the factor causing the atresia of the left vertebral artery or if this is a congenital abnormality.

Radiographs of this patient's cervical spine were made six years later. The odontoid view shows slight rotation of the axis to the left and narrowing of the joint space between the axis and atlas on the right side. Other views show partial calcification of the atlanto-occipital ligament, a loss of the forward curve, slight narrowing of the disc space at C4-5, slight forward slipping of C3 on C4 in flexion, calcification of the anterior longitudinal ligament at C5 and C6, backward slipping of C4 on C5 in hyperextension, foraminal narrowing at C5 and C6 on the left side and at C4 and C5 on the right side.

Certainly this patient does have vertebral artery insufficiency which is always aggravated by flexion of the neck, but she does have clinical evidence of nerve root irritation and radiographic changes, thus presenting complications concerning differential diagnosis.

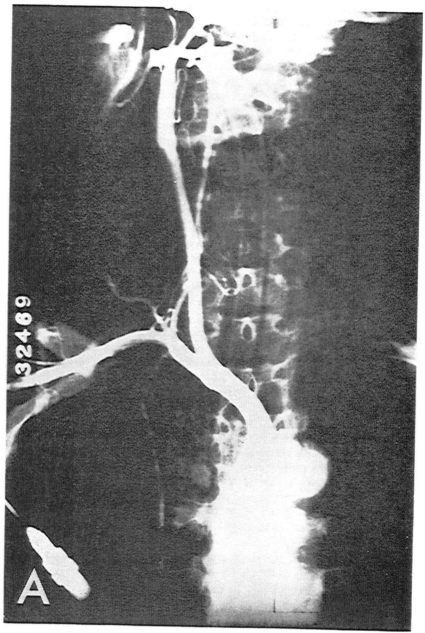

Figure 128A. Angiogram of the right carotid and vertebral arteries. The vertebral artery appears normal in size.

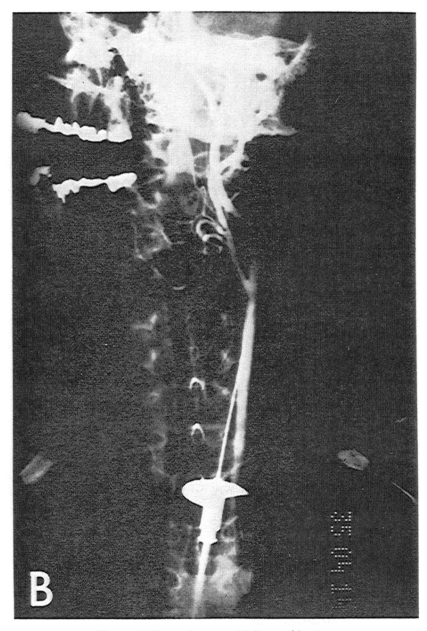

Figure 128B. Angiogram of left carotid artery.

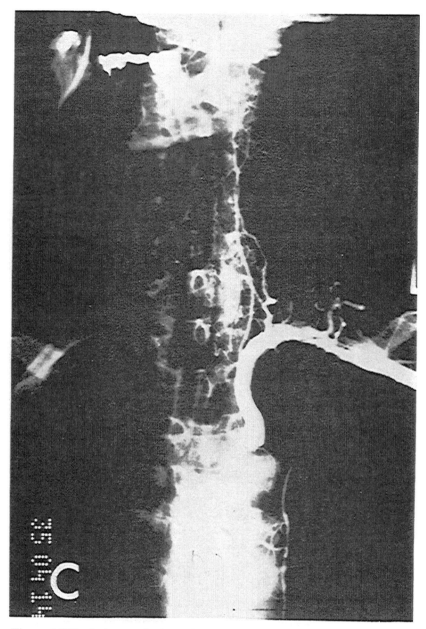

Figure 128C. Left vertebral angiogram shows marked narrowing of the artery throughout its course. Acute flexion of the neck caused a complete block at the suboccipital level.

OTHER CONDITIONS TO CONSIDER

Pancoast tumors or tumors of the superior pulmonary sulcus produce a characteristic group of symptoms and clinical findings which must be differentiated from lesions or disorders of the cervical spine. Pancoast defined such tumors as occurring at a definite location at the thoracic inlet, which produce pain in the areas of distribution of the eighth cervical and the first thoracic nerves.

Paulson states that bronchogenic carcinomas, which occur peripherally in the apex of the lung and invade the superior pulmonary sulcus, are frequently low-grade epidermoid carcinomas which grow slowly and metastasize late. Their location in the confines of the thoracic inlet permits them to invade the lower roots of the brachial plexus, the intercostal nerves, the stellate ganglion, adjacent ribs and vertebrae producing severe pain and a Horner's syndrome. Initially there is localized pain in the shoulder and along the vertebral border of the scapula. Later the pain extends along the ulnar nerve distribution to the elbow and finally to the ulnar surface of the forearm and the little and ring fingers. In some cases the spinal canal and spinal cord may be invaded or compressed, giving rise to symptoms and clinical findings of a spinal cord tumor. Paulson states, also, that pulmonary symptoms rarely constitute the presenting complaint and the patients are usually seen initially by an orthopaedist or neurologist.

In most cases the radiographs show an obvious tumor at the extreme apex of the lung. Certainly the orthopaedist, the neurologist and the neurosurgeon should be cognizant of such tumors and, if suspected, the patient should be referred promptly to a thoracic surgeon.

Temporomandibular joint dysfunction and orofacial pains must be differentiated from pain and muscle spasm which have their origin in the cervical spine. If there is any question concerning the origin of such pain syndromes, the patient should be referred to a dentist who is trained in differentiation and certainly the orthopaedist should be familiar with the publications of Shore and of Bell.

Summary

A differential diagnosis can usually be made if one remembers that irritation or compression of the cervical nerve roots with radiation of pain is accompanied by deep tenderness at the site of the painful areas. There may be segmental areas of deep tenderness that are not painful until palpated, which is further evidence of nerve root involvement. If there is doubt concerning the differential diagnosis, the simple procaine or local anesthetic injection test will dispel that doubt in most instances. Injection of a local anesthetic into myalgic areas which result from cervical nerve root irritation will reproduce momentarily the radicular pattern of pain and then give dramatic relief for days, weeks or months. Injection of a local anesthetic into a painful area where there is no associated tenderness will give fleeting relief of pain in that area and there will be no reproduction of the radicular pain at the time of injection. One should then look elsewhere for the lesion or lesions responsible for the pain. Visceral or somatic structures which have the same segmental nerve supply will be the offenders, in all probability.

These points in differential diagnosis are applicable to those patients who are known malingerers–those who are outright pervericators. The malingerer will deny any relief whatsoever from the injection of a local anesthetic into the alleged painful areas. The absence of muscle spasm, if the malingerer assumes an antalgic position and feigns limitation of motion, should arouse suspicion at least.

These points in differentiation should be useful in distinguishing the real from the exaggerated, also. Some highly emotional individuals who seem to magnify their symptoms are categorized often as psychoneurotics. If a traumatic incident has been experienced, these people are said to have developed a traumatic neurosis, which may be true and which may be very disabling.

The examiner's diagnostic ability and integrity may be questioned if he does not make every effort to establish the pathologic core of the patient's complaints.

Chapter 10

TREATMENT

TREATMENT OF ANY cervical spine disorder must be individualized, and it will depend on the etiology, the symptomatology, the clinical findings and the radiographic findings. Even the busiest physician must take the necessary time to evaluate the patient's complaints and their duration. If recent trauma has occurred, he should determine the mechanism of the injury. The physician must see the patient as a whole and not as "just another patient with a pain in the neck."

In the United States, each year between 55,000 and 57,000 people are killed on our highways and some 5½ million are injured. Should we in our placidity and disconcern consider this a method of preventing overpopulation of our country, or should we as physicians be concerned with ways and means of preventing such astronomical numbers of accidents? As Graffiti said "Don't gamble in traffic–the cars are stacked against you."

During my many years in the private practice of orthopaedics, I have seen more than 8000 patients with cervical spine disorders, and my records reveal that 85 to 90 percent has been the result of *injuries,* either single or multiple and of recent or remote origin.

PREVENTION OF INJURIES

The American Trauma Society was chartered in December of 1971 by twenty-five people who were interested in decreasing accidental deaths and injuries. Most of them had been working since 1966 to create an organization and to gain the support of other organizations to invest time, money and effort to conquer this "neglected disease of modern society–trauma." The American Trauma Society is now supported by many national organizations including The National Safety Council. It is supported also by many of the state safety organizations, insurance companies, automobile manufacturers and many other individuals.

The Stapp Car Crash Conferences sponsored by the Society of

269

Automotive Engineers, the United States Department of Transportation, the Trial Lawyers Association, the Motorcycle Safety Foundation, the Emergency Medical Services Conferences, the American Association of Automotive Medicine, the training programs for the personnel of the emergency ambulances in the proper handling and transportation of the injured, driver educational programs and courses and better protection for sports participants—all give us hope for a decline in injuries and deaths caused by accidents, as well as the socioeconomic benefits that will result.

As physicians we should be concerned especially with the problems involved in the prevention of injuries and deaths. Traffic laws and their enforcement are imperative and will surely help to reduce the injuries and deaths which occur on our streets and highways. Driver education and restrictions are imperative. It is the person behind the steering wheel who is responsible for most accidents and not the failure of the mechanisms of the vehicle he is driving.

The safety engineers of the Liberty Mutual Insurance Company several years ago designed and tested equipment for automobiles which, if properly utilized, would prevent injuries to the driver and the passengers (Fig. 129).

Inasmuch as the greatest percentage of cervical spine injuries occur as a result of rear-end collisions, although statistics may vary because they are not usually reported at the time of the accidents, the car of the future should be a well-padded capsule with proper restraining devices for the head and neck, as well as for the entire body. It should have unhampered visibility, bucket seats and proper head-protective devices for all passengers. The present seating arrangement in most cars provides for three or even four people to ride in each seat which, of course, adds greatly to body contact injuries in the event of a crash accident. The driver must not be crowded to the side of the car and from under the steering wheel if he is to have adequate control of the car—a potential vehicle of destruction. Family or lovers quarrels should not be executed in a car. Roadside parks should be provided for those who wish to make love while traveling.

Recently I saw the driver of a car pushed against the left-hand door by his female passenger who was beating him over the head, obviously in a fit of uncontrollable anger. The driver lost control of the car in his efforts to protect himself. The car hit not one but three other cars as they were waiting for a traffic signal.

My concept of the car of the future is shown in Figure 129D. It is provided with separate compartments for each passenger, an unbreakable heat resistant "bubble" or dome to provide complete visibility, properly positioned and padded head-rests at the rear of the seats and padded areas on the domes placed slightly higher than the head-rests to protect the forehead in the event of a head-on collision, inasmuch as we know the head and body are thrown upward in such an accident. Even proper harness restraints do not prevent lofting of the head and body in severe impacts. This car is provided with an intercommunication system to be used for speaking with the driver or passengers. The steering wheel is a half-round with hand grips at the ends of the half circle, such as is used in most airplanes, to give the driver better control of steering. Many other protective devices are incorporated in this somewhat fantastic, perhaps, car.

Seat or lap belts with shoulder harnesses and head-rests prevent many musculoskeletal injuries, but they do not assure that injury to the neck and/or head will not occur. Any sudden movement of the cervical spine is accompanied by a certain amount of torsion, which is an important factor in injuries of the neck.

The automatic self-inflating air bags have been tested and used in some cars, but there is much controversy concerning their value in the prevention of injuries. Certainly they will never become standard equipment.

Measures to prevent or decrease cervical spine injuries in industry and in sports must be encouraged and publicized.

The traction board used in emergency ambulances will assure, certainly, safer transportation for persons sustaining neck injuries and will prevent further injury by the protection it gives when properly utilized. The patient can be moved from the ambulance to the emergency room without fear of further injury, and radio-

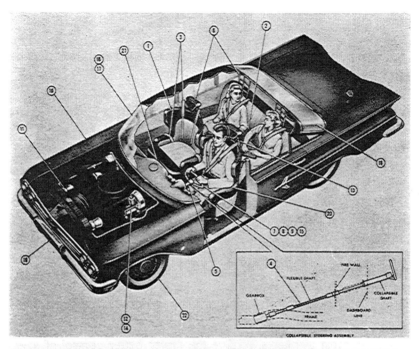

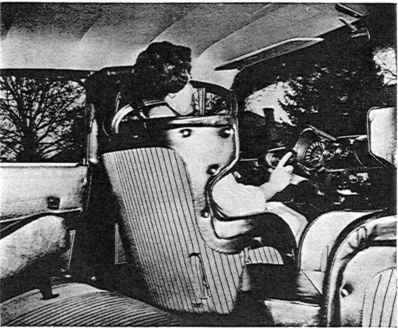

Figure 129A & B

Figure 129A. "Survival Car II." The basic principles of "Packaging the Passenger" which have been incorporated into the design of Liberty Mutual's Survival Car II are the result of more than eight years of research experimentation.

The drawing illustrates twenty-two important design considerations, all calculated to improve driver and passenger safety, increase visibility, reduce potential hazards and injury and conserve life. The numbers 1 through 22 show locations of these features.

(1) Capsule chairs, designed and tied to the floor so that they will restrain the driver and passenger in a 30MPH collision against a 5,000 pound blow and a deceleration force of 30g's in a front, rear or lateral crash. (2) Protection of passengers in rear seat against a 5,000 pound blow. (3) Restraining lap belts and shoulder harnesses on all seats. (4) Flexible steering shaft that will buckle in a crash situation. (5) Steering tube that telescopes a total of eight inches during a crash. (6) Whiplash protection on all seats to retain the head in the event of a rear-end crash. (7) Rectangular steering wheel to prevent breaking or bruising of kneecaps. (8) Steering wheel of reduced diameter for great visibility. (9) Improved maneuverability, faster turning ability and greater driving stability through utilization of special driving wheel. (10) Unit body construction with high energy absorption factor that will collapse and ruin car at moment of severe impact but protect passengers from bodily injury. (11) Automatic fire control system utilizing carbon dioxide. (12) Safety brake device. (13) Roll-over bars in capsule chairs for greater head protection. (14) Power brakes. (15) Power steering. (16) Laminated safety windshield with double-weight filler to afford greater resistance to penetration with no heavier blow upon the head. (17) Saflex interlayer windshield to eliminate 95 percent of ultraviolet rays. (18) Tinting of all glass windows reduces the heat load normally entering the car through the transparent glazing by approximately 30 percent. (19) Reflective license plates for greater visibility at night. (20) Support of arms to reduce driver and passenger fatigue. (21) Alert-O-Matic signal system to awaken driver if he falls asleep or stop the car if he does not awaken. (22) Micro-siping of tires to increase traction and reduce skidding possibilities on wet, icy and snow-covered roads. Additional features are side reflection mirrors for greater driver visibility and smooth hood over engine to reduce injury hazards to pedestrians, if hit. (Courtesy of Liberty Mutual.)

Figure 129B. Shoulder High . . . Specially designed capsule chairs in Liberty Mutual's Survival Car II afford maximum protection for driver and front seat passengers in front, rear, left or right hand crashes. Head rest on both front seats is designed to eliminate "whiplash" injuries in rear-end collisions. Both front seats can be rotated to permit easy access to and exit from the car. (Courtesy of Liberty Mutual.)

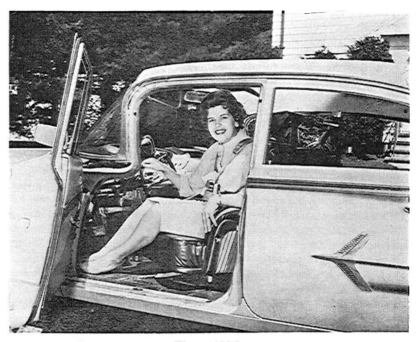

Figure 129C

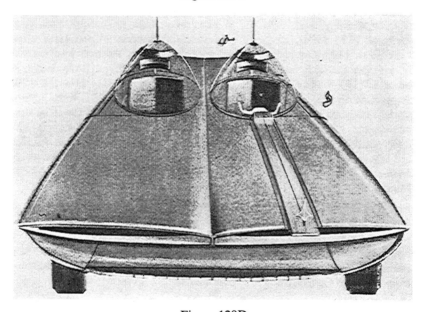

Figure 129D

Figure 129C. Seated in Safety . . . Driver and passengers in Liberty Mutual's Survival Car II all wear seat belts and cross-over shoulder harnesses, one of twenty-four built-in features of the insurance company's car designed to "package the passenger." Both harness and belt are held by an easily releaseable three-way buckle. Car's steering wheel, reduced in size and mounted on a collapsible shaft, permits easier steering and does away with possibility of severe face, chest or abdominal injuries from broken steering wheel or steering column in a head-on crash. (Courtesy of Liberty Mutual.)

Figure 129D. The car of the future.

graphs can be made without moving the patient to determine, to some extent, the seriousness of the injury of the cervical spine.

Every accident victim should have the benefit of a thorough orthopaedic and neurological examination. Many, too many, injured patients seen in the emergency rooms of many hospitals are given a cursory examination and then allowed to go home with one or several prescriptions for pain, muscle relaxation or tranquilizer medications, and advised to see their family doctor if the symptoms are not relieved in a few days. In many instances the symptoms do persist and the patient does consult his regular physician, who tells the patient that he has suffered a "whiplash" injury and that he will recover within a few days or weeks and gives him some other medications and advises him to use heat in some form and to "take it easy." After several visits to the doctor's office because of continued symptoms the patient is advised to see a specialist, and he may land in your office where he hopes to find the answer to his problems. Do not fail him, even if the medicolegal aspects may involve your candid opinion in the courtroom. This is your obligation to the patient who seeks your help, and any third party involvement should not concern you.

In some instances, although the clinical findings may not reveal the extent of the injuries immediately following an accident, it is much better to hospitalize the patient for observation and cervical traction and whatever tests may be indicated until one is certain of the extent of the injuries. To illustrate this contention the following case is of interest. A young man of nineteen was a passen-

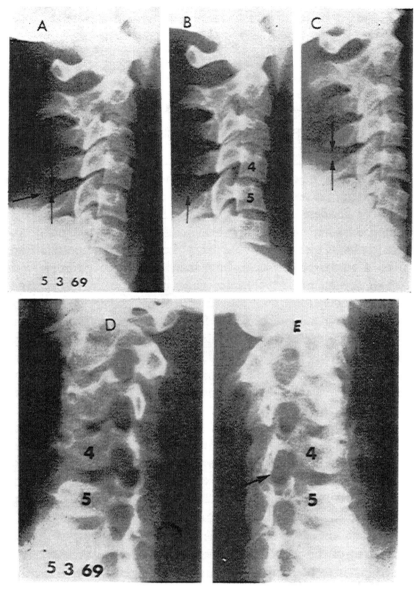

Figure 130. The initial radiographs show separation of the spinous processes of C4 and C5 in all positions and limitation of motion in flexion and extension. Note the posterior angulation at C4-5 on attempted flexion (B). The oblique views show a marked increase in the vertical diameters of the jntervertebral canals and distortion of their contours.

ger in a car which overturned when the driver failed to execute a sudden curve in the highway. He had immediate pain in his neck. He was transported to the nearest hospital where it was found that he had limitation of all neck motion and marked swelling of the soft tissue structures of his neck. Radiographs (Fig. 130) of his cervical spine were made, and he was transferred to another hospital under the care of an orthopaedic surgeon who ordered more radiographs and admitted him to the hospital for two days. Following his discharge from the hospital he was given heat and massage treatments twice each day for four days. He was allowed to return to school, and he was advised to limit his activities and to "take it easy." Eight months later he saw the doctor again because of persistent symptoms. Radiographs at that time showed rather marked malalignment of the fourth and fifth vertebrae.

A few months later he was sent to a neurosurgeon who made more radiographs. No treatment was recommended. Some sixteen months postinjury he was seen in my office, at which time radiographs showed increased displacement of the fourth vertebra on the fifth and sharp posterior angulation at that level.

Three years and twenty-one days postinjury the patient was having continued symptoms of pain in his neck and across his shoulders, aggravated by staying in one position for any length of time, and pain on the ulnar side of his hands. Radiographs made at that time are shown in Figure 131. Early recognition of the extent of this man's injury and the institution of proper treatment would have assured a more satisfactory result.

Another patient, an eighteen-year-old boy, was a passenger in a car which was speeding and which hit the railing of a bridge and was thrown from the car into a rock embankment. He was transported to a nearby hospital by ambulance where he was seen by a doctor in the emergency room. He was then transferred by ambulance to Dallas, a distance of some two hundred miles, where I saw him. Radiographs were made of the cervical spine without moving the patient from the ambulance carriage. Plate 4-1 shows the complete posterior displacement of the body of C5 into the spinal canal and the multiple fractures of the posterior elements. Needless to say, there was complete quadriplegia. Skull traction

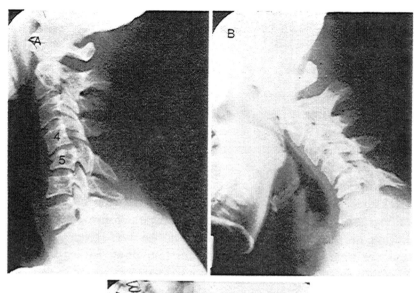

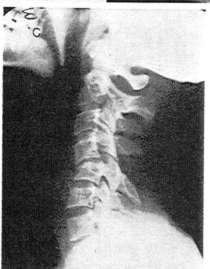

Figure 131

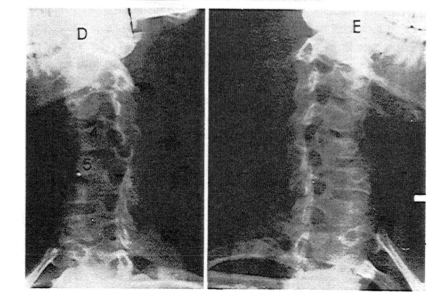

Figure 131. Radiographs made three years-and-twenty-one-days postinjury show increased posterior angulation at C4-5, narrowing of the disc between C4-5, compression of the anterior portion of the body of C5 with osteophytic formation. There is also backward slipping of C3 on C4 and of C5 on C6, as shown in C. Note, also, the much greater separation of the spinous processes of C4 and C5. The oblique views show much more distortion of the intervertebral canals.

←━

---

was instituted immediately; neurosurgical consultation was obtained and it was decided that there was no hope for recovery of the paralysis. The traction was maintained and the patient placed on a turning frame. He lived six months. An autopsy was done which revealed the extent of the injury of his spinal cord and the nerve roots, as shown in Plate 4-2.

It must be remembered that some eight hours had elapsed before he arrived in Dallas and he had been moved several times without the benefit of a traction board. Would more astute handling of this patient from the scene of the accident to his arrival in Dallas have prevented the amount of damage which resulted? Who can say, but certainly one wonders.

The extent of injuries suffered by any accident victim will, of course, determine the proper treatment, and if there is any question concerning the injury or injuries, it is advisable to hospitalize the patient for traction and further observation for at least forty-eight hours.

If there are no fractures and/or dislocations or other gross abnormalities, hospitalization may not be necessary. There are many treatment measures that should be utilized for relief of symptoms and to allow and aid in the healing of injured soft tissue structures, as well as for treatment of most other cervical spine disorders.

TREATMENT MODALITIES (NONSURGICAL)

Treatment should be designed for the relief of the symptoms, the restoration of function of the injured or disordered structures and the avoidance of further injury. It should be based on the severity of the injury, the causative factors and the clinical and radiographic findings.

Whatever the etiology, recent injury or other disorder, the most important part of the treatment is the establishment of a proper rapport between the patient and the physician, which cannot be accomplished by a computer.

Many treatment measures are at our employ. The following should be considered and used when indicated:

1. Heat and/or cold.
2. Massage.
3. Injection of a local anesthetic.
4. Traction.
   a. Motorized intermittent traction.
   b. Hand controlled intermittent traction.
   c. Continuous traction.
   d. Traction for home use.
5. Immobilization.
6. Correction of poor posture.
7. The cervical contour pillow.
8. Drugs.
9. Instructions to patients.
10. Exercises.
11. Manipulation.
12. Psychotherapy.

Heat and/or Cold

Heat is the most frequently used treatment for the relief of pain. It increases the blood supply and relieves some of the ischemia, pain and muscle spasm where applied. However, its prolonged use may aggravate rather than relieve the symptoms. It should be applied at the source of the irritation and is usually more efficacious when applied to the posterior area of the neck. It may be beneficial, however, if applied at the site of maximum pain and tenderness.

Diathermy, either microtherm or inductotherm, is the type of heat which is used most universally in office practice. However, hot moist packs are very gratifying to the patient. The Hydrocollator® affords a convenient method for the use of hot moist packs in office and hospital practices. Many patients prefer this type of heat. Between office treatments the patient should be instructed to use hot packs at home. A large bath towel placed over the neck and shoulders and hot water from a shower allowed to run on the towel for five or ten minutes will often give relief of pain and stiffness. This is a convenient and simple method of application of moist heat which is available to most patients.

Ultrasonic heat has been effective in the treatment of painful conditions, but it should be used with great care and by one who is fully trained in its use. It can do more damage than good if it is used excessively or if it aggravates the pain. Certainly no one can deny its value when used wisely.

In some instances cold packs or ice packs applied at the site of pain give relief. The Chattanooga Pharmical Company has for several years made cold packs which are excellent for the application of cold.

Caution in the use of too much heat or too much cold is advisable to prevent burns which may occur with either. The prolonged use of heat causes peripheral vascular dilation, whereas prolonged cold application causes vascular ischemia. The ethyl chloride spray (cold) is reputed to be of value for some painful conditions, but in my experience it has been most disappointing.

Massage

Massage following the application of heat may be beneficial. Some of the very mild cases may need no other treatment. Even deep pressure over a painful area may relieve localized pain in some instances, and massage will move the inflammatory products to relieve local stagnation and aid in the relaxation of muscle spasm and, to some extent, the pain. The effect is usually transitory but, at least, a welcome interval of relief.

Perhaps massage of the myalgic areas, which has been used for centuries, is comparable to acupressure as described by Cerney, who claims that pressure applied to painful points will give relief of many maladies. It is a "do it yourself version of acupuncture without needles." It may have some psychological merit and possibly some physiological merit inasmuch as we do not know all the pain pathways–who can say with certainty.

The Injection of a Local Anesthetic

The most dramatic relief of pain caused by irritation of the nerve roots is obtained by the injection of a local anesthetic into the painful, tender areas. This is particularly true if localized areas of pain have been present for twenty-four hours or longer. The local anesthetic breaks the pain reflex by paralyzing the pain receptors and conductors. It relieves muscle spasm and ischemia. Its effect may last for days, weeks or months.

The injection should be given at the site or sites of maximum deep tenderness. If the area of maximum tenderness is over the posterior articulations, the injection should be given there. One should be sure that the anesthetic material is placed in the posterior joint structures as well as in the posterior neck muscles. Frequently such an injection will relieve all the radicular pain. It is not necessary nor is it possible except by the anterolateral route to inject the nerve roots themselves.

However, if the point of maximum tenderness is in the supra-scapular muscles or at the superomedial angle of the scapula, the injection may be given in these areas or in any other myalgic area. The most important part of the procedure is the momentary reproduction of the radicular pain as the needle and local anesthetic enter the painful area. *If the pain is not momentarily aggravated*

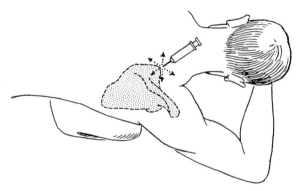

Figure 132. Injection of a local anesthetic in a stellate manner. The patient should be in a prone position with the head resting on the hands and with a folded pillow beneath the chest.

or reproduced the injection will be of little benefit. It *must* reproduce the radicular pain.

The anesthetic should be injected in a stellate manner from the site of maximum tenderness until all pain is relieved (Fig. 132). More than one injection may be necessary, but subsequent injections should not be given at the same site for several days, or until the full value of the original injection has been ascertained. Some residual soreness resulting from the injection may persist for one or two days, which, of course, is of a different character than was the original pain. At times, all the area of tenderness may not be reached, in which event the injection should be repeated after a few days.

It must be remembered, as already stated, that a local anesthetic injected into areas of pain which are reflexly referred from somatic or visceral structures or pain from cord and brain lesions will not reproduce or aggravate the pain and will be of little or no value in relieving such pain.

In some instances it may be necessary or advisable to block the sympathetic ganglia. Usually this procedure is not necessary unless paralysis of the sympathetic control seems essential. This can be done easily by the anterolateral route. Often, the injection will reproduce the radicular pain as the needle and solution enter the adjacent prevertebral muscles, or possibly the anterior primary ramus of the proximate cervical nerve.

The choice of the type of local anesthetic to be used should be considered. Procaine has been used more universally than any other local anesthetic. However, many patients have severe reactions following injections of this solution. During the past several years the author has used only *carbocaine* solutions and has had no undesirable reactions. The so-called long-lasting anesthetic agents and those with an oil base should not be used.

Certain precautions should be used to prevent the possibility of an undesirable reaction. The patient should be given a barbiturate fifteen or twenty minutes prior to the use of a local anesthetic. A 0.5% solution should be used rather than the usual 1.0, 1.5 or 2% solutions. Greater quantities of a 0.5% solution can be used without fear or trepidation. The inadvertent injection of a 0.5% solution into the blood stream or the spinal canal will not be disastrous, whereas a stronger solution might prove fatal. The injection should be done with the patient lying prone rather than in the upright position. An injectable barbiturate should be available in the event a severe reaction does occur. If, however, the reaction should be of the depressant type, a stimulant drug should be available. If there is any history of a previous sensitivity to a local anesthetic, a skin test should be made.

Traction

Traction has been used in the treatment of neck disorders for many decades. It may be employed as continuous traction or as intermittent traction.

Continuous traction assures a certain amount of immobilization of the cervical spine and relieves muscle spasm and pain. If correctly applied, it straightens the cervical spine and enlarges the intervertebral foramina (Fig. 134) to relieve compressive or irritative forces upon the nerve roots. We have demonstrated this by cinéradiography. However, the conventional method of continuous traction by a headhalter is not well tolerated because of the discomfort to the chin and lower jaw. The conventional amount of weight of five to ten pounds does nothing more than partially lift the weight of the head from the neck and keep the patient still to some extent. Fifteen to twenty pounds of traction is required to produce any distraction of the vertebrae.

Skull traction with head tongs is the most effective means of obtaining and maintaining constant traction, and any amount of weight up to forty or fifty pounds is well tolerated by the patient. However, this type traction is reserved for certain fracture-dislocation cases, usually, and requires hospitalization.

The use of motorized intermittent traction is supplanting all other methods of traction application except, of course, skeletal or skull traction when indicated. Intermittent traction relieves muscle spasm. It has a massagelike effect upon the muscles and the ligamentous and capsular structures. It reduces swelling and promotes better circulation in the tissues, thereby helping to quell the inflammatory reaction. It prevents the formation of adhesions between the dural sleeves of the nerve roots and the adjacent capsular structures. In some instances it may free the adhesions. In some chronic cases where adhesions have been present for some time, it may aggravate the symptoms of nerve root irritation because of the tug it places upon the adherent dural sleeves of the nerve roots.

Motorized Intermittent Traction

The most advantageous intermittent traction is that which can be controlled in the amount and in the duration and that which gives the maximum amount of traction with the minimum amount of discomfort to the patient's chin and jaw. This can be accomplished with motor operated apparatus. Numerous machines have been designed and manufactured since Griffith originated the idea some thirty years ago. Figure 133 illustrates the Tractolator® and the Tru-trac® machines. Anyone who treats cervical spine disorders should utilize motorized intermittent traction. Most machines cost less than a forty horse-power outboard motor. The units are adapted especially for office use and require a miminum amount of floor space.

J. E. Miller, M.D., Radiologist, and I have done cinéradiographic studies of the cervical spines of several patients during treatment with motorized intermittent traction. Ten to fifteen pounds of traction, as indicated on the scale of the machine, lifts the weight of the head from the neck but produces no visible distraction of the vertebrae. Twenty to twenty-five pounds of pull does produce visible distraction of the vertebrae and increases the size of the intervertebral foramina which can be demonstrated in the oblique position. With thirty-five pounds of pull, separation is still more marked, and the normal forward curve is completely straightened or reversed (Fig. 134).

Patients with postinjury and degenerative changes in the cervical spine show little or no actual distraction of the involved vertebrae. This is due to the thickening and fibrosis of ligamentous and capsular structures (Fig. 135). However, these patients do receive relief of symptoms, and traction should not be denied them.

Treatments should begin with fifteen to twenty pounds of traction and the pull gradually increased to thirty-five or forty pounds over a period of several treatments. Some heavy-muscled patients may require as much as fifty pounds of traction.

Judovich recommended injection of the anterior scalenus muscle with procaine immediately prior to the application of cervical intermittent traction, which I have not utilized as a routine mea-

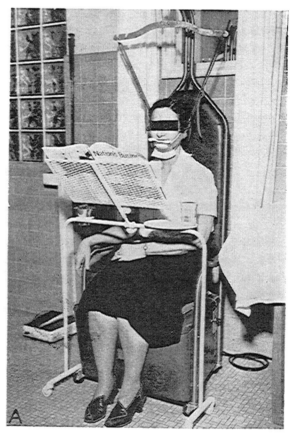

Figure 133A. Motorized intermittent traction (Tractolator), chair unit.

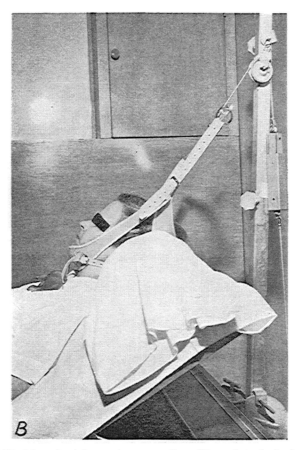

Figure 133B. Motorized intermittent traction (Tractolator), bed unit setup for office use. Patient is in a semi-jack-knife position for maximum comfort.

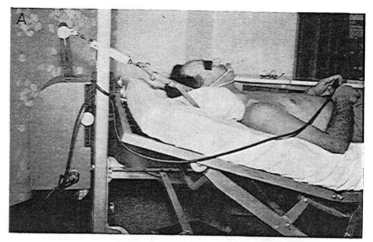

Figure 133C. Motorized intermittent traction, bed model.

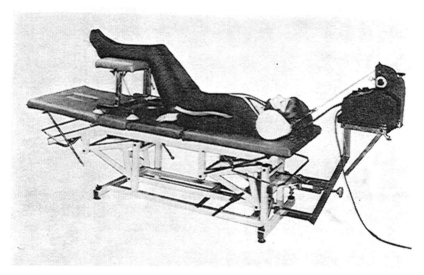

Figure 133D. Motorized intermittent cervical traction. Note the angle of
the pull, flexion of the hips, the Hydrocollator contoured hot pack, the
Cervipillo®. (The Tru-trac traction machine used on the variable-height
treatment-traction table.)

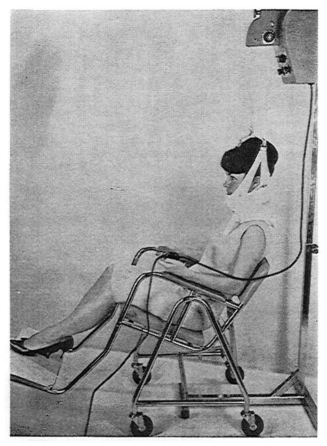

Figure 133E. Motorized intermittent traction. The chair is adjustable so that some forward pull is possible as illustrated, or the chair may be brought to the straight position if desired (Tru-trac).

sure. It may be necessary in selected cases where there is marked spasm of the scalene muscles, or in patients whose straight lateral films show marked reversal of the normal forward curve of the cervical spine, or in a patient whose radial pulse is obliterated when the arm is elevated.

Injection of other myalgic areas may be necessary prior to the administration of motorized intermittent traction. This should be determined by the severity and duration of the symptoms.

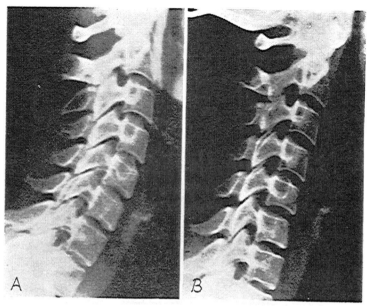

Figure 134. Radiographs of a cervical spine without traction is shown in A, and with thirty-five pounds of traction in B. With thirty-five pounds of pull the cervical spine is straightened and there is visible distraction of the vertebrae. The size of the intervertebral canals is definitely increased.

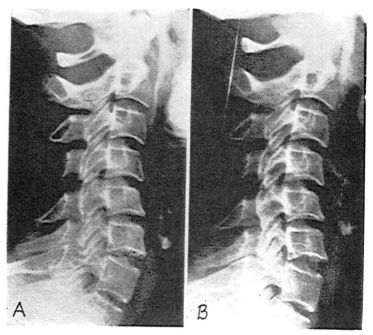

Figure 135. A straight lateral view of a cervical spine which had been in-jured ten months previously is shown in A. Note the reversal of the forward curve. Thirty-five pounds of traction produces very little distraction of the vertebrae and the reversed curve is slightly increased as shown in B. This is due to the thickening of the ligamentous and capsular structures and to their decreased elasticity, which follow sprain injuries.

Treatment schedules will vary somewhat for each individual. Some patients may require daily treatments for a week or two, after which the treatments should be given two or three times per week. As the symptoms decrease the treatments can be spaced farther apart unless the patient experiences an exacerbation of symptoms, in which event more frequent treatments may be necessary.

Hand-controlled Intermittent Traction

A type of intermittent traction which is hand controlled has been used in office practice. The patient is placed in a chair beneath a pulley on a hook in the ceiling. A head halter is applied to the patient. A rope is attached to the spreader of the halter and

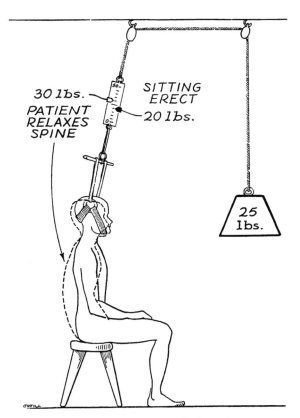

Figure 136. Hand-controlled traction.

placed through the pulley then through a second pulley which is placed in the ceiling twelve to twenty-four inches away. Weights may then be attached to the end of the rope for traction (Fig. 136). An assistant can lift or raise the weights at desired intervals. This is a rather crude method of intermittent traction application, but it can be used if no other method is available.

A few words of caution in the use of this apparatus is indicated. Inasmuch as the amount of pull varies with the friction of the ropes on the pulleys and the position of the patient, a scale to measure the amount of pull should be placed between the patient and first pulley (Fig. 136). The friction of the rope on the pulleys will alter the amount of actual traction so that twenty pounds of weight at the end of the rope will produce approximately fifteen pounds of traction. However, if the patient slumps or slides down in the chair the actual pull may be increased to twenty-five or thirty pounds without altering the position of the weights.

It is not advisable to use more than twenty pounds of weight with this type traction. Fifty pounds of weight has caused severe ligamentous and cord damage. It is unnecessary and dangerous to use that amount of traction. This traction should be used with the pulleys placed in front of the patient to assure a slightly forward direction of the pull.

Continuous Traction

If motorized intermittent traction is not available or if continuous traction is indicated, the patient should be hospitalized. This type traction requires constant supervision and its correct application is important. The direction of the pull should be in a straight line with the neck or above the neck so that the cervical spine is straightened or placed in slight flexion. The patient should be in a jackknife position for complete relaxation, and a cervical contour pillow should be placed beneath the neck (Fig. 137). A patient placed flat on a bed with traction applied to the neck suffers a great deal of abdominal distress but in the jackknife position this does not occur. If the traction is applied with the neck in hyperextension, the pain will usually be aggravated unless there are specific indications for hyperextension.

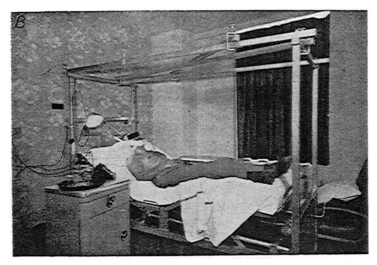

Figure 137. Continuous bed traction. Patient is in the semi-jack-knife position for maximum comfort.

The amount of weight should vary with the individual's tolerance. Most patients can tolerate eight to ten pounds of constant traction without too much discomfort from the head halter. If halter traction causes too much discomfort it may be necessary to use head tongs for skeletal traction.

It is important that the patient be sedated for twenty-four to forty-eight hours so that the maximum effects of the traction will be realized. As the symptoms subside the amount of weight may be reduced and then removed for short periods. The correct collar immobilization should be used when the patient is allowed to be ambulatory.

Traction for Use in the Home

It may be advisable to permit the patient to use traction at home. Many simple units are available for use on doors and on beds. The simpler the units the more likely they will be used. Specific instructions for the proper utilization of such units should be given and the doctor or a capable assistant should make certain that the patient understands thoroughly how and when the traction is to be used as well as the correct amount of weight or pull necessary. The patient should never be handed a traction appara- tus with the expectation that he will be able to use it properly and that he will be elated with the results when he returns for his next examination, if he returns at all.

Most on-the-door packaged units contain printed instructions which are often difficult to decipher. Many of them contain illus- trations which show the model with his back to the door. This position is incorrect. The patient should *face* the door and should

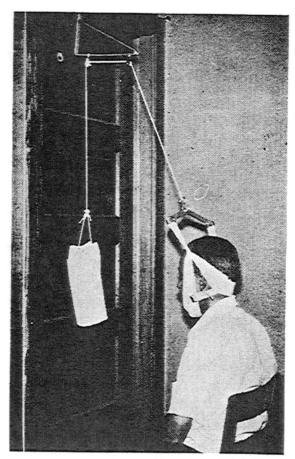

Figure 138A. On-the-door traction, which the patients can use at home.

sit in line with the first pulley but not directly under it. The line of pull should be forward at approximately twenty degrees, as shown in Figure 138.

The initial amount of pull or weight should be fifteen pounds and should be increased gradually to twenty and thirty pounds. The patient should sit in a straight chair with arm rests, and the traction should be used for fifteen to twenty minutes. It is

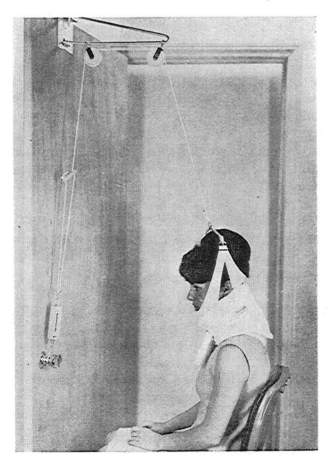

Figure 138B. On-the-door traction for home use (Tru-eze Model). The scale indicates the amount of pull, which the patient can see and adjust. The Hydrocollator pack supplies heat during traction and is recommended for home use.

much more advantageous to use the maximum pull for short periods than to use a small amount of weight for longer periods. We must not forget that ten to fifteen pounds of pull only lifts the head from the neck and does not effect any appreciable traction on the neck itself. The traction can be made intermittent by raising the weight for short periods.

Lead or iron weights, sandbags and waterbags are difficult to handle without assistance. Therefore, a scale placed in the down-rope with a hook for securing it to the doorknob makes it possible to dispense with the cumbersome weights, as shown in Figure 138B. With this arrangement the patient can make the traction intermittent by leaning forward, which releases the pull, and then by assuming the original position the pull is in force again, and in the prescribed amount.

There are no contraindications to cervical traction if it is properly used. In rare instances it may aggravate the sumptoms at first. Patients who have had previous injuries to the lower back may experience pain in that area when receiving cervical traction. This is due to an adherent dura or to an adherent dural sleeve of a nerve root at that level.

Correctly controlled motorized intermittent traction in my experience has given the best results and has reduced greatly the need for hospitalization.

Comments: A few words about head halters and their proper use are in order at this point. Many varieties are available. The most satisfactory halter is one which does not require a strap to join the occiput and chin pieces. If a strap is necessary, it should be placed near the angle of the mandible so that no pressure is applied to the carotid arteries, and not at the carotid sinus certainly. Such pressure from the straps may never occur when traction is given to the thin-necked patients, but the pressure which occurs on the soft tissue structures of a thick-necked person may produce sudden syncope, which if noted promptly may be not too hazardous—but certainly frightening.

The halters illustrated in Figure 138 are recommended, although there may be others of equal safety and comfort. The ideal halter is one which produces minimum pressure to the chin and maximum pull on the back of the head.

During traction, the patient should be instructed to keep the teeth apart to prevent uncomfortable pressure on the temporo-mandibular joints and on the teeth themselves.

Rotation of the head during traction should be avoided. Why? Rotation of the head during traction causes tightening of the guy ligaments at the atlantoaxial level on one side and relaxation of these ligaments on the other side. A pull on the taut ligaments, and capsules too, may cause undue stretching of these structures and produce a traumatic inflammatory reaction and increased symptoms. Gentle, constant or rhythmic traction on all the soft tissue structures will relieve pain and muscle spasm and will help dissipate the inflammation.

Immobilization

Immobilization of the cervical spine with a proper brace or collar is essential in the treatment of acute injuries and often for chronic conditions. Collars or braces should be designed to hold the neck in the optimum position for healing of the injured skeletal, ligamentous and capsular structures. This position must be with the neck straight and the chin "tucked in." Braces which hold the neck in hyperextension are completely wrong in principle and should not be used for the treatment of sprain injuries unless there is definite disruption of the posterior ligaments (Fig. 139). Immobilization in hyperextension causes further stretching of the anterior longitudinal ligament and allows the posterior ligamentous structures to heal in a shortened position and causes narrowing of the intervertebral canals, especially if there is ligamentous and capsular instability.

Also, we should be cognizant of the joint changes induced by immobilization in hyperextension. Compressive forces on the articular cartilage of joints may result in fibrillation of the cartilage which is subjected to prolonged pressure. In hyperextension, the posterior portion of the capsules and the posterior ligamentous structures results in shortening of these tissues. If the anterior structures are traumatized, stretched or sprained as is the case often, they heal in the extended position resulting in anterior instability. Therefore, the optimum position of immobilization is with all the structures relaxed, which is the same principle we fol-

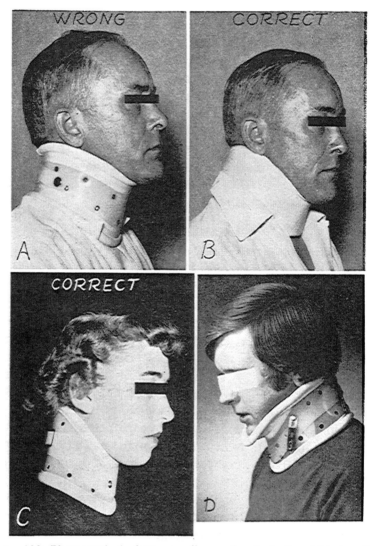

Figure 139. Photograph A shows a collar made of plastic which is adjust-able and which is used frequently in the treatment of sprain injuries of the neck. This collar gives good immobilization but is much too high in front and causes hyperextension of the neck. The collar in B is made of felt. It keeps the neck straight and gives adequate immobilization in most in-stances. The collar in C is made of plastic, it is adjustable and it prevents hyperextension of the neck. The plastic collar in D has adjustments and a chin rest for better immobilization. (C & D are made by the Florida Mfg. Corp.)

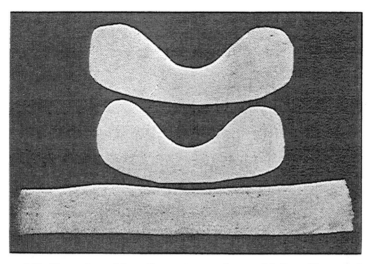

Figure 140. To make a felt collar, cut two pieces of felt as illustrated, and one piece of four-inch Stockinet. Place the smaller piece on the larger piece and pull both pieces through the stockinet. The ends of the stockinet can be secured by safety pins or clips when the collar is applied, as shown in Figure 139B. This collar is adequate and gives sufficient immobilization for most sprain injuries of the neck.

low in the treatment of other joint injuries and disorders. Furthermore, the position of hyperextension decreases the anteroposterior and the vertical diameters of the intervertebral canals to crowd the nerve roots and give rise to radicular symptoms.

Those who insist on collars or braces which hold the head and neck backward would be somewhat amazed at the relief obtained by changing to a straight or chin-tucked-in position, which is physiologically, mechanically and comfortably the position of choice in most instances.

In my clinic we have made radiographs of the cervical spines of patients wearing collars which hold their necks in hyperextension and whose symptoms were aggravated or prolonged by these collars. Next we made radiographs of the same patients wearing collars which held their necks in the straight position and who had relief of symptoms by use of these collars. This has been true in those with acute symptoms following injuries and in those with chronic symptoms.

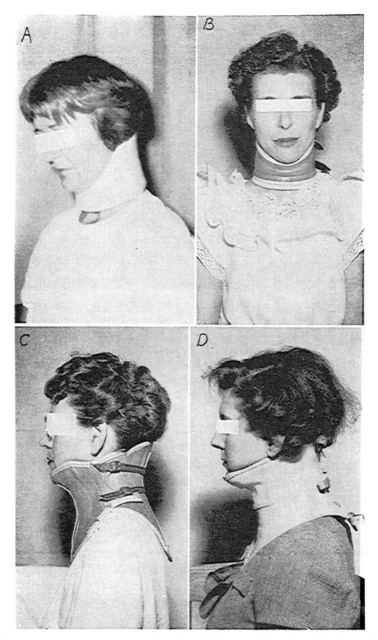

Figure 141. Collars for immobilization of the cervical spine. The Tru-*FLEX* felt collar covered with stockinet is shown in A. Collar made of sponge rubber and covered with soft white leather which is reinforced with a piece of stiff leather is shown in B. The collar in C is a molded leather collar which is made in two parts, and the collar in D is made of elastic.

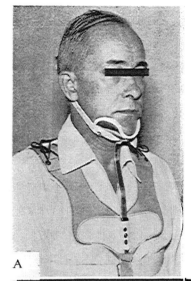

Figure 142A. The Miller neck brace, which is an excellent support when rigid immobilization is indicated.

Figure 142B & C. This brace is made in two pieces and is adjustable. It is of minimum weight and affords adequate immobilization for treatment of many cervical spine disorders.

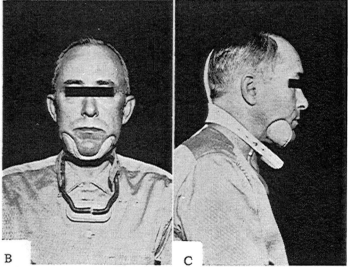

The illustrations shown in Figure 143 support my contention that hyperextension collars or braces are contraindicated in the treatment of most neck injuries and disorders. Patients with acute fractures of the articular facets, with marked compression fractures of the vertebral bodies and those who have suffered marked disruption of the posterior ligamentous structures may require

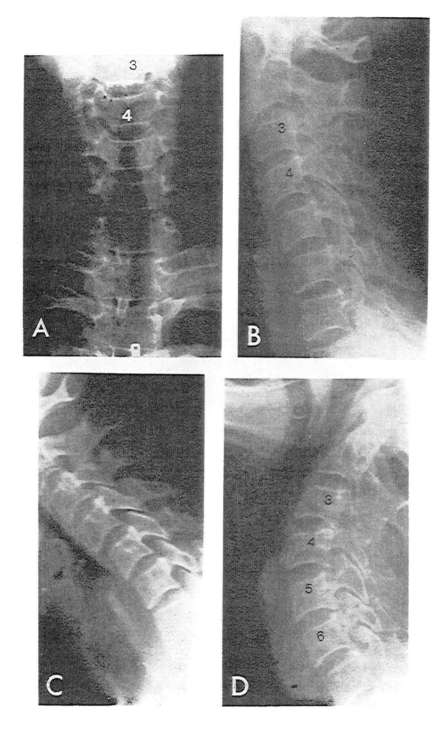

←‑‑‑

Figure 143A. Anteroposterior radiograph of the cervical spine of woman, age forty, who was involved in a rear-end collision twelve years previously. She received heat and massage treatments for one year but had continued right-sided intermittent symptoms which were aggravated by hyperextension of the neck. Note the changes at the lateral interbody joints at C3-4 and rotation of C3 to the right side.

Figure 143B. Lateral view shows straightening of the forward curve, osteophytic changes at the posterolateral aspect of C3 vertebral body and narrowing of the disc space at C3-4.

Figure 143C. Lateral flexion view showing narrowed intervertebral canal at C3-4 and slight forward slipping of C4 on C5 and of C5 on C6.

Figure 143D. Hyperextension lateral view showing backward slipping of C3 on C4, C4 on C5 and long kissing spinous processes of C3-4-5.

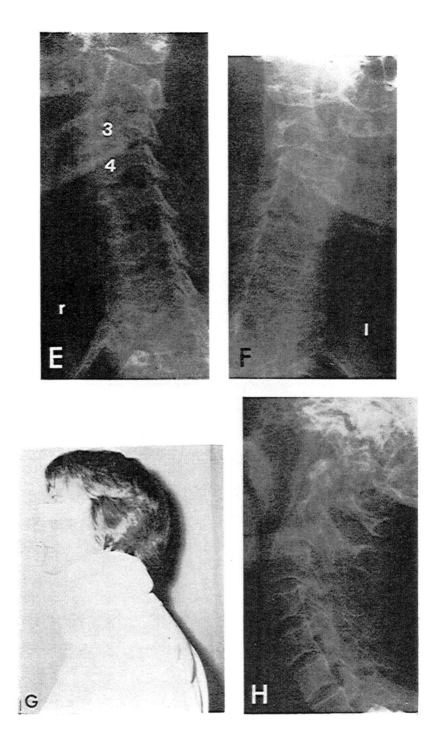

←⋘

Figure 143E. Right oblique view which shows narrowing of the intervertebral canal at C3-4.

Figure 143F. Left oblique view showing no narrowing of the intervertebral canal at C3-4.

Figure 143G & H. Photograph of patient wearing a plastic hyperextension collar and a lateral radiograph which shows backward slipping of C3 on C4 and of C4 on C5.

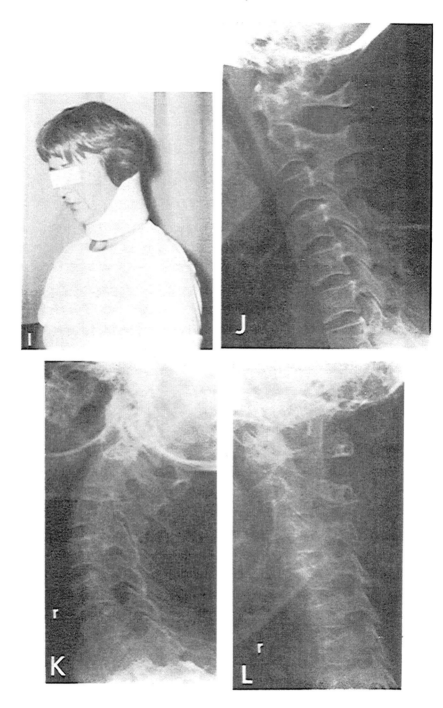

←▦

Figure 143I & J. Photograph of patient wearing a Tru-*FLEX* felt collar and a lateral radiograph which shows no forward curve and is comparable to B which is nature's way of protecting the nerve roots by enlarging the intervertebral canals and relieving undue pressure on the joint structures.

Figure 143K. Right oblique radiograph made with the patient wearing the hyperextension collar. There is marked narrowing of the canal at C3-4 and overriding of the facets at C4-5 and C5-6.

Figure 143L. Right oblique radiograph made with the patient wearing the Tru-*FLEX* collar. Note minimal narrowing of the canal at C3-4.

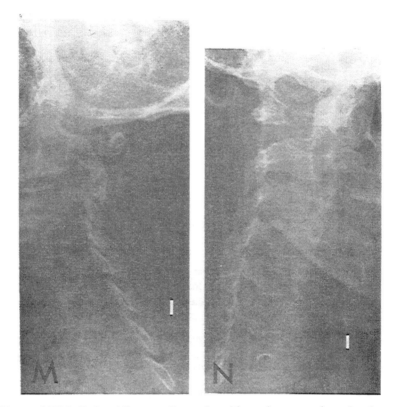

Figure 143M. Left oblique radiograph with patient wearing the hyper-extension collar. There is narrowing of the canal at C3-4, and patient had left-sided symptoms following the making of the photographs and radiographs with the neck in hyperextension.

Figure 143N. Left oblique radiograph made with the patient wearing the Tru-*FLEX* collar. There is no narrowing of the canal at C3-4, and the patient's symptoms were relieved.

bracing the neck in hyperextension. In some instances where complete immobilization of the cervical spine is indicated, the Halo-cast may be necessary.

In acute injuries immobilization should be continued for three to eight, or more, weeks, or until the sprained or fractured structures have healed. Chronic cases may need immobilization only for short intervals.

If it is necessary to apply a collar or brace for immobilization its use should be continued until the symptoms have subsided and then it should be discontinued gradually at short intervals until the patient learns to adjust his activities to his neck or his neck to his activities.

Some of the collars and braces which I have used are shown in Figures 139, 140, 141, 142 and 143. The degree of immobilization needed will determine the type collar to be used.

Posture Correction

Correction of poor posture and of poor postural habits is of utmost importance in the treatment program, and all corrective measures should be directed toward straightening the cervical spine. Drooping of the shoulders, which causes a compensatory hyperextension of the neck, can usually be corrected by the use of some type shoulder brace (Fig. 144). The brace should be worn until the patient becomes posture conscious and is able to hold the shoulders up and back without the assistance or reminder of any restrictive brace. When the correct position of the shoulders is maintained the cervical spine is held in a more normal relation-

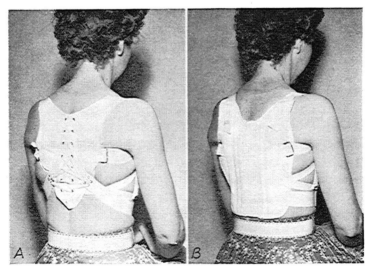

Figure 144. Shoulder braces to correct round shoulders and, hence, to straighten the cervical spine.

ship and hyperextension of the neck is obliterated. This position does not obstruct the so-called cervicothoracic outlet.

In some instances shoulder braces will relieve the pain associated with cervical nerve root irritation and no other treatment may be needed.

Many individuals sit, stand and walk as if they were falling apart, or as if they were too tired or too lazy to maintain any semblance of correct postural attitudes. However, with persistence on the part of the doctor these poor postural habits can be corrected. Corrective exercises may be necessary but the most essential corrective measure is the determination of the patient to help himself. Braces and supports for posture improvement are only crutches. They should be used intelligently and discontinued as soon as possible.

The Cervical Contour Pillow

Inasmuch as many patients complain of increased pain and discomfort at night, the correction of poor sleeping posture should be considered in all instances. Many people sleep on one or more pillows which causes prolonged flexion of the neck and aggravation of pain. Sleeping without any pillow aggravates the symptoms. Some patients think they cannot sleep unless they are in the prone position. This keeps the neck rotated and laterally bent for long periods.

By a process of trial and error, the Cervical Contour Pillow* was developed (Fig. 145). This pillow is eighteen inches long, and eight inches in diameter. It should be stuffed with feathers and down or with dacron as are the current ones. It is smaller in the center than at its ends so that the neck rests on the proper amount of support for comfort. This leaves a bulge on either side which prevents too much rotation and lateral bending. If the patient sleeps on his side the bulge at either end gives adequate support to assure comfort and to keep the neck straight.

Lateral radiographs of the cervical spine made without any pillow under the neck, with a regular pillow beneath the head and

---

* The Cervipillo® (TRU-EZE Mfg. Co., Inc.).

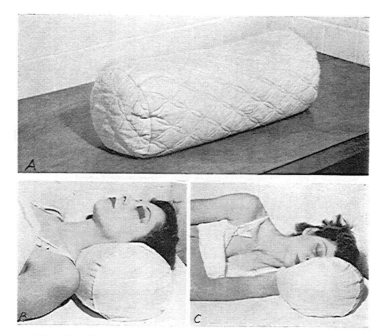

Figure 145. The Cervical Contour Pillow (Cervipillo®). Designed by me for correct sleeping posture.

with the neck upon a Cervical Contour Pillow illustrate well the advantage of this pillow (Fig. 146).

The Cervical Contour Pillow has been one of the greatest adjuncts in the treatment of cervical spine disorders, and in many cases no other treatment is needed.

Drugs

Drug therapy is indicated in many disorders of the cervical spine. It is of definite value in the acute cases. Following an injury of the neck, analgesics for relief of pain, one of the proteolytic enzyme preparations for the relief of swelling and inflammation but given in double the dosage usually recommended, muscle relaxant drugs for the relief of muscle spasm and perhaps a sedative are the drugs of greatest value. One must keep in mind that many of the muscle relaxing drugs do not relax skeletal muscle spasm

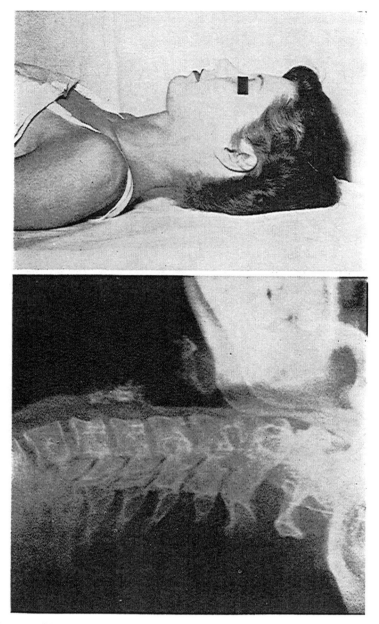

Figure 146A. Photograph and radiograph of a neck with no pillow beneath it. Rotate the book ninety degrees to see the position of the cervical vertebrae.

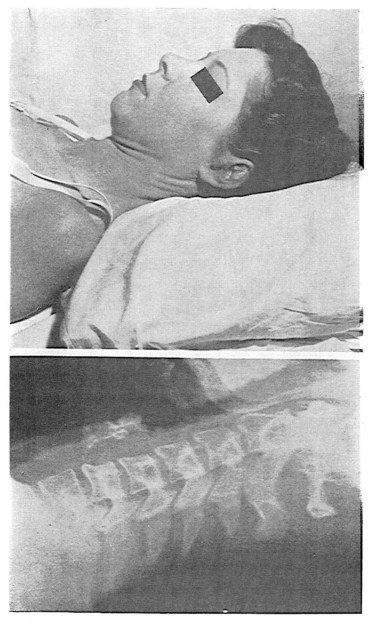

Figure 146B. The same neck with an ordinary pillow beneath it. Rotate the book again to see the position of the vertebrae.

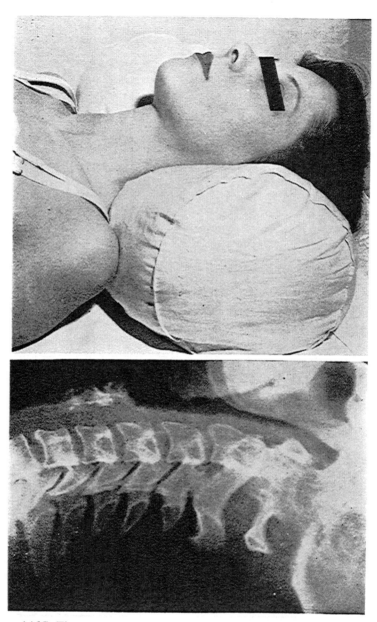

Figure 146C. The same neck with a Cervical Contour Pillow beneath it. In the horizontal position the neck appears to be in hyperextension. Rotate the book ninety degrees to see that there is only a normal forward curve of the neck and no hyperextension. This is the most comfortable sleeping or supine position.

but act primarily as sedatives. Diazepam (Valium®) in correct dosage has, in my practice, proven to be the most efficacious, with orphenadrine citrate (Norflex®) a close second. If only two drugs were available, I would choose an analgesic and an enzyme preparation for treating the acute postinjury cases. Also, time-release vitamin C, 500 mg twice daily, aids the healing process.

The subacute and chronic cases, or those showing the so-called degenerative changes in the cervical joints, respond well to phenylbutazone (Butazolidin®), colchicine or salicylates. Steroids should not be given unless there are specific indications for them. There are numerous other nonsteroid anti-inflammatory drugs available, which, of course, should be used with proper discrimination.

If marked osteoporosis is present, injections of vitamin B_{12} give some relief of pain. Injections of estrogen and androgen combinations may be indicated. Their value is questionable.

If the symptoms in women are aggravated during the premenstrual period due to hormonal imbalance, treatment should be directed toward the correction of premenstrual tension and edema.

Instructions to Patients

Each patient is supplied with a brief and simple written explanation of the anatomy and physiology of the cervical spine and instructions designed to teach the patient how to protect the neck in his everyday activities so that he can control to some extent the unpleasant symptoms and can avoid aggravation of such symptoms. It is impossible to cover all the activities which should be restricted or guarded, but those which are listed should serve as helpful guides—keeping in mind that backward bending of the neck, prolonged forward and side bending of the neck and repeated or prolonged rotation of the neck are the movements to be avoided.

The instructions and the illustrations are as follows:

Reclining

Always lie or sleep on a hard bed. If the mattress is not quite firm, put a bedboard between the mattress and the springs.

When lying down, sit on the edge of the bed and lie down side-

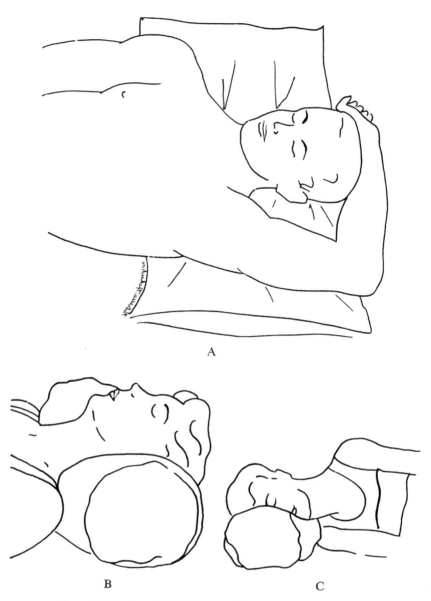

A

B   C

Figure 147A through Z'. Illustrated instructions for patients.

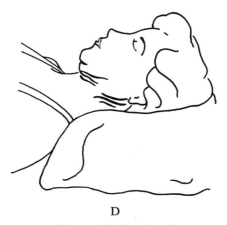

D

Figure 147 *Continued*

ways. When getting up, turn on your side and put your feet on the floor, then push yourself to a sitting position by using your elbow on the side to which you have turned. This will keep your neck and back straight and will prevent any undue strain on your neck.

Lie or sleep on your back or on your side. Never sleep on your abdomen because this keeps your head turned to one side at the maximum position of rotation and puts a constant strain on the neck for long periods of time, or until you change positions.

Do not sleep with one or both arms above your head. This may cut off the circulation of blood to your arm or arms (Fig. 147A).

Sleep on a soft round pillow (a contour pillow) which assures proper positioning of the neck if you lie on your back or on your side (Figs. 147B and C).

Avoid sleeping on hard or thick pillows or sponge rubber pillows. Such pillows raise your head too high and cause your neck to be bent forward which puts a strain on the structures at the back of your neck (Fig. 147D).

Writing

Do not slump over a desk when you are writing (Fig. 147E). Sit straight and look down at what you are writing and do not keep your head forward or backward. Choose a chair and desk of proper height so that you can see what you are doing without hav-

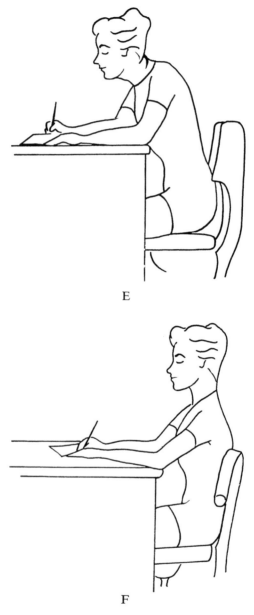

E

F

Figure 147 *Continued*

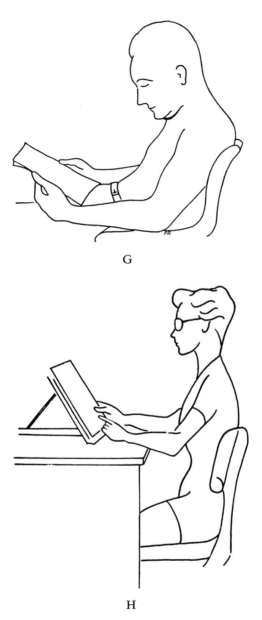

G

H

Figure 147 *Continued*

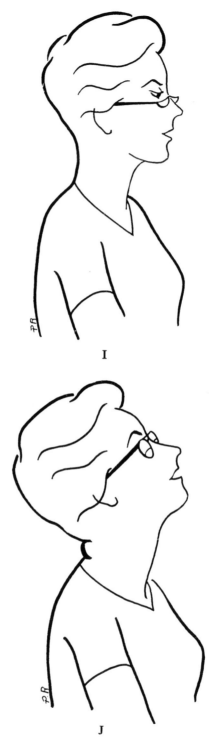

I

J

Figure 147 *Continued*

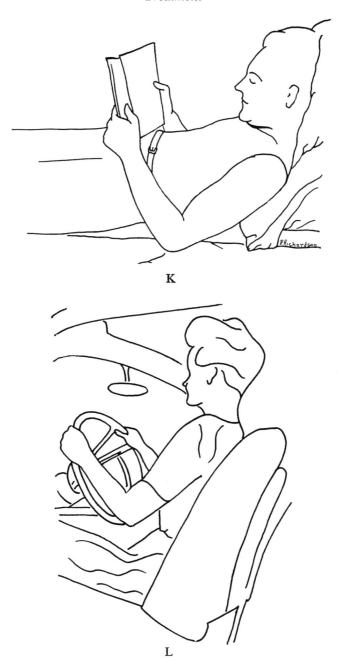

K

L

Figure 147 *Continued*

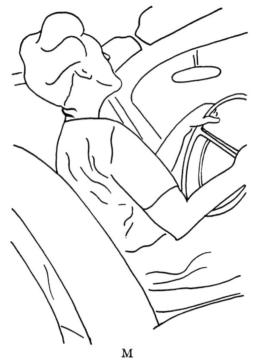

M

Figure 147 *Continued*

ing to hold your head in a forward or backward position (Fig. 147F). A tilt-top desk is of great advantage.

Reading

Do not slump in your chair when you are reading (Fig. 147G). Try to sit erect and keep your reading material as near eye level as possible. A reading stand to hold your book or magazine is of real advantage (Fig. 147H).

Use reading glasses rather than bifocal glasses (Fig. 147I) or have the reading portion of the lenses enlarged or placed at a higher level so that you will not have to put your head backward in order to read (Fig. 147J).

Do not read in bed unless you have the proper backrest. It is difficult to sit erect in bed, and, if you try to read, you will soon find yourself slumped over and your head and neck thrust forward (Fig. 147K).

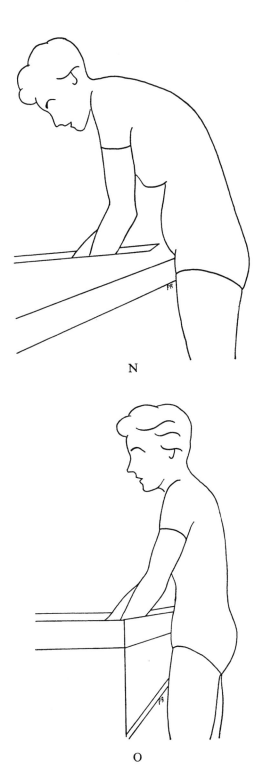

N

O

Figure 147 *Continued*

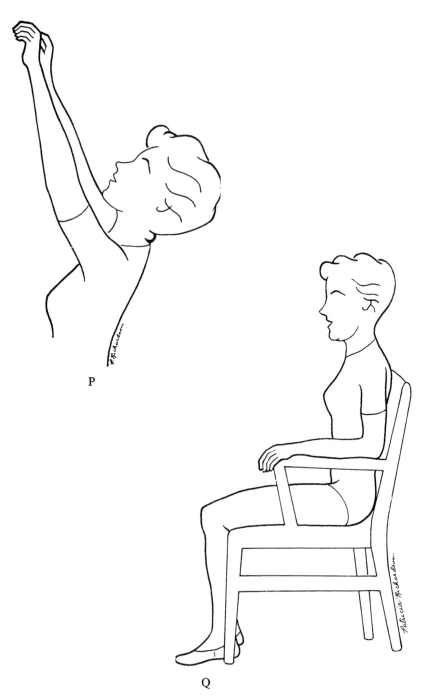

P

Q

Figure 147 *Continued*

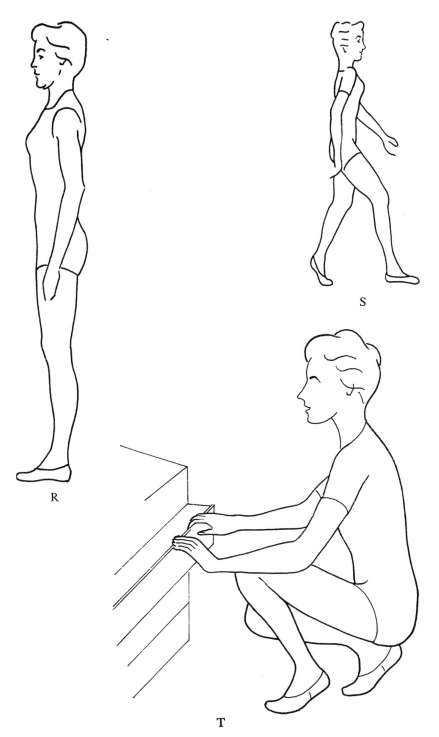

R

S

T

Figure 147 Continued

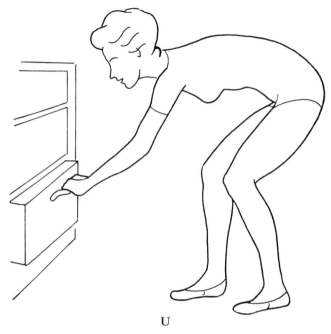

U

Figure 147 *Continued*

Driving

Keep your car seat as close to the steering wheel as possible. This helps you to sit straight and keeps you from putting your head backward in order to see over the steering wheel and the hood of the car (Figs. 147L and M). Adjustable bucket seats are the most comfortable, and four-way adjustments are desirable.

Arm rests at the proper height add to your comfort. Do not lean on the window frame because this makes you sit to the left of the steering wheel. Avoid riding with three people on the seat, especially if this forces or crowds you against the door and away from the steering wheel. Avoid driving for more than an hour at one time. Stop the car, get out and walk around for a few minutes.

Working

When working, avoid keeping your head held forward, backward or turned to one side (Figs. 157N, O and P). Sit straight, stand straight and walk straight (Figs. 147Q, R and S). Avoid

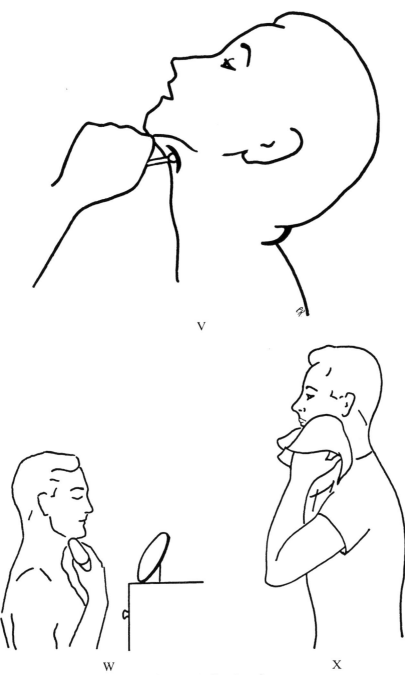

V

W   X

Figure 147 *Continued*

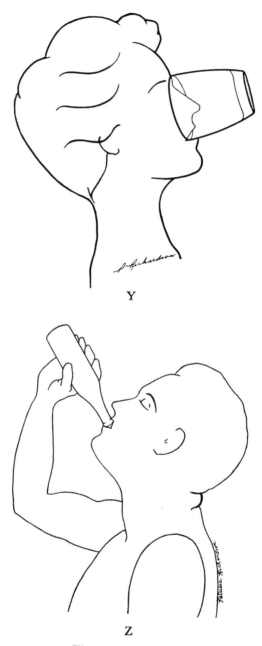

Y

Z

Figure 147 *Continued*

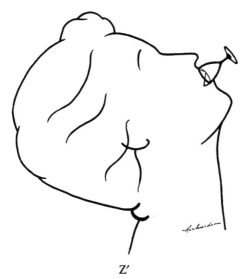

Z'

Figure 147 *Continued*

working with your arms above your head. Use a step-stool or a ladder so that whatever work you are doing is near eye level.

Stooping

Learn to squat to pick up things (Fig. 147T). Do not stoop (Fig. 147U). When one stoops over, the head and neck go backward automatically.

Shaving

Do not put your head backward when shaving under your chin (Fig. 147V). Avoid stooping over the lavatory to wash your face after you have shaved. Use a wash cloth or try conscientiously to keep your chin tucked in if you do stoop (Figs. 147W and X).

Drinking

Avoid drinking from bottles, cans or narrow-mouthed glasses (Figs. 147Z and Z'). Use wide-mouthed glasses or cups so that you will not need to tilt your head backward to drink (Fig. 147Y).

The illustrations in Figure 147 are visual aids designed to give the patient a better understanding of some of the problems involved, so that he can avoid aggravation of his symptoms while engaging in everyday activities.

Exercises

Exercise to increase mobility of the cervical spine is recommended by many who treat disorders of this portion of the spine. Based on my personal and patient experience, it is my opinion that exercises are unnecessary and in most instances do more harm than good. Painful joints are best treated by rest until the pain subsides, following which movement is necessary for restoration of function and to prevent joint stiffness. However, movement of an injured or deranged joint should not be forced beyond its functional tolerance. If function of such joints is continued within their limits of tolerance, they will be useful joints and much less painful. This may sound like heresy to those who believe that exercise, passive and active, is the answer to most joint problems. However, pain in the capsular structures, which are richly innervated, cannot be relieved by constant movement beyond their restricted tolerance. Therefore, motion should not be encouraged beyond the subpain level, otherwise the muscles which activate the joints will go into spasm to protect the joints.

In the cervical spine, the proximity of the nerve roots to the posterior joints and to the lateral interbody joints makes them susceptible to irritation from movement. The inherent great range of motion in the cervical spine is not dependent on movement between any two segments but on the composite movement of all the joints, and loss of motion between any two segments affects very little the overall movement. Strengthening the neck muscles by passive and/or active exercises is of little value in the relief of pain. Inasmuch as the special sense organs are housed in the head, the activities of everyday living will provide adequate exercise of the neck. In fact, patients with neck disorders get more relief from limiting neck activity, especially hyperextension and prolonged flexion, than is afforded by any attempt to move the neck beyond its functional tolerance. Isometric exercises and resistive exercises are preferred and should be encouraged.

Carrying a book on the head, as suggested by DePalma, is

probably the best neck exercise for the relief of pain in certain neck disorders. In order to walk with a book balanced on the head, one must straighten the cervical spine which gives the nerve roots maximum clearance within their canals.

Manipulation

Mennell states that joint dysfunction is the result of loss of movement which is involuntary, and that movement can only be restored by being reproduced by the manipulator who restores normal function by the use of normal movement. There are many manipulators who manipulate the cervical spine and who claim excellent results.

My experience with manipulation of the cervical spine has been limited to the cases of unilateral subluxation of the posterior joints, and then only after the injection of a local anesthetic into the painful joint structures. When the pain has been relieved by anesthesia the neck can be gently and passively moved through a full range of motion. However, after the anesthetic effect is dissipated, the muscles go into spasm to prevent motion in the painful joint structures. The muscle spasm does not subside until the inflammatory reaction has abated.

Manipulation of the cervical spine should not be undertaken by any person who is not well versed in the anatomy of this very complex structure. Neck popping has resulted in severe neurological problems, some near fatal and others fatal.

Psychotherapy

Inasmuch as concussions of the brain often occur with necklash injuries, some of these patients develop so-called psychogenic changes. Many patients seeking relief have visited so many doctors that they have been labeled neurotics. Psychotherapy may be needed before satisfactory results are obtained.

Emotional stress and strain, anxieties and frustrations may aggravate the symptoms. In many instances a simple explanation of this fact will give the patient a better understanding of his symptoms and may help to relieve the tension associated with emotional problems.

TREATMENT OF SPECIFIC CONDITIONS

Strains

A strain of the neck usually requires nothing more than the intermittent application of heat to the neck, a mild analgesic, a few motorized intermittent traction treatments and perhaps a soft collar for a few days. Strains do not require extensive treatment. The symptoms subside within a few days to three weeks and leave no residual disability. If the symptoms do not subside at the end of three weeks, the patient has suffered a more serious injury.

Sprains

It is often difficult to differentiate between a strain and a sprain immediately following a traumatic experience, in which event it is better to err in overtreatment than undertreatment. It is always wise to suspect that an accident victim has suffered a sprain until proved otherwise by the rather prompt subsidence of the symptoms and clinical findings.

It is not necessary to hospitalize a patient who has a sprain of the neck. In fact, hospitalization should be discouraged except for traction and observation for no more than two or three days or when no other treatment is available.

If no skeletal injuries are evident, the neck should be immobilized with a collar or brace which allows minimal movements of the injured joint structures. This will give protection to the joints and yet allow slight motion to prevent joint fibrosis. The collar or brace should be worn night and day for a period of six to eight weeks to allow maximal healing of the injured structures. During this period, some form of heat and motorized intermittent traction should be given daily for a few days and then three times each week for two or three weeks and then reduced to once or twice each week until the symptoms have abated. No more than fifteen pounds of traction should be used initially, followed by a gradual increase to thirty or thirty-five pounds. If motorized intermittent traction is not available, continuous traction with fifteen to twenty-five pounds of weight for short periods may be used. If localized areas of tenderness persist, they should be injected with a local anesthetic.

Medication during this time should be used wisely. Oversedation and overtranquilization should be avoided. A proteolytic enzyme to reduce swelling and inflammation in the injured tissues and an analgesic, as well as time-release vitamin C, should be provided for several days. Muscle relaxants in proper dosage are usually beneficial, but their prolonged use should be discouraged.

After six or eight weeks, the collar or brace should be discontinued gradually and movements of the neck within tolerance encouraged, but avoidance of hyperextension and prolonged or repeated flexion, rotation and lateral bending is imperative.

If this treatment program is followed, the symptoms will subside within three to six months usually. However, some treatment may be necessary in some cases over a longer period of time but usually at irregular intervals. No two patients respond exactly the same, and no two patients may be able to follow in the same degree the instructions listed above.

This treatment program will prevent the patient from wandering from one doctor to another seeking relief of his symptoms which he had been told would subside within a few weeks, but did not, and he will avoid the label of psychoneurosis. Also, it is my opinion, based on many years of experience, that the treatment outlined here will delay and perhaps lessen the inevitable joint changes which occur following trauma.

The Acute Unilateral Subluxation

Unilateral subluxation, or the "crick" in the neck, which is diagnosed easily when the patient walks into the doctor's office, should be treated by injecting a local anesthetic about and into the posterior joint at the site of maximum tenderness. The severe pain will subside immediately and then gentle manual traction should be applied and the head and neck moved passively through the usual range of motion. Heat and motorized intermittent traction should be given then, followed by the application of a properly designed collar which should be worn for several weeks. Heat and motorized traction should be given at regular intervals until all symptoms have subsided.

The Posttraumatic Chronic Cases

Oftentimes the orthopaedist sees patients who have had neck injuries and who have had little or no treatment and whose symptoms have persisted well beyond the anticipated time.

The same treatment as outlined for the acute neck injury or sprain should be utilized to give the patient relief of his symptoms. These patients will be most grateful that something is being done to give them relief. They will be relieved of worry and anxiety, and at last they will know that they have an explainable reason for their symptoms and that they are not "just neurotics."

Fractures and Dislocations

Skeletal injuries of the cervical spine require hospitalization for skull traction usually. If one or both vertebral arches or one or both posterior articular processes are fractured, with or without displacement of the vertebral body, skull traction is indicated. The amount of weight will depend on the injury, and may vary from twenty to forty pounds. It is necessary usually to keep the neck in some hyperextension to achieve and maintain proper alignment.

Traction should be continued for eight to twelve weeks or until sufficient healing has occurred to prevent loss of alignment. Then rigid brace or cast immobilization should be applied while the traction is maintained. The traction is then removed and the brace or cast continued until there is radiographic evidence of complete healing. The postimmobilization treatment is then the same as for any fracture near or involving joints. The soft tissue structures suffer the penalty of long immobilization, and never should the cast or brace be removed and the patient discharged as cured. He is not cured, although the fracture or fractures may be well healed. Gradual mobilization of the joint structures, which are contracted and stiff and sore, by proper physical therapy modalities should follow. Sudden release of the injured structures does not assure immediate restoration of function.

The Halo-traction cast, as recommended originally by Perry for paralysis of the cervical muscles, has become a popular method of traction in many institutions where complete immobilization is indicated. It has the advantage of rigid immobilization and early ambulation of the patient.

For an anterior dislocation of one set of facets on their mates, without fractures, skull traction should be applied with the neck in flexion, and once the dislocated facets are shown by a lateral radiograph to be above their proximate distal facets, the direction of the traction pull should be changed so that hyperextension is achieved and the dislocated facets resume their normal position. The amount of weight should then be reduced to a minimum and maintained until the soft tissue injuries have healed sufficiently to permit brace immobilization of the neck and ambulation of the patient.

Nerve root compression or irritation and in some cases cord compression will subside during the treatment, depending on the severity of the injury to these structures. However, if cord compression is present and if it does not respond to traction within a reasonable period of time, decompression by laminectomy may be indicated. If there is central cord compression, decompression may be of little or no value.

Fractures of the Atlas and Axis

Many fractures of the axis and atlas may not be recognized in the immediate postinjury radiographs. However, one should follow the first rule in the treatment of sprains, which is immobilization for six to eight weeks. After this length of time, the radiographs will, in all probability, reveal evidence of healing fractures.

Displaced fractures should be treated with skull traction. Each individual case will present its own problems and no one method of treatment is applicable to all. Rigid immobilization should follow the traction and continue until the fracture or fractures are well healed. Some fractures of the atlas may be difficult or impossible to reduce because of the soft tissue damage.

Spondylitis of Nontraumatic Origin

The joints of the cervical spine are not usually the initial site of nontraumatic inflammatory conditions. The treatment of such joint conditions which involve the cervical joints differs little from the treatment of other joints. Immobilization in the optimum position, traction and appropriate medication are indicated.

Associated Conditions

Cervical spine disorders are often responsible for secondary involvement of the shoulder, elbow and hand. The painful shoulder which has some degree of limitation of motion should be injected with a local anesthetic at the site or sites of maximum tenderness, followed by the intelligent use of heat and, when the pain has subsided, exercises to mobilize the joint. In some instances, the injection of 25 mg of Hydrocortone® into the shoulder capsule will speed recovery. The pain may be aggravated by the injection after the effect of the anesthetic has subsided, and an appropriate analgesic should be supplied in the event it is needed and to avoid a telephone call in the middle of the night.

The frozen shoulder may require manipulation under a general anesthetic. However, conservative measures should be tried first because the postmanipulation convalescence requires a long period of active treatment and because dislocation of the shoulder sometimes occurs during or after manipulations. If manipulation is necessary, immobilization of the shoulder with the arm in ninety degrees or more of abduction should be maintained for ten days. During this time the brace may be removed daily for pendulum exercises of the shoulder. At the end of ten days, active exercises should be started and continued until full mobilization is restored.

If a calcium deposit is present in one of the tendons of the shoulder cuff, it should be removed by aspiration under a local anesthetic and the area irrigated with saline solution until all the deposit has been removed, then 25 mg of Hydrocortone Acetate® may be injected through the same needle. This gives dramatic relief of pain and the patient usually has full, painless motion within two or three days.

Epicondylitis or tendinitis at the elbow associated with cervical nerve root irritation is best treated by injection of 5 cc of local anesthetic at the site of maximum tenderness. Through the same needle, 0.5 cc of Hydrocortone Acetate may then be injected if indicated. The pain will be relieved immediately following this treatment. However, a few hours later the discomfort at the epicondyle may be severe for twelve to twenty-four hours. Usually by the second morning after the injection the patient awakens completely free of pain and with full restoration of function.

The injection of a steroid with the local anesthetic is done routinely by some doctors. My own experience has shown that this is rarely, if ever, of more value than the use of the local anesthetic if done properly. A nonsteroid anti-inflammatory drug taken orally for a few days is usually beneficial.

Fibrotic changes in the palmar fascia, resembling Dupuytren's contractures, can be relieved if irreversable changes have not occurred, by blocking the stellate ganglion to paralyze the vasoconstrictors and improve the blood supply. Oral administration of a vasodilator and 500 mg of time-release vitamin C two or three times daily slows and even relieves the process.

Blurring of vision and loss of balance can be relieved with intermittent traction usually. Several patients who have had uncontrolled Mèniére's disease have been completely relieved by the use of intermittent traction. Some cases may require injections of a local anesthetic and immobilization of the neck before relief of symptoms is obtained. In some instances, it may be necessary to differentiate vertebral lesions from central ones, in which event electronystagmography is indicated.

Those patients who have headaches which are of cervical nerve root origin will, in many instances, obtain complete relief of head pain following one or two intermittent traction treatments. Others may require the injection of a local anesthetic at the level of C2, C3 and C4, or at the point of maximum tenderness over the occiput, which is the point where the main trunk of the posterior ramus of the second cervical nerve pierces the semispinalis capitis and the trapezius muscles to supply the scalp as the greater occipital nerve. Many patients are relieved of their headaches by sleeping on the Cervipillo®, whereas others may require a properly designed collar for part-time wear.

AN OVERVIEW OF OTHER TREATMENT MODALITIES

We are now living in a pain conscious era, as evidenced by the establishment of numerous Pain Clinics and the various and even devious methods of relieving pain syndromes. Health quackery devices are, according to the *National Migraine Foundation Newsletter* of April, 1976, extorting millions of dollars annually from the gullible, the sick and the desperate.

Suddenly all major ills are being treated by acupuncture, auriculotherapy, acupressure, hypnosis and transcendental meditation, as well as various electrical nerve stimulation and destructive devices. Biofeedback, the process of furnishing the brain automatically with information concerning some bodily functions so that the intensity or frequency of such functions can be changed, has become another widely used tool for the relief of pain. Intraspinal hypothermia is being used to control pain. Intraspinal and intradiscal steroid injections are being done with the hope that they will relieve pain syndromes.

It has been my privilege to follow many patients who have been subjected to such methods of would-be pain control without relief. It is my belief, based on my many years of experience, that we as physicians are obligated to search diligently for the causative factors of the patient's symptoms, keeping in mind always the psychogenic aspects which may be involved. This requires time, patience and a thorough clinical analysis.

The computerization of symptoms and clinical findings which give us, supposedly, the answers to painful conditions has done much to destroy the art of medical practice. Can we conscientiously revert to methods used some five thousand years ago which have no medically scientific background, or do we go forward to relatively new methods which lack the same scientific credibility, or do we perform more and more surgical procedures without having utilized adequate conservative measures because they are time consuming?

SURGERY

Steindler often said "There are those who wish to go non-stop, and in their haste pass by the stations of indications and diagnosis, to arrive at specific operative techniques. No doubt they will be disappointed." There has been a rash of surgical procedures for cervical spine disorders during the past two decades. How many operations should really have been done we will never, in all probability, know.

Cervical laminectomies should be reserved for those cases which have positive evidence of cord compression from subarachnoid space occupying lesions.

Anterior interbody fusions should be reserved for those cases showing marked skeletal and/or ligamentous instability where there is danger of spinal cord compression. Severe osteophytic lesions which sometimes occur on the posterior aspect of vertebral margins and cause cord compression can be removed by the anterior approach usually, and an interbody fusion should be done.

Facetotomies for the removal of intervertebral canal osteophytic encroachment and for freeing of adhesions about the dural sleeve of the adjacent nerve root are indicated when there is persistent and resistant nerve root involvement (Plate 5). Osteophytes at the margins of the lateral interbody joints can be removed by the anterior approach in some instances, but this does not always free the nerve roots and hence the symptoms.

Surgical operations on the cervical spine should not be undertaken lightly, and there should be very definite and positive indications for such procedures before they are contemplated. Interscapular pain is not sufficient reason for disc removal and interbody fusion by the anterior approach, nor is a small amount of ligamentous instability sufficient indication for fusion, nor is the persistence of radicular pain sufficient indication for fusion. When, then, should fusion be done? Certain fracture-dislocations with marked instability may need fusion (Fig. 148). Marked ligamentous instability with spinal cord irritation, or if there is danger of cord involvement, may indicate the necessity for fusion.

Congenital absence of the odontoid process or the presence of a rudimentary disc between the body of the axis and the odontoid with definite instability may require posterior fusion of the occiput to the first and second vertebral arches.

This is true if there has been a disruption of the transverse liga-

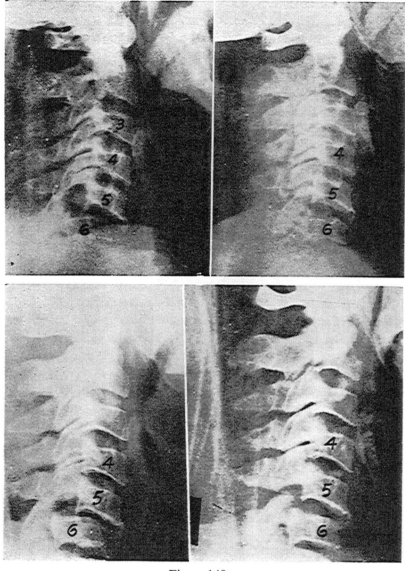

Figure 148

ment of the atlas by trauma, or by a collagen disorder such as rheumatoid arthritis, in order to protect the spinal cord from compression.

Fusion of two or more vertebrae places a greater strain on the

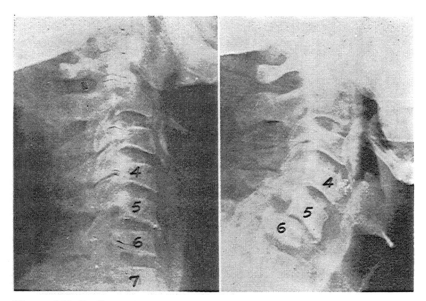

Figure 148. Radiographs of the cervical spine of a man who was injured in an automobile accident. There was marked forward displacement of the fifth vertebra on the sixth. This patient had walked some distance from the scene of the accident to his home, and when first examined several hours later only minimal neurologic changes were found. Fractures of the facets could not be demonstrated and the dislocation was due to marked ligamentous instability. Forty pounds of skull traction resulted in fairly adequate reduction, and the traction was reduced to twenty pounds which allowed the dislocation to recur as shown in the subsequent film. Twenty pounds of weight was added and reduction accomplished again. The patient was allowed to go home in a hospital bed with the forty pounds of traction and with the promise that he would remain in traction in bed for eight weeks.

The next illustrations show the reduction at five weeks postinjury and when the patient returned for a check-up at the end of eight weeks. Obviously, the patient did not stay in traction. However, the neurologic changes were very minimal and he had no complaints. This patient should have had either an anterior interbody fusion or a posterior fixation and fusion. (He has not been seen since six months after the injury.)

adjacent movable vertebral joints to give rise to continued symptoms and the necessity, apparently, for further fusions.

Overriding spinous processes which are responsible for limitation of motion, pain in the neck and the irritation of nerve roots in some instances may require removal for relief of symptoms.

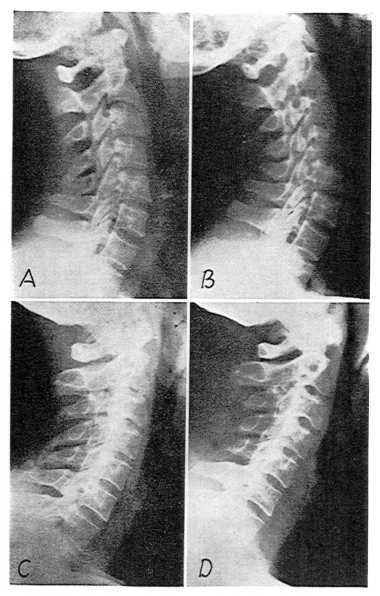

Figure 149. Lateral radiographs of two cervical spines (A & C) which show overriding of the fourth and fifth spinous processes. The overriding processes were removed and the films in B and D show the postoperative range of hyperextension. (O'Donoghue's cases.)

O'Donoghue has reported good results following this procedure. Two of his cases are shown in Figure 149.

One of my cases of overriding spinous processes which was completely relieved by removal of the fifth and sixth spinous processes is shown in Figure 150. This patient had had an operation for "a ruptured disc" two years previously. No "disc" was found, and the patient had continued to have the same pain in the upper rhomboid area which he had had before the disc operation. The relief which he received from removal of the overriding spinous processes was most gratifying.

In rare instances it may be necessary to resect a portion of the greater occipital nerve to relieve persistent headaches. This should be done in those very few cases which obtain relief from their headaches for only a few hours after the injection of the nerve

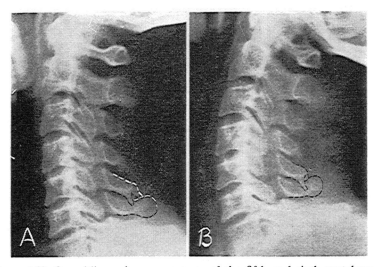

Figure 150. Overriding spinous processes of the fifth and sixth vertebrae. A straight lateral view (A) and a hyperextension view (B). A partial facetectomy was done in 1955 to relieve nerve root compression of the sixth nerve root on the right side. The patient was not relieved of the pain in the posterior muscles of the right shoulder. He was treated in my clinic in 1957 with motorized intermittent traction, injections of a local anesthetic and with a collar to hold his neck in a straight or slightly flexed position, with good results. However, when treatment was stopped his symptoms returned. Removal of the overriding spinous processes gave him complete relief.

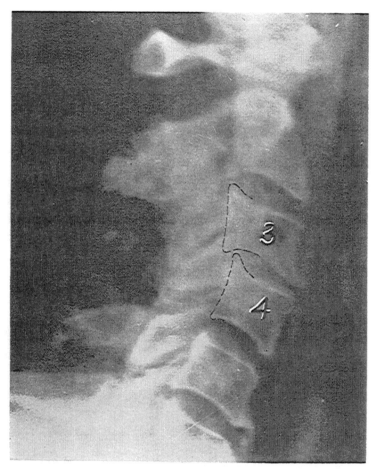

Figure 151. A lateral radiograph of a patient who had an exploratory oper-ation at the third and fourth vertebrae, in 1950. This man had had diving injuries and falls on several occasions during the previous twenty years. Prior to the surgery he had noticed some numbness of his hands which oc-curred while he was mowing a lawn. He had difficulty with fine movements of his hands. Following surgery he had a very stormy convalescence for some four or five months. In 1957, he could not use his hands as well as he did prior to the operation, and he had developed signs of cord compression due to the posterior subluxation of C-3 on C-4 and the inevitable increasing hypertrophic changes.

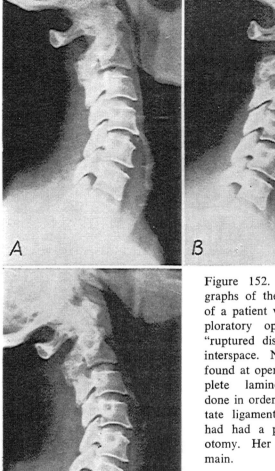

Figure 152. Lateral radiographs of the cervical spine of a patient who had an exploratory operation for a "ruptured disc" at the fifth interspace. No "disc" was found at operation, but complete laminectomies were done in order to cut the dentate ligaments. This patient had had a previous scalenotomy. Her symptoms remain.

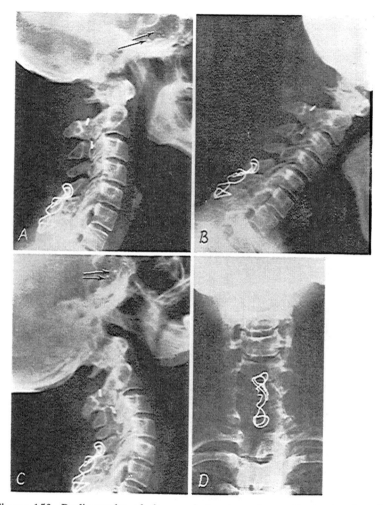

Figure 153. Radiographs of the cervical spine of a patient who first had symptoms of cervical nerve root irritation in 1950. After a short six days of traction failed to relieve the pain in her right shoulder and arm, the fifth, sixth and seventh vertebrae were fused. Several months later, following myelographic studies, a "ruptured disc" was removed between the sixth and seventh vertebrae on the right side. Several months later the upper portion of the cervical spine was explored and screws were used across the joints for fixation. Eight months later the screws were removed and a cordotomy was done. In 1957, the patient still had irritation of the cervical nerve roots, plus a stiff neck and complete loss of sensation on the right side!

with a local anesthetic. The operation should be done under local anesthesia to facilitate the exact localization of the nerve. The patient can tell the operator the exact instant the needle pierces the nerve. The syringe should be removed from the needle then, leaving the needle in place. With another needle and syringe the surrounding tissues should be infiltrated and the incision made at the site of the previously placed needle to expose the nerve. The

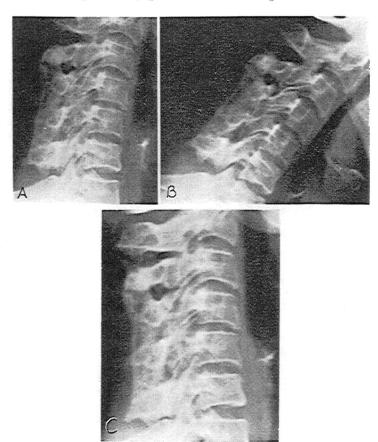

Figure 154. Lateral radiographs of a patient who had an exploratory operation of the fourth left nerve root and a spinal fusion of the third, fourth, fifth and sixth vertebrae, three years previously. She had been in an automobile accident seven years prior to surgery and had had symptoms of nerve root irritation for six months. In 1957, her symptoms of nerve root irritation were still present and she had the added burden of a stiff neck.

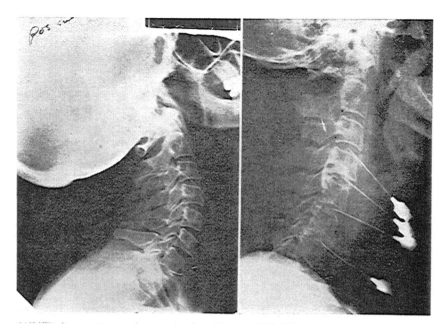

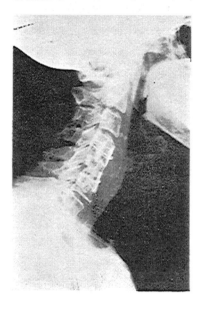

Figure 155. The radiograph at the upper left was made with the neck in hyperextension and shows posterior slipping of the fourth vertebra on the fifth and of the fifth vertebra on the sixth. The next film shows the result of the discogram—extravasation of the radiopaque material at the fourth and fifth and at the fifth and sixth interspaces. The lower left film shows the interbody fusion at these levels.

This patient first experienced pain on the right side of her neck in 1953 while eating lunch. She was hospitalized for cervical traction, following which she experienced some relief but had continued attacks of intermittent pain. One year later, she was hospitalized again for traction. She then developed pain which radiated to her right suprascapular area and right arm. In 1956, she suffered a rear-end collision while stopped in her car at a traffic light. She was "knocked out" for a few minutes, following which her symptoms were greatly aggravated and she was hospitalized again for traction. (No medical-legal involvement.) Her symptoms continued and she developed numbness of the right arm and difficulty using it, as well as severe occipital headaches. Myelographic studies revealed no evidence of a space occupying lesion. In 1958, she was referred to my clinic. Treatment consisted of collar immobilization, motorized intermittent traction, home traction, injections of local anesthetic and finally resection of overriding spinous processes at the second and third vertebrae and resection of the occipital nerve on the right side. The symptoms abated following the surgery for several months. Then, the patient painted her bathroom and the shoulder and arm symptoms recurred but were relieved by injections of a local anesthetic. Several weeks later, she slipped and jerked her neck, following which nothing relieved her pain and she developed a burning type pain over the shoulder area, the lateral surface of the arm and at the wrist. Finally, the patient was referred elsewhere for consultation. The discogram was made and this was followed by anterior fusion.

The patient received some relief of her symptoms for a few months following the surgery and then they recurred. All conservative measures failed to have any lasting effect, and she was returned to the surgeon who had operated on her previously. Discograms were made again and fusion of the third and fourth and of the sixth and seventh vertebrae was done. She improved somewhat for a short time following the second operation, but soon the symptoms recurred. Again, conservative measures gave only temporary relief and the patient has gone from bad to worse. In 1977 X-rays show marked arthritic changes at C2-3 and severe osteoporosis of all cervical vertebrae. Her symptoms persist.

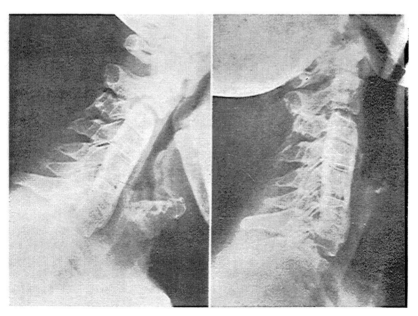

Figure 155D & E. Lateral bending films show solid bone fusion from the third vertebra through the seventh.

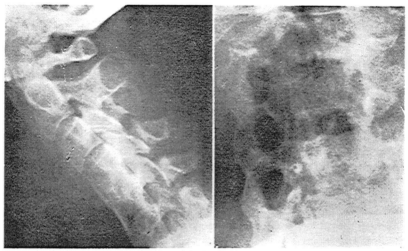

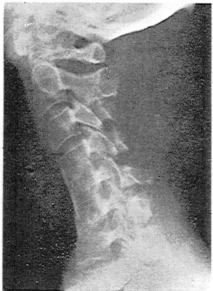

Figure 156. Postoperative radiographs of a patient, age forty-one, who had episodes of pain in the neck since childhood. In 1956, she developed right arm and shoulder pain after washing some venetian blinds. In 1957, while walking on the street she developed severe pain in her neck and right arm to the fingers. Conservative treatment consisting of traction and a collar gave some relief. In 1958, she received x-ray therapy following a negative myelogram. In 1959, she developed severe headaches, weakness of the right arm, suprascapular pain and experienced "black-out" sensations. Lateral radiographs of the cervical spine revealed some ligamentous instability at the fifth vertebra. Conservative treatment in my clinic gave some relief, but not enough to satisfy the patient and her husband. She was referred elsewhere for consultation. Discography was done and an anterior interbody fusion of the fifth and sixth vertebrae followed. She improved somewhat until her neck was jerked in a rear-end automobile collision. Conservative measures failed to give relief of the severe symptoms which fol-

←━━

lowed the collision. Discography and fusion of the fourth and fifth and of the sixth and seventh vertebrae were done three months after the injury. Two months later her symptoms were so severe that she could not get out of bed and was unable to hold up her head. Lateral bending films, five months post-operation, revealed motion at the sixth and seventh vertebrae. Facetotomies were recommended for exploration of the nerve roots on the right side. This was done and bone grafts were used for posterior fusion of the sixth and seventh vertebrae. In due course, the symptoms abated somewhat and the patient was able to do some of her housework and to drive her car. However, as time went on the symptoms recurred and grew progressively worse, so that when she returned to my clinic in 1963 she was unable to hold up her head without support and she suffered unbearable headaches and pain in the suprascapular area. A is the lateral radiograph which shows the area of fusion, the forward position of the neck and overriding spinous processes of the second, third and fourth vertebrae. The oblique view shows the enlarged intervertebral foramina following the facetotomies. Resection of the spinous processes which were overriding and of the right occipital nerve were done. This enabled the patient to straighten the neck somewhat and to hold up her head again, and the headaches were relieved. However, she continued to have pain in and about the right shoulder. C shows that the patient was able to hold up her head following the removal of the spinous processes.

---

nerve can be resected easily after it has been freed from the accompanying occipital artery.

Removal of the first rib for the all too frequently diagnosed *thoracic outlet syndrome* has become a popular surgical procedure. In my experience conservative measures have relieved the symptoms and clinical findings, and surgical intervention has been unnecessary. Posture correction, traction and the injection of the scalene muscles with a local anesthetic give relief.

The simple tilting of the head to the side of the symptoms relaxes the scalene muscles and relieves pressure on the vertebral artery and tension on the brachial plexus. All people carry their heads tilted to one side because this is the position that seats the cervical joints and is the position of comfort and ease. Would you believe that such a simple change of habit could save the patient unnecessary surgery?

Figures 151 through 158 are representative cases which were not relieved by surgical procedures. There are many more.

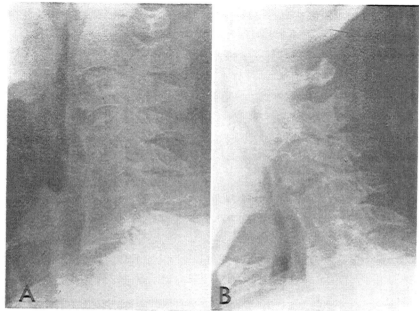

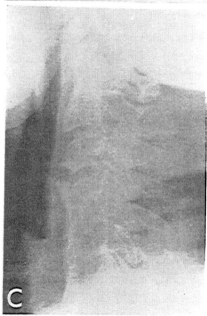

Figure 157. Patient injured in rear-end collision in 1965. Initial radiographs showed degeneration of discs at C5 and C6 and at C6 and C7. The patient was treated conservatively and returned to work. A few months later symptoms were worse and the patient stopped working and was, at his request, referred to a neurosurgeon who did myelograms and discograms, followed by an anterior interbody fusion at C4, C5, C6 and C7. His symptoms were not relieved and he could not work. In 1974 he was involved in another rear-end collision while driving a Volkswagen. The radiographs made following this injury are shown here and indicate injury above C4. The patient's symptoms were increased, although conservative measures gave some relief, the patient sought acupuncture therapy. His symptoms persist. Note the marked osteophytic changes at the anterosuperior margin of C4.

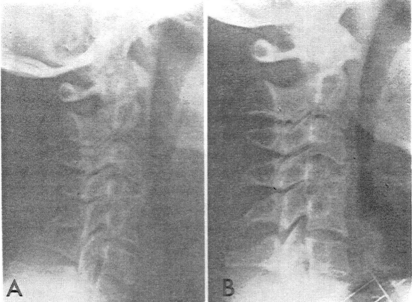

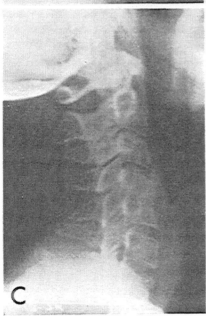

Figure 158. At age 34, in 1967, the patient was involved in a car accident when the car in which she was a passenger skidded, spun around and the rear end of the car hit a tree. The seat was torn loose and the patient was thrown into the back seat. She was treated with skull traction for two weeks for a fracture of the anterosuperior portion of the body of C4 and posterior subluxation of C4 on C5. An anterior interbody fusion was done. Postoperative radiographs showed that the graft which was used for the interbody fusion was displaced anteriorly. She returned to work two weeks postoperatively. One week later she tried to prevent a ledger from falling from her desk and following this she had immediate pain in her neck and between her shoulder blades, for which her doctor prescribed medication. No radiographs were made. Three and one-half months later radiographs showed a triangular-shaped graft between C4 and C5 which was displaced anteriorly to the vertebral bodies by one-quarter of an inch and there was backward settling of C4 on C5 and foraminal narrowing on the right side at C4 and C5. The patient was involved in another car accident in 1973. Radiographs, as shown here, show fusion at C4 and C5 with an osteophytic formation extending proximally from the body of C4. The backward displacement of C4 on C5 is obvious and there is backward slipping of C5 on C6 also.

CONCLUSIONS

In conclusion it must be stressed again that treatment should be definitive and individualized. Good results can be obtained by conservative measures but the problem of permanent damage to the ligamentous and capsular structures of the joints, as well as to the intervertebral discs, remains.

It is impossible to estimate the exact amount of residual disability, but it can be stated with certainty that these joints will be intolerant of unusual stress or strain. They will be subject to further damage on even slight provocation. Patients should be taught the importance of proper usage and protection of their necks to prevent recurrent attacks of pain and disability. The resulting disability will be dependent upon the functional demands made upon the cervical spine, and upon the ability of the patient to adjust to, and to tolerate, the limitations imposed upon his activities. Even with guarded usage degenerative changes are inevitable. However, early recognition and treatment of sprain injuries of the neck may minimize or delay the late degenerative changes.

Surgery should be avoided unless there are absolute and definite indications for it, otherwise the results from operative procedures will be disappointing and the symptoms may be worse than they were before surgery was done. These cases are treatment cases which require time, patience and understanding, but the results will be gratifying.

The surgeon who believes that his scalpel can cure the ills of the cervical spine should take time to live with his patients before and after surgery. If he does this, he would be more cautious in the selection of patients for cervical spine surgery. The most beautiful surgical technique may fail if there is not the proper indications for its execution. The patient's future must be of prime concern.

Steindler has stated that patience as well as study are required in the treatment of the complex cervical spine disorders. The deplorable trend to short-circuit these responsibilities by precipitate operations, the disdaining of conservative efforts as useless wastes of time and the uncompromising attitude of generalizing operative indications has done nothing to establish a wholesome equilibrium between radical action and conservative expectation, but, on the contrary, has contributed much to cloud the issue.

The importance of cervical investigation in any patient with head, neck, chest, shoulder and arm pain cannot be overemphasized. The usual diagnosis of arthritis, bursitis, neuritis, muscular rheumatism, fibrositis, fasciitis, tendinitis, pseudo-angina, migraine, etc. should not be made until cervical nerve root irritation has been ruled out entirely, if that is possible–which it usually is.

BIBLIOGRAPHY

Abel, M. S.: Occult fractures of the cervical spine: roentgenologic diagnosis and clinical significance. *Clin Med, 8:*647-655, April, 1961.

Abel, M. S.: *Occult Traumatic Lesions of the Cervical Vertebrae.* St. Louis, Green, 1970.

Abel, M. S. and Harmon, P. H.: Stress studies of the cervical spine for diagnosis of discopathy. Scientific Exhibit, *Am Acad Orthop Surgeons,* Chicago, Illinois, January, 1964.

The acute inflammatory response. *Ann NY Acad Sci, 116:*747-1084, August 27, 1964.

Adson, A. W.: Cervical rib—a new approach. *Ann Surg, 85:*839, June, 1927.

Against cervical discography (letters to the editor): *JAMA, 189:*1033, September 28, 1962.

Albertson, P.: Physiological benefit found in transcendental meditation. *Med Tribune, 15:*23, June 19, 1974.

Alexander, L.: Differential diagnosis between psychogenic and physical pain; the conditional psychogalvanic reflex as an aid. *JAMA, 181:*855-861, September 8, 1962.

Allaben, R. D., Posch, J. L. and Larsen, R. D.: An experimental evaluation of the efficacy of chymotrypsin in the reduction of edema in crushed extremities. *J Bone Joint Surg, 44A:*41-48, January, 1962.

Anderson, G. V. W.: The mechanism of the costo-clavicular syndrome. *East Afr Med J, 34:*269-276, June, 1957.

Anderson, L. D. and D'alonzo, R. T.: Fractures of the odontoid process of the axis. *J Bone Joint Surg, 56A:*1633-1674, December, 1974.

Arias, B. A., Cascino, J. P. and Carney, A.: Pitfalls in the diagnosis of cranio-cerebral trauma. *J Int Coll Surg Bull, 37:*343-362, April, 1962.

Ashkenazy, M.: Migraine—a diagnostic dilemma? or wastebasket syndrome? *South Med J, 56:*247-251, March, 1963.

Austin, G. M.: The significance and nature of pain in tumors of the spinal cord. *Surg Forum, 10:*782-785, 1960.

Bailey, R. W.: Observations of cervical intervertebral-disc lesions in fractures and dislocations. *J Bone Joint Surg, 45A:*461-470, April, 1963.

Bailey, R. W. and Badgley, C. E.: Stabilization of the cervical spine by anterior fusion. *J Bone Joint Surg, 42A:*565-594, June, 1960.

Bardenwerper, H. W.: Serum neuritis from tetanus antitoxin. *JAMA, 179:*763-766, March 10, 1962.

Barnes, W. P., Jr.: The use of blade-guides in intervertebral-body bone-grafting. *J Bone Joint Surg, 40A:*461-464, April, 1958.

Barnett, C. H., Davies, D. V. and MacConaill, M. A.: *Synovial Joints: Their Structure and Mechanics.* Springfield, Thomas, 1961.

Basmajian, J. V.: *Muscles Alive: Their Functions Revealed by Electromyography.* Baltimore, Williams & Wilkins, 1962.

Bauer, R., Sheehan, S. and Meyer, J. S.: Arteriographic study of cerebrovascular disease. II. Cerebral symptoms due to kinking, tortuosity, and compression of carotid and vertebral arteries in the neck. *Arch Neurol,* 4:119-131, February, 1961.

Beatson, T. R.: Fractures and dislocations of the cervical spine. *J Bone Joint Surg, 45B:*21-35, February, 1963.

Behan, Richard J.: *Pain.* New York, Appleton, 1914.

Bell, B. T., Viek, P. and Santangelo, S. C.: A problem in the diagnosis of traumatic lesions of the lower cervical spine. *Orthopedics, 2:*130-135, June, 1960.

Bell, G. E., Jr. and Goldner, J. L.: Compression neuropathy of median nerve. *South Med J, 49:*966-972, September, 1956.

Bell, W. E.: *Orofacial Pains—Differential Diagnosis.* Dallas, Denedco, 1973.

Bennett, Sir Wm.: Some clinical aspects of pain. *Br Med J, 2:*1-4, 1904.

Benson, O. O., Jr. and Campbell, P. A.: Developments in aerospace medicine and association with preventive medicine. *JAMA, 174:*939-941, October 22, 1960.

Bernstein, S. A.: Acute pain with soft tissue calcium deposition anterior to the interspace of the first and second cervical vertebrae. *J Bone Joint Surg, 57A:*426-428, April, 1974.

Bick, E. M.: Vertebral osteophytosis in the aged. *Clin Orthoped, 26:*50-53, 1963.

Bickerstaff, E. R.: Basilar artery migraine. *Lancet, 1:*15-17, January 7, 1961.

Billig, H. E., Jr.: Bone and joint changes following injury. *J Int Coll Surg, 19:*760-762, June, 1953.

———: Traumatic neck, head, eye syndrome. *J Int Coll Surg, 20:*558-560, November, 1953.

———: The mechanism of whiplash injuries. *Int Rec Med, 169:*3-7, January, 1956.

———: Head, neck, shoulder and arm syndrome following cervical injury: the mechanism of injury and the symptoms and signs involved. *J Int Coll Surg, 32:*287-297, September, 1959.

Bingham, R.: Treatment of sprains with ethyl chloride spray. *Milit Surg, 96:*170-174, February, 1945.

Bjorksten, J.: The crosslinkage theory of aging; clinical implications. *Comp Ther, 2:*65-74, February, 1976.

Blair, R. D. G. and Lee, G.: Dorsal column stimulation. *Arch Neur, 32:* 826-829, December, 1975.

Blashy, M. R. M.: Manipulation of the neuromuscular unit via the periphery of the central nervous system. *South Med J, 54:*873-879, August, 1961.

Blumberg, B. S.: Joint lubrication. *Bull Rheum Dis, 9:*169-170, October, 1958.

Blumer, D.: Psychiatric disorders of the spine. In Rothman and Simeone (Eds.): *The Spine,* Vol. 2. Philadelphia, Saunders, 1975, pp. 871-905.

Bogoch, S. and Dreyfus, J.: The broad range of use of diphenylhydantoin. *The Dryfus Med Found Lib of Cong,* Vol 1, 1970; Vol 2, 1975.

Bonica, J. J. and Clawson, D. K.: Management of chronic pain. *Inst Course, A.A.O.S.,* January 1974.

Boucher, H. H.: A method of spinal fusion. *J Bone Joint Surg, 41B:*248-259, May, 1959.

Bovill, E. G., Jr. and Drazek, J. A.: Anatomic study of cervical spine based on clinical-roentgenologic concept of etiology of brachiaglia. *U Mich Med Bull, 16:*387-398, December, 1950.

Boylston, B. F.: Oblique roentgenographic views of the cervical spine in flexion and extension, an aid in the diagnosis of cervical subluxations and obscure dislocations. *J Bone Joint Surg, 39A:*1302-1309, December, 1957.

Braaf, M. M. and Rosner, S.: Symptomatology and treatment of injuries of the neck. *NY State J Med, 55:*237-242, January 15, 1955.

———: Whiplash injury of the neck: symptoms, diagnosis, treatment, and prognosis. *NY J Med, 58:*1501-1507, May 1, 1958.

———: More recent concepts on treatment of headache. *Headache, 5:*38-44, July, 1965.

Braham, J. and Herzberger, E. E.: Cervical spondylosis and compression of the spinal cord. *JAMA, 161:*1560-1562, August 18, 1956.

Brain, R.: Cervical spondylosis. *Ann Intern Med, 41:*439, 1954.

Brannon, E. W.: Congenital malformation of the atlantoaxial joint with dislocation. *J Bone Joint Surg, 42A:*1377-1380, December, 1960.

Brashear, H. R., Jr. et al.: Fractures of the neural arch of the axis. *J Bone Joint Surg, 57A:*879-887, October, 1975.

Breasted, James Henry: The Edwin Smith surgical papyrus. *U Chicago Pr, 1:*319-323, 1930.

Bucy, P. C. and Oberhill, H. R.: Pain in the shoulder and arm from neurological involvement. *JAMA, 169:*798-803, February 21, 1959.

Bull, J. W. D.: Discussion on rupture of intervertebral disc. *Proc R Soc, 41:*513, 1948.

Bunts, A. T.: The surgical treatment of spasmodic torticollis. *Am Surg, 26:* 560-563, August, 1960.

———: The mimicry of tumors of the spinal cord. *Am Surg, 26:*630-633, September, 1960.

Calandruccio, R. A. and Gilmer, W. S., Jr.: Proliferation, generation, and repair of articular cartilage of immature animals. *J Bone Joint Surg, 44A:* 431-455, April, 1962.

Cameron, B. M.: The C-6-7 fusion of the cervical spine. *Am J Orthoped, 6:* 191-193, August-September, 1964.

————: The lawyer and the rear-end collision. *Am J Orthoped, 6:*177, August-September, 1964.

———— and Cree, C. M. N.: A critique of the compression theory of whiplash. *Orthopedics, 2:*127-129, June, 1960.

Camosso, Maria E. and Marotti, G.: The mechanical behavior of articular cartilage under compressive stress. *J Bone Joint Surg, 44A:*699-709, June, 1962.

Camp, W. A. and Wolff, H. G.: Studies on headache; electroencephalographic abnormalities in patients with vascular headache of the migraine type. *Arch (Chicago) Neurol, 4:*475-485, May, 1961.

Campbell, A. M. G., and Phillips, D. G.: Cervical disk lesions with neurological disorder; differential diagnosis, treatment and prognosis. *Br Med J, 2:*481-485, August 13, 1960.

Campbell, B. J.: The automotive crash injury research program of Cornell University. *J Iowa Med Soc, 51:*760-762, December, 1961.

Campbell, H. E.: And shoulder straps, too. (letter to the editor). *Med Tribune, 4:*11, January 25, 1963.

Campbell, J. A. and Campbell, R. L.: Angiographic diagnosis of traumatic head and neck lesions. *JAMA, 175:*761-768, March 4, 1961.

Cantrell, J. R.: Acupuncture: a form of psychological healing. *South Med J, 63:*14-17, 1975.

Cave, A. J. E. et al.: Osteoarthritis deformans of Luschka joints. *Lancet, 1:* 176, 1955.

Cerney, J. V.: *Acupuncture without Needles.* West Nyack, Parker, 1974.

Chapman, L. F., Ramos, A. O., Goodell, H. and Wolff, H. G.: Neurohumoral features of afferent fibers in man: their role in vasodilatation, inflammation, and pain. *Arch Neurol (Chicago), 4:*617-650, June, 1961.

Chapple, R. V. and Singher, H. O.: *The Use of the Enzyme Plasmin (Fibrinolysin) in Clinical Therapy.* Paper presented at the 108th annual meeting, AMA, June 8-12, 1959.

Chen, K. K.: Newer synthetic analgesics. *Med Clin North Am, 34:*369-378, March, 1950.

Chin, W. J. and Derrick, W. S.: Acupuncture indications, techniques and preliminary clinical results. *Tex Med J, 77:*66-73, January, 1975.

Clippinger, F. W., Goldner, J. L. and Roberts, J. M.: Use of the electromyogram in evaluating upper-extremity peripheral nerve lesions. *J Bone Joint Surg, 44A:*1047-1060, September, 1962.

Cloward, R. B.: Cervical diskography; technique, indications and use in diagnosis of ruptured cervical disks. *Am J Roentgen, 79:*563-574, April, 1958.

———: The anterior approach for removal of ruptured cervical disks. *J Neurosurg, 15:*602-617, November, 1958.

———: Vertebral body fusion for ruptured cervical discs; description of instruments and operative technic. *Am J Surg, 98:*722-727, November, 1959.

———: Cervical diskography; a contribution to the etiology and mechanism of neck, shoulder and arm pain. *Ann Surg, 150:*1052-1064, December, 1959.

———: The clinical significance of the sinu-vertebral nerves of the cervical spine in relation to the cervical disk syndrome. *J Neurol Neurosurg Psychiat, 23:*321-326, November, 1960.

Cohen, A., Scott, G. E., Turner, R. F. and Rose, I.: Intra-articular and paravertebral injection of cortisone in osteoarthritis of spine. *JAMA, 159:*1724-1727, December 31, 1955.

Cohn, A. M.: Evaluation and management of the dizzy patient. *South Med J, 68:*548-590, May, 1975.

Collins, H. R.: An evaluation of cervical and lumbar discography. *Clin Orthop, 107:*133-138, 1975.

Compensation complex: *Physicians Bull, 1:*60-61, Summer, 1951.

Compere, E. L. and Keyes, D. C.: Roentgenological studies of the intervertebral disc. *Am J Roentgen, 29:*774-795, June, 1933.

Compere, E. L., Tachjian, M. O. and Kernahan, W. T.: The Luschka joints; their anatomy, physiology and pathology. *Orthopedics, 1:*159-163; 166-167, May, 1959.

Coppola, A. R.: Neck injury. *Intern Surg, 50:*510-515, December, 1968.

Cordrey, L. J.: Trauma in arthritis of the spine. *Orthopedics, 2:*137-139, June, 1960.

Crane, C. and Johnson, R.: Nerve conduction velocity and doppler evaluations of thoracic outlet syndrome. *South Med J, 67:*269-270, March, 1974.

Crawford, E. S., DeBakey, M. E. and Fields, W. S.: Roentgenographic diagnosis and surgical treatment of basilar artery insufficiency. *JAMA, 168:*509-514, October 4, 1958.

Crock, H. V.: Post-traumatic erosions of articular cartilage. *J Bone Joint Surg, 46B:*530-538, August, 1964.

Crowe, H.: A new diagnostic sign in neck injuries. *Calif Med, 100:*12-13, January, 1964.

Crue, B. L., Pudenz, R. H. and Shelden, C. H.: Observations on the value of clinical electromyography. *J Bone Joint Surg, 39A:*492-500, June, 1957.

Cunningham, D. J.: *Cunningham's Textbook of Anatomy,* 10th ed. G. J. Romanes, ed. London, New York, Oxford, 1964.

Davis, A. G.: Injuries of the cervical spine. *JAMA, 127:*149-156, January 20, 1945; *127:*936, April 7, 1945.

Defense Research Institute: *The Continuing Revolt Against "Whiplash."* Milwaukee, Defense Research Institute, 1964.

DeJong, R. N.: *The Neurologic Examination.* 2nd ed. New York, Hoeber, 1958.

Delmas, J., Laux, G. and Guerrier, Y.: Comment atteindre les fibres préganglionaires. *Gaz Méd France, 54:*703, 1947.

Denny-Brown, D. and Russell, W. R.: Experimental cerebral concussion. *Brain, 64:*93-164, September, 1941.

DeWeese, D. D.: *Dizziness; An Evaluation and Classification.* Springfield, Thomas, 1954.

Drackman, D. A.: What's new and important in dizziness. *Med Tribune, 7,* December 25, 1974.

Duchenne, G. B. A.: *Physiology of Motion Demonstrated by Means of Electrical Stimulation and Clinical Observation and Applied to the Study of Paralysis and Deformities.* Philadelphia, Lippincott, 1949.

Dugan, Mildred C., Locke, S. and Gallagher, J. R.: Occipital neuralgia in adolescents and young adults. *N Engl J Med, 267:*1166-1172, December 6, 1962.

Dunn, E. J.: Techniques of fusion in treatment of fractures and dislocations of cervical spine. *Orthop Rev, 11:*17-24, April, 1973.

Durman, D. C.: Trauma in the causation and aggravation of arthritis. *J Int Coll Surg, 34:*674-678, November, 1960.

Dyck, P. J. et al.: Clinical vs quantitative evaluation of cutaneous sensation. *Arch Neurol, 33:*651-657, September, 1976.

Eagle, W. W.: The symptoms, diagnosis and treatment of the elongated styloid process. *Am Surg, 28:*1-5, January, 1962.

Editorial: Chinese medicine—acupuncture statement of the AMA delegation. *Dallas Med J, 60:*429-430, September, 1974.

Ellis, W. G., Green, D., Holzaepfel, N. R. and Sahs, A. L: The trampoline and serious neurological injuries; a report of five cases. *JAMA, 174:* 1673-1676, November 26, 1960.

Epstein, J. A., Epstein, B. S. and Lavine, L. S.: Cervical spondylotic myelopathy. The syndrome of the narrow canal treated by laminectomy, foramenotomy, and the removal of osteophytes. *Arch Neurol (Chicago), 8:*307-317, March, 1963.

Evaluating back injuries. *Spectrum, 9:*54-57, Summer, 1961.

Evans, D. K.: Reduction of cervical dislocations. *J Bone Joint Surg, 43B:* 552-555, August, 1961.

Evans, J. A.: Reflex sympathetic dystrophy. *Ann Intern Med, 26:*417-426, March, 1947.

Eyzagiurre, Carlos: *Physiology of the Nervous System.* Chicago, Year Bk Med, 1965.

Fang, H. C. H.: Cerebral arterial innervations in man. *Arch Neurol (Chicago), 4:*651-656, June, 1961.

Fang, H. S. Y. and Ong, G. B.: Direct anterior approach to the upper cervical spine. *J Bone Joint Surg, 44A:*1588-1604, December, 1962.

Fazekas, J. F., Alman, R. W. and Sullivan, J. F.: Vertebral-basilar insufficiency; management of patients with vertebral-basilar insufficiency. *Arch Neurol (Chicago), 8:*215-220, February, 1963.

Feric, D. C. et al.: Surgical treatment of the symptomatic unstable cervical spine in rheumatoid arthritis. *J Bone Joint Surg, 57A:*349-354, April, 1974.

Fielding, J. W.: Cineroentgenography of the normal cervical spine. *J Bone Joint Surg, 39A:*1280-1288, December, 1957.

Fielding, J. W. et al.: Disorders of the cervical spine. *Clin Orthop, 109:*2-102, June, 1975.

Fielding, J. W. et al.: Tears of the transverse ligament of the atlas. *J Bone Joint Surg, 56A:*1683-1691, December, 1974.

Fields, A.: The autonomic nervous system in whiplash injuries. *Int Rec Med, 169:*8-10, January, 1956.

Fineman, S., Borrelli, F. J., Rubinstein, Berta, M., Epstein, H. and Jacobsen, H. G.: The cervical spine; transformation of the normal lordotic pattern into a linear pattern in the neutral posture. A roentgenographic demonstration. *J Bone Joint Surg, 45A:*1179-1183, September, 1963.

Font, J. H.: Otorhinolaryngological considerations on the temporal arteritis syndrome. *JAMA, 174:*853-856, October 15, 1960.

For cervical discography. (letters to the editor). *JAMA, 189:*1032, September 28, 1964.

Ford, L. T. and Key, J. A.: The differential diagnosis of shoulder, upper back and neck pain and the conservative treatment of cervical disc lesions. *South Med J, 47:*961-968, October, 1954.

Forsyth, H. F., Alexander, E., Jr., Davis, C., Jr. and Linderdal, R.: The advantage of early spine fusion in the treatment of fracture-dislocation of the cervical spine. *J Bone Joint Surg, 41A:*17-36, January, 1959.

Fowlks, E. W.: A new approach to the treatment of cervical osteoarthritis with radiculitis. *Arch Phys Med, 35:*765-772, December, 1954.

Freeman, G. E., Jr.: Correction of severe deformity of the cervical spine in ankylosing spondylitis with the halo device. A case report. *J Bone Joint Surg, 43A:*547-552, June, 1961.

Friedenberg, Z. B. and Miller, W. T.: Degenerative disc disease of the cervical spine. A comparative study of asymptomatic and asymptomatic patients. *J Bone Joint Surg, 45A:*1171-1178, September, 1963.

Friedenberg, Z. B., Broder, H. A., Edeiken, J. E. and Spencer, H. N.: Degenerative disk disease of cervical spine; clinical and roentgenographic study. *JAMA, 174:*375-380, September 24, 1960.

Friedenberg, Z. B., Edeiken, J. and Spencer, H. N.: Degenerative changes in the cervical spine. *J Bone Joint Surg, 41A:*61-70, January, 1959.

Friedman, A. P., Finley, K. H., Graham, J. R., Kunkle, E. C., Ostfeld, A. M. and Wolff, H. G.: Classification of headache (The Ad Hoc Committee on Classification of Headache). *Arch Neurol (Chicago), 6:*173-176, March, 1962.

Froimson, A.: Stockinet head halter. *J Bone Joint Surg, 43A:*1241-1242, December, 1961.

Garretson, H. D. and Elvidge, A. R.: Glossopharyngeal neuralgia with asystole and seizures. *Arch Neurol (Chicago), 8:*26-31, January, 1963.

Gay, J. R. and Abbott, K. H.: Common whiplash injuries of the neck. *JAMA, 152:*1698-1704, August 29, 1953.

Gayral, L. and Neuwirth, E.: Oto-neuro-ophthalmologic manifestations of cervical origin; posterior cervical sympathetic syndrome of Barrè-Lieou. *NY J Med, 54:*1920-1926, July 1, 1954.

Geissendörfer, R.: Über die Kompression der Halsnerven in den Wirbellöchern and ihre Behandlung. *Arch Klin Chir, 276:*123-140, 1953.

Georgiade, N., Georgiade, R., Eiring, A., Stocker, F. W. and Matton-Von Leuven, M. T.: The prolonged preservation of tissues in a viable state. *Am Surg, 28:*6-12, January, 1962.

Gershon-Cohen, J., Budin, E. and Glauser, F.: Whiplash fractures of cervicodorsal spinous processes: resemblance to shoveler's fracture. *JAMA, 155:*560-561, June 5, 1954.

Gessel, A.: *Biofeedback in Pain Management.* Biomonitoring Applications Inc., 1975.

Gillman, E. L.: Congenital absence of the odontoid process of the axis; report of a case. *J Bone Joint Surg, 41A:*345-348, March, 1959.

Goff, C. W., Aldes, J. H. and Alden, J. O.: *Traumatic Cervical Syndrome and Whiplash.* Philadelphia, Lippincott, 1964.

Goldner, J. L.: Suprascapular nerve block for painful shoulder. *South Med J, 45:*1125-1131, December, 1952.

Gordan, G. S.: Osteoporosis: diagnosis and treatment. *Tex J Med, 57:*740-747, September, 1961.

Gordon, E. J.: Stellate ganglion block in treatment of bursitis and tendinitis of the shoulder. *South Med J, 45:*1131-1138, December, 1952.

Graham, W. and Rosen, P.: The shoulder-hand syndrome. *Bull Rheum Dis, 12:*277-278, April, 1962.

Greenwood, J., Jr.: Optimum vitamin C intake as a factor in preservation of disc integrity. *Med Ann DC, 33*(6): June 1964.

Gregorius, F. K. et al.: Cervical spondylitic radiculopathy and myelopathy. *Arch Neurol, 33:*618-625, September, 1976.

Grollman, A.: How drugs work: the analgesics. *Consultation, 14:*77-79, March, 1974.

Gurdjian, E. S. and Webster, J. E.: *Head Injuries; Mechanisms, Diagnosis, and Management.* Boston, Little, 1958.

Gurdjian, E. S., Lissner, H. R. and Patrick, L. M.: Protection of the head and neck in sports. *JAMA, 182:*509-512, November 3, 1962.

Gurdjian, E. S., Lissner, H. R., Evans, F. G., Patrick, L. M. and Hardy, W. G.: Intracranial pressure and acceleration accompanying head impacts in human cadavers. *Surg Gynecol Obstet, 113:*185-190, August, 1961.

Gurdjian, E. S., Lissner, H. R., Latimer, F. R., Haddad, B. F. and Webster, J. E.: Quantitative determination of acceleration and intracranial pressure in experimental head injury; preliminary report. *Neurology (Minneap), 3:*417-423, June, 1953.

Gustafson, G. E.: Cinéradiography in the diagnosis and prognosis of cervical injuries. Personal communication, January, 1974.

Hackett, G. S., Huang, T. C. and Raftery, A.: Prolotherapy for headache: pain in the head and neck, and neuritis. *Headache, 2:*20-28, April, 1962.

Hadley, L. A.: *The Spine Anatomico-Radiographic Studies: Development and the Cervical Region.* Springfield, Thomas, 1956.

————: Development and congenital anomalies of the cervical vertebrae. *Clin Orthop, 24:*12-21, 1962.

Hadley, Lee A.: *Anatomico-Roentgenographic Studies of the Spine.* Springfield, Thomas, 1964.

Hall, M. C. and Selin, G.: Spinal involvement in gout. A case report with autopsy. *J Bone Joint Surg, 42A:*341-343, March, 1960.

Hall, M. C.: *Luschka's Joint.* Springfield, Thomas, 1965.

Hamel, H. A. and James, O. E., Jr.: Acute traumatic cervical syndrome (whiplash injury). *South Med J, 55:*1171-1177, November, 1962.

Hanflig, S. S.: Pain in the shoulder girdle, arm and precordium due to foraminal compression of nerve roots. *Arch Surg (Chicago), 46:*652-663, May, 1943.

Hanson, T. A. et al.: Subluxation of the cervical vertebrae due to pharyngitis. *South Med J, 66:*427-430, April, 1973.

Haynes, A. L. and Lissner, H. R.: Experimental head impact studies. *Proceedings of the Fifth Stapp Automotive Crash and Field Demonstration Conference,* 1961, pp. 158-170.

Health quackery devices. *N.M.F. Newsletter, 16:*1, April, 1976.

Heard, G. E., Holt, J. F. and Naylor, B.: Cervical vertebral deformity in von Recklinghausen's disease of the nervous system. A review with necropsy findings. *J Bone Joint Surg, 44B:*880-885, November, 1962.

Hendry, N. G. C.: The hydration of the nucleus pulposus and its relation to intervertebral disc derangement. *J Bone Surg, 40B:*132-144, February, 1958.

Hermann, R.: How auto crash research would lessen the toll. Scientists press for more seat belts, want car that's like armor. *Nat Observer, 2:*1, 14, December 2, 1963.

Hilding, D. A. and Tachdjian, M. O.: Dysphagia and hypertrophic spurring of the cervical spine. *N Engl J Med, 263:*11-14, July 7, 1960.

Hohl, M.: Soft tissue injuries of the neck in automobile accidents. *J Bone Joint Surg, 56A:*1675-1682, December, 1974.

Hollander, J. L. (Ed.): *Arthritis and Allied Conditions,* 6th ed. Philadelphia, Lea, 1960.

Hollander, J. L.: Environment and musculoskeletal diseases. *Arch Environ Health (Chicago), 6:*527-536, April, 1963.

Holt, E. P., Jr.: Fallacy of cervical discography; report of 50 cases in normal subjects. *JAMA, 188:*799-801, June 1, 1964.

————: Further reflections on cervical discography. *JAMA, 231:*613-614, 1975.

Horton, W .G.: Further observations on the elastic mechanism of the intervertebral disc. *J Bone Joint Surg, 40B:*552-557, August, 1958.

Horwich, H. and Kasner, D.: The effect of whiplash injuries on ocular functions. *South Med J, 55:*69-71, January, 1962.

Hubbard, J. H.: The management of pain of spinal origin. In Rothman, R. H. and Simeone, F. A. (Eds.): *The Spine,* Vol. 2. Philadelphia, Saunders, 1975, pp. 837-869.

Humphrey, J. S. and Shy, G. M.: Diagnostic electromyography: clinical and pathological correlation in neuromuscular disorders. *Arch Neurol (Chicago), 6:*339-352, May, 1962.

Husni, E. A. et al.: Mechanical occlusion of the vertebral artery. *JAMA, 196:*475-478, May 9, 1966.

Hussey, H. H.: Cardiac pain. *GP, 8:*41-51, September, 1953.

Iraci, G. and Ruberti, R.: Intraspinal tumors of the cervical spinal tract. *Int Surg, 46:*154-167, August, 1966.

Jackson, J. D. and Schindel, W.: *Cervical Spondylosis.* Scientific Exhibit, Am Acad Orthop Surgeons, Chicago, Illinois, January, 1964.

Jackson, Ruth: The cervical syndrome as a cause of migraine. *J Am Med Wom Assoc, 2:*529-534, December, 1947.

————: The cervical syndrome. *Clin Orthop, 5:*138-147, 1955.

————: The structural injuries. *Arch Phys Med, 40:*383-386, September, 1959.

————: The syndrome of cervical nerve root compression. In Hollander, J. L. (Ed.): *Arthritis and Allied Conditions,* 6th ed. Philadelphia, Lea & Febiger, 1960, pp. 1162-1180.

————: Neck injuries. *Trauma, 1:*7-85, February, 1960.

————: Whiplash injuries of the neck. Editorial. *Dallas Med J, 46:*502, October, 1960.

————: Preface to symposium: Disorders of the cervical spine. *Clin Orthop, 24:*9-11, 1962.

————: Die konservative Behandlung bei Verletzungen der Halswirbelsäule. *Sonderdruck ous Verhandlungen der Deutschen Orthopädischen Gesellschaft, 50th Congress, Munich, September 19-22, 1962.* Stuttgart, Enke, 1963.

————: The positive findings in alleged neck injuries. *Am J Orthop, 6:* 178-181; 184-187, August-September, 1964.

————: Injuries of the upper portion of the cervical spine. *Lawyers Med Cyclopedia,* supplement, *8:*53-60, 1965.

————: Nonsurgical therapeutic aims. Cervical Pain. *Wenner-Gren Center, Int Sym Series, 19:*113-144, January, 1971.

————: The syndrome of cervical nerve root compression. In Hollander, J. L. (Ed.): *Arthritis,* 8th ed. Philadelphia, Lea & Febiger, 1972, 1444-1460.

Jacobs, B. et al.: Cervical spondylosis with radiculopathy. *JAMA, 211:* 2135-2139, March 30, 1970.

Judovich and Bates: *Pain Syndromes.* Philadelphia, Davis, 1953.

Judovich, B. D.: Herinated cervical disc; a new form of traction therapy. *Am J Surg, 84:*646-656, December, 1952.

Jung, A. and Brunschwig, A.: Recherches histologiques sur l'innervation des articulations des corps vertébraux. *Presse Med, 40:*316-317, February 27, 1932.

Kambin, P., Smith, J. M. and Hoerner, E. F.: Myelography and myography in diagnosis of herinated intervertebral disk; use in confirming clinical findings. *JAMA, 181:*472-475, August 11, 1962.

Kaplan, E. B.: Anatomy of recurrent meningeal branch of spinal nerves. *Bull Hosp Joint Dis, 8:*108, April, 1947.

Kaplan, L. and Kennedy, F.: Effect of head posture on the manometrics of cerebrospinal fluid in cervical lesions. *Brain, 73:*337-345, September, 1950.

Karlen, A.: Congenital hypoplasia of the odontoid process. *J Bone Joint Surg, 44A:*567-570, April, 1962.

Karpati, S. et al.: Multiple peripheral entrapments of peripheral nerves. *Arch Neurol, 31:*418-422, 1974.

Kaslow, A. L.: *A Primer on Electro-acupuncture without Needles.* Bio Instr, Inc., 1974.

Kawamura, B. and Hosome, S.: Scalenus syndrome and its causation. *J Jap Ortho Surg Soc, 31:*1611, February, 1958.

Kayfetz, D. O.: Occipitocervical (whiplash) injuries treated by prolotherapy. *Med Trial Techn Q, 9:*9-29; passim, June, 1963.

Keggi, K. J. et al.: Vertebral insufficiency secondary to trauma and osteoarthritis of the cervical spine. *Yale J Bio Med, 38:*471-478, April, 1966.

Kelly, M.: Does pressure on nerves cause pain? *Med J Aust, 1:*118-121, January 23, 1960.

Keplinger, J. E. and Bucy, P. C.: Paraplegia from treatment with sclerosing agents. *JAMA, 173*(12): July 23, 1960.

Kerr, F. L.: The etiology of trigeminal neuralgia. *Arch Neurol (Chicago), 8:*15-25, January, 1963.

Kerr, F. W. L. and Alexander, S.: Descending autonomic pathways in the spinal cord. *Arch Neurol (Chicago)*, *10:*249-261, March, 1964.

Kerr, F. W. L. and Brown, J. A.: Pupillomotor pathways in the spinal cord. *Arch Neurol (Chicago)*, *3:*262-270, March, 1964.

Keyes, D. C.: Personal Communication.

Kirgis, H. D. and Buchtel, B. C.: *Traumatic Cervical Myelopathy: Etiology, Evaluation and Treatment.* AMA Exhibit, June, 1968.

Kishan, Chand: Cervical spine and rheumatoid arthritis. *Int Surg, 57:*721-726, 1972.

Köhler, A.: *Borderlands of the Normal and Early Pathologic in Skeletal Roentgenology,* 10th ed. completely revised by E. A. Zimmer. New York, Grune & Stratton, 1956.

Kolondy, A. L.: Double-blind evaluation of asperkinase, a new proteolytic enzyme. *Orthopedics, 5:*234-235, August, 1963.

Korkis, F. B.: The treatment of Bell's palsy by cervical sympathetic block. *J Int Coll Surg, 35:*42-46, January, 1961.

Kory, M.: Serotonin. *Physician's Bull, 28:*43-47, August, 1963.

Kosoy, J. and Glassman, A. L.: Audiovestibular findings with cervical spine trauma. *Tex Med J, 70:*66-71, October, 1974.

Kraus, H.: Evaluation and treatment of muscle function in athletic injury. *Am J Surg, 98:*353-362, September, 1959.

Kremer, R. M. and Alquist, R. E.: Thoracic outlet compression syndrome. *Am J Surg, 130:*612-615, November, 1975.

Krusen, E. M.: Acute injuries of the neck. *Mod Med, 28:*200-215, September 15, 1960.

Kubala, M. J. and Millikan, C. H.: Diagnosis, pathogenesis and treatment of "drop attacks." *Arch Neurol (Chicago), 11:*107-113, August, 1964.

Kuhn, R. A.: Successful radiographic demonstration of the human circle of Willis. *JAMA, 175:*769-772, March 4, 1961.

Kulowski, Jacob: Motorist injuries and motorist safety. *Clin Orthop, 9:* 251-344, Philadelphia, Lippincott, 1957.

Kuntz, A.: The anatomical basis of reflex vasomotor activity and pain of vascular origin. *South Med J, 48:*338-344, April, 1955.

Kuntz, Albert: Afferent innervation of peripheral blood vessels through the sympathetic trunks. *South Med J, 44:*673-778, 1951.

LaFratta, C. W. and Porterfield, J. B.: A review of the "fibrostitis" question. *South Med J, 54:*1242-1247, November, 1961.

Lagos, J. L.: Current concepts in diagnosis: electromyography in the diagnosis of neuromuscular disease. *South Med J, 66:*823-829, July, 1973.

Langley, R. W.: Painful conditions simulating heart disease. *Ann West Med Surg, 6:*49-52, January, 1952.

Leuernieux, J.: *Les Tractions Vertebrales Expansion.* Paris Scientifique Francaise, 1960.

Lewis, R. C. and Coburn, D. F.: The vertebral artery; its role in upper cervical and head pain. *Missouri Med, 53:*1059-1063, December, 1956.

Lin, T. H.: Paraplegia caused by epidural hemorrhage of the spine. *J Int Col Surg, 36:*742-749, December, 1961.

Linenthal, A. J.: Effects of carotid sinus reflex on cardiac impulse formation and conduction. *Circulation, 20:*595-601, October, 1959.

Lipow, E. G.: Whiplash injuries. *South Med J., 48:*1304-1310, December, 1955.

Lipow, E. G. and Fulcher, O. H.: *Traumatic Affections of the Cervical Spine.* Washington, D.C., Georgetown University School of Medicine, 1960.

Lipow, E. G. and Fulcher, O. H.: Traumatic disorders of cervical spine. *Mod Med, 30:*103-112, July 9, 1962.

Lipscomb, P. R.: Cervico-occipital fusion for congenital and post-traumatic anomalies of the atlas and axis. *J Bone Joint Surg, 39A:*1289-1301, December, 1957.

Livingston, M. C. P.: Spinal manipulation causing injury. *Clin Ortho, 81:* 82-86, November-December, 1971.

Lockhart, R. D., Hamilton, G. F. and Fyfe, F. W.: *Anatomy of the Human Body.* Philadelphia, Lippincott, 1959.

Loeser, J. A. et al.: Relief of pain by transcutaneous stimulation. *J Neurosurg, 42:*308-314, 1975.

Lourie, H. et al.: The syndrome of central soft disk herniation. *JAMA, 226* (No. 3):302-305, October 15, 1973.

Love, J. G. and Rivers, M. H.: Spinal cord tumors simulating protruded intervertebral disks. *JAMA, 179:*878-881, March 17, 1962.

Macnab, Ian: Acceleration injuries of the cervical spine. *J Bone Joint Surg, 46A:*1797-1799, December, 1964.

————: Acceleration extension injuries of the cervical spine. In Rothman and Simeone (Eds.): *The Spine,* Vol. 2. Philadelphia, Saunders, 1975, pp. 515-528.

Magee, K. R. and DeJong, R. N.: Paralytic brachial neuritis; discussion of clinical features with review of 23 cases. *JAMA, 174:*1258-1262, November 5, 1960.

Magill, C. D.: Letter to the editor. *JAMA, 236* (No. 6):562, August, 1976.

Maigne, R.: *Orthopaedic Medicine. A New Approach to Vertebral Manipulation.* Springfield, Thomas, 1972.

Majno, G. and Palade, G. E.: Studies on inflammation. I. The effect of histamine and serotonin on vascular permeability: an electron microscopic study. *J Biophys Biochem Cytol, 11:*571-605, December, 1961.

Majno, G., Palade, G. E. and Schoefl, G. I.: Studies on inflammation. II. The site of action of histamine and serotonin along the vascular tree: a topographic study. *J Biophys Biochem Cytol, 11:*607-626, December, 1961.

Major Types of Chronic Headache; A Study of Their Etiology and Management. St. Louis, Dios Chemical Company, 1951.

Malingering: *Therapeutic Notes, 68:*271-275, October, 1961.

Mannick, J. A., Suter, C. G. and Hume, D. M.: The "subclavian steal" syndrome: a further documentation. *JAMA, 182:*254-258, October 20, 1962.

Manning, G. C., Jr.: The estimation of disability following injury. *J Int Coll Surg, 33:*471-481, April, 1960.

Mansour, J. M., Ph.D.: The permeability of articular cartilage under compressive strain and at high pressures. *J Bone Joint Surg, 58A:*509-516, June, 1976.

Marar, B. C.: Hyperextension injuries of the cervical spine. *J Bone Joint Surg, 56A:*1655-1662, December, 1974.

————: The pattern of neurological damage as an aid to the diagnosis of the mechanism in cervical spine disorders. *J Bone Joint Surg, 56A:*1648-1654, December, 1974.

Marinacci, A. A. and Courville, C. B.: Radicular syndromes simulating intra-abdominal surgical conditions. *Am Surg, 28:*59-63, February, 1962.

Markolf, K. L. and Morris, J. M.: Structural components of the intervertebral disc. *J Bone Joint Surg, 56A:*675-687, June, 1974.

Martin, G. J.: Proteolytic enzymes and inflammation. *Ex Med Int Cong Series, 82:*90-97, September, 1974.

Master, A. M.: The spectrum of anginal and noncardiac chest pain. *JAMA, 187:*894-899, March 21, 1964.

McBride, E. D.: Examination of the back, a diagnostic outline for standardized routine. *South Med J, 39:*867-876, November, 1946.

McCarroll, J. R., Braunstein, P. W., Cooper, W., Helpren, M., Seremetis, M., Wade, P. A. and Weinberg, S. B.: Fatal pedestrian automotive accidents. *JAMA, 180:*127-133, April 14, 1962.

McCracken, D. M.: Survival car II. *Med Mat, 5:*30-31, 1963.

McFarland, R. A.: The epidemiology of motor vehicle accidents. *JAMA, 180:*289-300, April 28, 1962.

Mennell, J. McM.: *Back Pain: Diagnosis and Treatment Using Manipulative Techniques.* Boston, Little, 1960.

Meyer, J. S., Gotoh, F., Tazaki, Y., Hamaguchi, K., Ishikawa, S., Nouailhat, F. and Symon, L.: Regional cerebral blood flow and metabolism in vivo. Effects of anoxia, hypoglycemia, ischemia, acidosis, alkalosis, and alterations of blood PCO_2. *Arch Neurol (Chicago), 7:*560-581, December, 1962.

Michele, A. A., Davies, J. J., Krueger, F. J. and Lichtor, J. M.: Scapulocostal syndrome (fatigue-postural paradox). *NY J Med, 50:*1353-1356, June 1, 1950.

Microscope shows whiplash injuries unseen on x-ray. Seventh Annual Stapp Car Crash Conference. *Med Tribune, 4:*3, December 30, 1963.

Miller, D. and Bleasel, K. F.: Cervical nerve root compression and "shoulder-hand syndrome." *Med J Aust, 25:*448-450, September 22, 1956.

Milligan, P. R.: The neck-shoulder-arm syndrome. *Rocky Mountain Med J, 56:*63-67, September, 1959.

Mones, R. J., Christoff, N., and Bender, M. B.: Posterior cerebral artery occlusion. A clinical and angiographic study. *Arch Neurol (Chicago), 5:*68-76, July, 1961.

Moore, M. E. and Burke, S.: Acupuncture in arthritis treatment. *Ortho Rev, 5:*55-56, 1976.

Morgan, E. H.: Pain in the shoulder and upper extremity; visceral causes considered by the internist. *JAMA, 169:*804-808, February 21, 1959.

Morgan, E. H. and Hill, L. D.: Objective identification of chest pain of esophageal origin. *JAMA, 187:*921-926, March 21, 1964.

Morrison, A.: Hyperextension injury of the cervical spine with rupture of the oesophagus. *J Bone Joint Surg, 42B:*356-357, May, 1960.

Munro, D.: Relation between spondylosis cervicalis and injury of the cervical spine and its contents. *N Engl J Med, 262:*839-846, April 28, 1960.

Musser, J. H.: Pain of obscure origin simulating neuritis, neuralgia, or organic lesions. *Penn Med J,* 1905.

Nachlas, I. W.: The broad symptomatologic spectrum in injuries of the cervical spine. *Southwest Med, 39:*93-97, February, 1958.

Nathan, H.: Osteophytes of the vertebral column. An anatomical study of their development according to age, race, and sex with considerations as to their etiology and significance. *J Bone Joint Surg, 44A:*243-268, March, 1962.

Nelson, P. A.: Physical treatment of the painful arm and shoulder. *JAMA, 169:*814-817, February 21, 1959.

Nelson, Peter: Mayo study contradicts gate theory of pain. *Med Tribune,* 20, March 26, 1975.

Neuwirth, E.: The vertebral nerve in the posterior cervical syndrome. *NY J Med, 55:*1380, May 1, 1955.

————: Current status of spinal traction. *J Lancet, 77:*243-246, July, 1957.

————: Current concepts of the cervical portion of the sympathetic nervous system. *J Lancet, 80:*337-338, July, 1960.

———— and Gayral, L.: The shoulder-hand syndrome, syndrome of Barré-Lieou, and osteoarthritis of the cervical spine. *J Lancet, 79:*172-173, April, 1959.

Neviaser, J. S. and Eisenberg, S. H.: Giant cell reparative granuloma of the cervical spine. *Bull Hosp Joint Dis, 20:*73-78, April, 1954.

Nicholson, J. T. and Wieder, H. S., Jr.: Shoulder pain. *JAMA, 169:*809-814, February 21, 1959.

Nodine, J. H. and Moyer, J. H. (Eds.): *Psychosomatic Medicine.* Philadelphia, Lea & Febiger, 1962.

Norman, A.: The use of tomography in the diagnosis of skeletal disorders. *Clin Orth, 107:*139-145, 1975.

Norrell, H. H.: Fractures and dislocations of the spine. In Rothman, R. H. and Simeone, F. A. (Eds.): *The Spine,* Vol. 2. Philadelphia, Saunders, 1975, pp. 529-557.

North Carolina Highway Safety Research Center: Age and sex factors in the control of automobiles. February, 1972.

North Carolina Symposium on Highway Safety: Vol. 5, 1971 and Vol. 6, 1972.

Norton, W. L.: Fractures and dislocations of the cervical spine. *J Bone Joint Surg, 44A:*115-139, January, 1962.

O'Donoghue, Arch F.: Personal communication.

Ogden, H. D. and Schockett, L.: Controlled studies of chlorzoxazone and chlorzoxazone plus acetaminophen in the treatment of myaglia associated with headache. *South Med J, 53:*1415-1418, November, 1960.

Okubo, Jin: Study of the upper cervical spine by means of panoramic tomography. *Bull Tokyo Med, 20:*105-119, 1973.

Olsson, S.: Controlled paravertebral injection of hydrocortisone in cervical rhizopathy. *Acta Rad, 51:*439-442, June, 1959.

Oppenheimer, A.: The swollen atrophic hand. *Surg Gynecol Obstet, 67:*446-450, October, 1938.

Orofino, C., Sherman, Mary S. and Schechter, D.: Luschka's joint—a degenerative phenomenon. *J Bone Joint Surg, 42A:*853-858, July, 1960.

Ostrowski, A. Z., Hardy, W. G., Lindner, D. W., Thomas, L. M. and Gurdjian, E. S.: Retrograde brachial vertebral-basilar angiography: an analysis of angiographic visualization of the vertebral-basilar system and branches. *Arch Neurol (Chicago), 4:*608-616, June, 1961.

Ostrowski, J. P.: Carisoprodol (Soma) in orthopedic practice. *Orthopedics, 2:*7-9, January-February, 1960.

Overton and Grossman: Anatomic variations in the axiocervical articulations. *West Orthop Assoc,* 1950.

Palmer, D. M.: Abnormal mental reactions following trauma not involving the nervous system. *J Int Coll Surg, 34:*237-245, August, 1960.

Pancoast, H. K.: Superior pulmonary sulcus tumors. *JAMA, 99:*1391, 1932.

Patrick, L. M.: *Caudo-cephaled Static and Dynamic Injuries to the Vertebrae.* Proceedings of the Fifth Stapp Automotive Crash and Field Demonstration Conference, 1961, pp. 171-181.

Paulos, E. et al.: Experience with the subclavian steal syndrome. *Tex Med, 71:*74-79, 1975.

Paulson, D.: Carcinomas in the superior pulmonary sulcus. *J Thor Cardiovas Surg, 70:*1095-1104, December, 1975.

Perret, G.: Experimental and clinical investigations of peripheral nerve injuries of the upper extremities. *JAMA, 146:*556-560, June 9, 1951.

Peterson, C. R.: Electrodiagnosis in peripheral nerve lesions. *Tex J Med, 61*:18-21, January, 1965.

Peterson and Graham: Stiff neck. *West Orthop Assoc,* 1956.

Pettigrew, J. A.: Who has a brain tumor? *Am Surg, 28*:604-605, September, 1962.

Pierce, D. S.: Electrodiagnosis in orthopaedic surgery. *Clin Ortho Surg, 107*:25-35, 1975.

Poalo, D. J. et al.: The injured cervical spine, immediate and long-term stabilization with the halo. *JAMA, 224*:591-594, 1973.

Poser, C. M., Snodgrass, R. G. and Faris, A. A.: Radiologic visualization of neck vessles in cerebrovascular insufficiency. *JAMA, 182*:126-131, October 13, 1962.

Potes, J., McDowell, F. and Wells, C. E.: Electroencephalogram in brain stem infarction. *Arch Neurol (Chicago), 5*:21-27, July, 1961.

Prinzmetal, M. and Massumi, R. A.: The anterior chest wall syndrome—chest pain resembling pain of cardiac origin. *JAMA, 159*:177-184, September 17, 1955.

Proceedings of Conferences of the Am Assoc for Automotive Med, 1974, 1975, 1976.

Prolo, D. J. and Hanberry, J. W.: Cervical stabilization-traction-board. *JAMA, 224*:615, 1973.

Pruce, A. M.: Whiplash injury: what's new? *South Med J, 57*:332-337, March, 1964.

Rabinovitch, Reuben: *Diseases of the Intervertebral Disc and Its Surrounding Tissues.* Springfield, Thomas, 1961.

Rainer, W. G. et al.: Surgical considerations in the treatment of vertebro-basilar arterial insufficiency. *Am J Surg, 120*:594-597, November, 1970.

Rand, R. W. and Crandall, P. H.: Central spinal cord syndrome in hyperextension injuries of the cervical spine. *J Bone Joint Surg, 44A*:1415-1422, October, 1962.

Rawlings, M. S.: The "rib syndrome." *Dis Chest, 41*:432-441, April, 1962.

Rawls, W. B., Evans, W. L., Jr., Mistretta, C. V. and D'Alessandro, F. M.: Nocturnal or recumbency muscle cramps. *Med Times, 87*:818-828, June, 1959.

Reischauer, F. (Ed.): *Die cervikalen Vertebral-Syndrome.* Stuttgart, Thieme, 1955.

Rhoads, J. E. and Howard, J. M.: *The Chemistry of Trauma.* Springfield, Thomas, 1963.

Ritvo, M.: *Bone and Joint X-ray Diagnosis.* Philadelphia, Lea & Febiger, 1955.

Roaf, R.: A study of the mechanics of spinal injuries. *J Bone Joint Surg, 42B*:810-823, November, 1960.

———: Lateral flexion injuries of the cervical spine. *J Bone Joint Surg, 45B*:36-38, February, 1963.

Robbins, S. L.: *Textbook of Pathology with Clinical Applications,* 2d ed. Philadelphia, Saunders, 1962, pp. 62-89.

Robinson, R. A.: Fusion of the cervical spine. *J Bone Joint Surg, 41A:*1-6, January, 1959.

————: The result of anterior interbody fusion of the cervical spine. *J Bone Joint Surg, 44A:*1569-1587, December, 1962.

————: The problem of referred pain in abnormal intervertebral function-decompression rarely helps. *Braces Today,* May, 1964, pp. 2, 3, 4.

Robinson, R. A. and Southwick, W. O.: Indications and technics for early stabilization of the neck in some fracture dislocations of the cervical spine. *South Med J, 53:*565-579, May, 1960.

Robinson, R. A., Walker, E., Ferlic, D. C. and Wieckling, D. K.: The results of anterior interbody fusion of the cervical spine. *J Bone Joint Surg, 44A:*1569-1587, December, 1962.

Robinson, W. D.: Current status of the treatment of gout. *JAMA, 164:*1670-1674, August 10, 1957.

Rogers, L.: The surgical treatment of cervical spondylotic myelopathy. Mobilization of the complete cervical cord into an enlarged canal. *J Bone Joint Surg, 43B:*3-6, February, 1961.

Rogers, W. A.: Fractures and dislocations of the cervical spine; an end-result study. *J Bone Joint Surg, 39A:*341-376, April, 1957.

Rose, D. L.: The conservative management of the painful shoulder. *South Med J, 44:*1063-1066, November, 1951.

————: The whiplash injury. *Orthopedics, 2:*141-144, June, 1960.

Rose, G. K.: Prolapsed intervertebral disc. *Med Illustrated, 9:*219-232, April, 1955.

Rosenberg, S.: *Biofeedback: Clinical Application and Research.* Biomonitoring Applications, Inc., 1974.

Roth, D. A.: Cervical analgesic discography: a new test for diagnosis of the painful disc syndrome. *JAMA, 235:*1713-1714, April, 1976.

Rothman, R. H. and Simeone, F. A. (Eds.): *The Spine.* Philadelphia, Saunders, 1975.

Rubin, D.: Cervical radiculitis: diagnosis and treatment. *Arch Phys Med, 41:*580-586, December, 1960.

Rubin, W. and Norris, C. N.: *Electronystagmography.* Springfield, Thomas, 1974.

Rudin, L. N.: Physical therapy for pain in the neck. *Curr Med Dig, 24:*58-61, December, 1957.

Ruedemann, Albert D.: Automobile safety device headrest to prevent whiplash injury. *JAMA, 164:*1889, August 24, 1957.

Ruskin, S .L.: The control of muscle spasm and arthritic pain through sympathetic block at the nasal ganglion and the use of the adenylic nucleotide. Contributions to the physiology of muscle metabolism. Part II. *Am J Dig Dis, 13:*311-320, October, 1946.

————: A newer concept of arthritis and the treatment of arthritic pain and deformity by sympathetic block at the sphenopalatine (nasal) ganglion and the use of the iron salt of the adenylic nucleotide. "The dynamics of muscle tonus." Part IV. *Am J Dig Dis, 16:*386-401, November, 1949.

Sadler, T. R. et al.: Thoracic outlet compression. *Am J Surg, 130:*704-706, December, 1975.

Sahs, A. L.: Extracerebral neurovascular disease. A short review. *Arch Neurol (Chicago), 6:*87-95, February, 1962.

Sassard, W. R. et al.: Posterior atlantoaxial dislocation without fracture. *J Bone Joint Surg, 56A:*625-628, April, 1974.

Scherbel, A. L. and Gardner, W. J.: Infections involving the intervertebral disks. Diagnosis and management. *JAMA, 174:*370-374, September 24, 1960.

Schiff, D. C. and Parke, W. W.: The arterial supply of the odontoid process. *J Bone Joint Surg, 55A:*1450-1456, October, 1973.

Schmorl, G. and Junghanns, H.: *The Human Spine in Health and Disease.* New York, Grune & Stratton, 1959.

Schneider, R. C., Papo, M. and Soto Alverez, C.: The effects of chronic recurrent spinal trauma in high-diving; a study of Acapulco's divers. *J Bone Joint Surg, 44A:*648-656, June, 1962.

Schneider, R. C., Reifel, E., Crisler, H. O. and Oosterbaan, B. G.: Serious and fatal football injuries involving the head and spinal cord. *JAMA, 177:*362-367, August 12, 1961.

Schubert, H. A.: Peripheral nerve conduction studies; diagnostic value. *Tex J Med, 61:*10-17, January, 1965.

Schwan, H. P. and Carstensen, E. L.: Advantages and limitations of ultrasonics in medicine. *JAMA, 149:*121-125, May, 1952.

Seegmiller, J. E., Howell, R. and Malawista, S. E.: The inflammatory reaction to sodium urate; its possible relationship to the genesis of acute gouty arthritis. *JAMA, 180:*469-475, May 12, 1962.

Segal, J.: Biofeedback as a medical treatment. *JAMA, 232:*179-180, April, 1975.

Seletz, E.: Death on the highway and in sports. *J Int Coll Surg, 40:*41-44, September, 1963.

Selvin, B. and Howland, W. S.: New concepts of the physiology of the carotid sinus reflex. *JAMA, 176:*12-15, April 8, 1961.

Shannon, E. W.: Post traumatic neuroses. *Insurance Counsel J, 28:*472-475, July, 1961.

Shealy, C. N.: Disc syndrome termed vast clinical wasteland. *Med Tribune,* August 15, 1973, p. 1.

Sheehan, S.: Syndromes of basilar and carotid artery insufficiency: diagnosis and medical therapy. *South Med J, 54:*465-470, May, 1961.

Sheehan, S., Bauer, R. S. and Meyer, J. S.: Vertebral artery compression in cervical spondylosis. Arteriographic demonstration during life of vertebral artery insufficiency due to rotation and extension of the neck. *Neurology (Minneap)*, *10:*968-986, November, 1960.

Shenkin, H. A., Tatsumi, T. and Bantley, D.: Simplified method for total cerebral angiography. *JAMA*, *182:*132-135, October 13, 1962.

Shore, N. A.: *Occlusal Equilibration and Temporomandibular Joint Dysfunction.* Philadelphia, Lippincott, 1959.

Shore, N. S.: The symptomatology of temporomandibular joint dysfunction. *J NY Dent Assoc, 31:*10-15, September, 1959.

Silver, Carroll et al.: Orthopaedic management of affections of the temporomandibular joint. Scientific Exhibit, A.A.O.S., 1965.

Silver, D. J.: Cervical discography: is surgery necessary? *JAMA, 236(6):* 562, August, 1976.

Silver, M. and Steinbrocker, O.: The musculoskeletal manifestations of systemic lupus erythematosus. *JAMA, 176:*1001-1003, June 24, 1961.

Silverstein, A., Gilbert, H. and Wasserman, L. R.: Neurologic complications of polycythemia. *Ann Intern Med, 57:*909-916, December, 1962.

Smith, G. W. and Robinson, R. A.: The treatment of certain cervical spine disorders by anterior removal of the intervertebral disc and interbody fusion. *J Bone Joint Surg, 40A:*607-624, June, 1958.

Smith, H.: Painful shoulders; periarthritis. *J Tenn Med Assoc, 44:*330-334, August, 1951.

Smith, H. W. and Hubbard, O. E.: *Doing Scientific Justice: Psychological Reactions to Traumatic Stimuli.* U Illinois Law Forum, Summer, 1962.

Smith, L. A.: The pattern of pain in the diagnosis of upper abdominal disorders. *JAMA, 156:*1566-1573, December 25, 1954.

Smulker, N.: Arthritic disorders of the spine. In Rothman, R. H. and Simeone, F. A. (Eds.): *The Spine,* Vol 2. Philadelphia, Saunders, 1975, pp. 764-774.

Smyth, M. J. and Wright, V.: Sciatica and the intervertebral disc. An experimental study. *J Bone Joint Surg, 40A:*1401-1418, December, 1958.

Sokoloff, L.: Experimental studies of degenerative joint disease: *Bull Rheum Dis, 14:*317-318, September, 1963.

Sorensen, L. B.: The pathogenesis of gout. *Arch Intern Med (Chicago), 109:*379-390, April, 1962.

Southwick, W. O. and Robinson, R. A.: Surgical approaches to the vertebral bodies in the cervical and lumbar regions. *J Bone Joint Surg, 39A:*631-644, June, 1957.

Spigelman, L., and Lerman, M.: Wire frame cervical brace. *JAMA, 166:* 1985, April 19, 1958.

Spurling, R. Glen: *Lesions of the Cervical Intervertebral Disc.* Springfield, Thomas, 1956.

Stein, B. M., McCormick, W. F., Rodriguez, J. N. and Taveras, J. M.: Postmortem angiography of cerebral vascular system. *Arch Neurol (Chicago), 7:*545-559, December, 1962.

Stein, F., Bloch, H. and Kenin, A.: Nontraumatic subluxation of the atlanto-axial articulation; report of a case. *JAMA, 152:*131-132, May 9, 1953.

Steindler, A.: *The Cervical Pain Syndrome.* Instructional Course Lectures, Ann Arbor, Edwards, 1957.

Steindler, Arthur: *Lectures on the Interpretation of Pain in Orthopedic Practice.* Springfield, Thomas, 1959.

Stewart, D. Y.: Anterior approach to degenerative disk disease of the cervical spine. *NY J Med, 61:*3083-3096, September 15, 1961.

Stimson, B. B. and Swenson, P. C.: Unilateral subluxations of cervical vertebrae without associated fracture. *JAMA, 104:*1578-1579, May 4, 1935.

Stoeckle, J. D. and Davidson, G. E.: Bodily complaints and other symptoms of depressive reaction; diagnosis and significance in a medical clinic. *JAMA, 180:*134-139, April 14, 1962.

Stookey, B.: Compression of the spinal cord due to ventral extradural cervical chondromas. *Arch Neurol Psych, 20:*275-290, 1928.

Stowell, A.: Diagnosis and treatment of neck-shoulder-arm syndromes with medicolegal considerations. *Am Surg, 25:*59-64, January, 1959.

Straight, W. M., Edwards, R. V., Belle, M. S. and Cooke, F. N.: Occlusion of the internal carotid artery. *South Med J, 54:*1085-1092, October, 1961.

Suhr, V. W.: Are simulated autos "doing the job" in training our future drivers? *Safety Education, 36:*14-16, November, 1957.

Sunderland, Sydney: A classification of peripheral nerve injuries producing loss of function. *Brain, 74:*491-516, 1953.

Swartz, N.: The rheumatoid factor and its significance. *JAMA, 177:*50-54, July 8, 1961.

Symposium and inflammation and role of fibrin in the rheumatic diseases. *Bull Rheum Dis, 14:*323-326, November, 1963.

Talbert, O. R. and Pettit, H. S.: Neurologic manifestations in cervical spondylosis. *South Med J, 54:*1093-1100, October, 1961.

Taub, A.: The myth of acupuncture anesthesia. *Surg Team, 4:*26-33, 1975.

Tbachnick, N.: Sexual aspects of the automobile. *Med Asp Human Sexuality, 5:*138-161, September, 1973.

Teng, P.: Spondylosis of the cervical spine with compression of the spinal cord and nerve roots. *J Bone Joint Surg, 42A:* 392-407, April, 1960.

Tenicela, R. and Cook, D. R.: Treatment of whiplash injuries by nerve block. *South Med J, 65* (No. 5):572-574, May, 1972.

Thomas, A.: Whiplash, a misnomer. *Trial, 1:*27-30, February-March, 1965.

Thompson, H.: The "halo" traction apparatus. A method of external splinting of the cervical spine after injury. *J Bone Joint Surg, 44B:*655-661, August, 1962.

Thompson, W. A. L. and Kopell, H. P.: Peripheral entrapment neuropathies of the upper extremities. *N Engl J Med, 260:*1261-1265, June 18, 1959.

Timken, K. R.: Biofeedback—a brief review. *Dallas Med J, 60* (No. 9): 432-436, September, 1974.

Tinel, J.: *Le Système Nerveux Végétatif.* Paris, Masson, 1937.

Toole, J. F. and Tucker, S. H.: Influence of head position upon cerebral circulation. Studies on blood flow in cadavers. *Arch Neurol (Chicago), 26:*616-623, June, 1960.

Torg, J. S. et al.: Collision with spring-loaded football tackling and blocking dummies. *JAMA, 236* (No. 11):1270-1271, September 13, 1976.

Torres, F. and Shapiro, S. K.: Electroencephalograms in whiplash injury. A comparison of electroencephalographic abnormalities with those present in closed head injuries. *Arch Neurol (Chicago), 5:*28-35, July, 1961.

Toward a generation of safer drivers. *Atlantic Month, 197:*25-29, February, 1956.

Traffic deaths: *Consumer Bull, 46:*19-21, September, 1963.

Trueta, J.: Trauma and the living cell. *Bull Am Coll Surg, 46:*73-77, May-June, 1961.

Turkington, R. W. and Stiefel, J. W.: Sensory radicular neuropathy. *Arch Neurol (Chicago), 12:*19-24, January 11, 1965.

Van Buskirk, C. and Davidson, M.: Vascular insufficiency of the spinal cord. *South Med J, 53:*162-169, February, 1960.

Van Citters, R. L., Wagner, B. M. and Rushmer, R. F.: Architecture of small arteries during vasoconstriction. *Circ Res, 10:*668-675, April, 1962.

Von Hagen, K. O.: Common neurological diseases seen in general practice. *JAMA, 148:*1269-1273, April 12, 1952.

Von Luschka, H.: *Die Halbergelenke des Menschlechen Korpers.* G. Reimer, 1858.

von Torklus, D. and Gehle, W.: *The Upper Cervical Spine.* New York, Grune, 1972.

Wallack, E. M. et al.: Hemiparesis in cervical spondylosis. *JAMA, 236:* 2524-2525, November 29, 1976.

Wartenberg, R.: Some useful neurological tests. *JAMA, 147:*1645-1648, December 22, 1951.

Washington, E. R.: Non-traumatic atlanto-occipital and atlanto-axial dislocation; a case report. *J Bone Joint Surg, 41A:*341-344, March, 1959.

Webb and Woodhall: *Peripheral Nerve Injuries.* Philadelphia, Saunders, 1945.

Weiss, T. E. and Segaloff, A.: *Gouty Arthritis and Gout.* Springfield, Thomas, 1959.

White, A. A. et al.: An experimental study of the immediate load bearing capacity of three surgical constructions for anterior spine fusion. *Clin Ortho 91:*21-29, 1973.

Wilkins, R. H.: Neurosurgical relief of pain: recent developments. *Tex Med, 70:*53-61, October, 1974.

Williams, D. and Denny-Brown, D.: Cerebral electrical changes in experimental concussion. *Brain, 64:*223-238, December, 1941.

Wilson, G. D.: Fibrositis. *South Med J, 42:*387-391, May, 1949.

Wolf, R. A.: The discovery and control of ejection in automobile accidents. 792 lives may be saved yearly if properly constructed door locks are utilized in automobiles. *JAMA, 180:*220-224, April 21, 1962.

Wolff, H. G.: Man's nervous system and disease. *Arch Neurol (Chicago), 5:*235-243, September, 1961.

Wolff, Harold G. and Wolf, Stewart: *Pain,* 2d ed. Springfield, Thomas, 1958.

Wright, R. S. and Edwards, W. H.: Extrathoracic surgical correction of proximal subclavian and vertebral occlusive disease. *South Med J, 66:* 1019-1025, September, 1973.

Young, W. M., Jr.: *Psychotherapy and Organic Brain Disease.* Paper read at the twenty-fourth annual meeting of the Medical Society of St. Elizabeth's Hospital, Washington, D.C., 1961.

INDEX

Vulnerability of uninjured adjacent structures, 139

W

Wagging of head, 174
Wallerian degeneration, 187
Water, loss of, 127
Weakness, 163
  arms, 163
  grip, 163, 183

muscles, 163, 183-184, 248, 250-251
  neck muscles, 163
Weather changes, effect of, 132
Webster, J. E., 4
Weir, T. J. Jr., 145
Whiplash injuries, 88-93, 101, 122-123, 130, 168, 207, 275
Working, instructions for, 323-326, 329
Writing, instructions for, 317-322
Writing, position for, 112